Introduction to Research for Midwives

Introduction to Research for Midwives

Fourth Edition

ROWENA DOUGHTY, PHD, MSC, BA (HONS), ADM, RM, RGN

Lead Midwife for Education
The Leicester School of Nursing and Midwifery
Midwifery and Paramedicine
De Montfort University
Leicester, UK

DIANE MÉNAGE, PHD, MBA, BSC (HONS), RM

Senior Lecturer in Midwifery
The Leicester School of Nursing and Midwifery
Health and Life Sciences
De Montfort University
Leicester, UK

ELSEVIER

First edition 1997
Second edition 2003
Third edition 2011

Notices

Practitioners and researchers must always rely on their own experience and knowledge in evaluating and using any information, methods, compounds or experiments described herein. Because of rapid advances in the medical sciences, in particular, independent verification of diagnoses and drug dosages should be made. To the fullest extent of the law, no responsibility is assumed by Elsevier, authors, editors or contributors for any injury and/or damage to persons or property as a matter of products liability, negligence or otherwise, or from any use or operation of any methods, products, instructions, or ideas contained in the material herein.

ISBN: 978-0-7020-8003-6

Printed in Poland
Last digit is the print number: 9 8 7 6 5 4 3 2 1
Content Strategist: Poppy Garraway
Content Project Manager: Arindam Banerjee
Design: Ryan Cook
Marketing Manager: Belinda Tudin

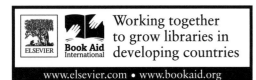

Working together to grow libraries in developing countries

www.elsevier.com • www.bookaid.org

CONTENTS

FOREWORD

The Future Midwife standards of proficiency (2019) were developed through an extensive and rigorous process of evidence review. They reflect contemporary national and international evidence on the health, well-being, needs of women and newborn infants (Nursing and Midwifery Council (NMC, 2019: 7)).

Critiquing and using evidence is one of the essential components of safe and effective midwifery care and importantly being able to:

1.5 Use share and apply research findings and lesson to promote and inform best midwifery policy and practice and to support women's evidence-informed decision-making (NMC, 2019: 14).

This introductory, step-by-step, text to research will be a very useful addition to a student midwife's reading list and for midwives who want to refresh or further develop their skills, particularly when supporting students in practice.

This text will also be helpful to novice researchers as well as those who want to adopt a systematic approach to critiquing research in their midwifery practice.

This new updated edition of *Introduction to Research for Midwives* continues to be presented in an accessible style with useful bullet-point summaries and tables to promote understanding.

The authors provide useful examples from midwifery practice and research so that the principles can be applied. The definitions are clear and the reader is directed to earlier sections in the text if they need reminding of the concepts already covered. Reflective prompts promote review and consideration of what has been read and could be useful for revalidation evidence gathering.

This text has appeal for different audiences whether it be the student midwife being introduced to research or preparing their dissertation or a resource for midwives wanting to ensure their research skills are kept up to date.

DR JACQUI WILLIAMS
SENIOR MIDWIFERY ADVISOR (EDUCATION)
NURSING AND MIDWIFERY COUNCIL
UK

Nursing and Midwifery Council, 2019. Standards of Proficiency for Midwives. [online] Nursing and Midwifery Council. Available at: https://www.nmc.org.uk/globalassets/sitedocuments/standards/standards-of-proficiency-for-midwives.pdf.

ACKNOWLEDGEMENTS

We would like to express our gratitude to Poppy Garraway and Arindam Banerjee at Elsevier, for their patient support while we updated this fourth edition. It was not meant to take as long as it did but many events conspired to delay us, one of which was a global pandemic!

We both owe a great deal to the support and encouragement of our husbands and families who were always there for us and a very big thank you goes to them. A special acknowledgement goes to Dr Laura McFarlane, lecturer (statistics specialism), at De Montfort University for her invaluable support with Chapter 13: Statistics in Research; we are very grateful for her input. We are of course ultimately grateful to Colin Rees for writing what has become a 'must have' book on research for midwives and for trusting us to take it forward.

Thank you to all the midwives and students who we have had the pleasure of teaching. Understanding what you need from an up-to-date research textbook that is midwifery focused has been essential to us. In this fourth edition, we have tried to include all the best aspects of the previous editions and make new additions. We have endeavoured to make it fresh and relevant to the current context of maternity care. Research literacy is a crucial aspect of professional development and we hope this book helps you to write great assignments and dissertations, provide evidence-based midwifery care and support you in your research projects. However, you use it, this is for you.

ROWENA DOUGHTY AND DIANE MÉNAGE

Throughout this book we use the words woman and mother. However, it is written in the spirit of inclusivity, acknowledging that not all people who are pregnant and give birth identify as women.

ABOUT THE AUTHORS

ROWENA DOUGHTY

Dr Rowena Doughty is a committed and passionate registered midwife, whose career has spanned across many areas of midwifery, including practice, management and education. Currently, she is the Lead Midwife for Education at De Montfort University in Leicester. Her professional interests are varied and include research, additional care needs and care of the compromised mother/foetus/neonate, including resuscitation, and the promotion of breast-feeding. She has a particular interest in obesity both outside of pregnancy and during childbearing. Her PhD, completed in 2019 at De Montfort University, was entitled: '*An Interpretive Exploration of the Experiences of Mothers with Obesity and Midwives Who Care for the Obese Mother during Childbearing*'.

DIANE MÉNAGE

Dr Diane Ménage is a senior lecturer in midwifery at De Montfort University in Leicester, UK, where she teaches on a variety of subjects, including research skills, evidence-based practice and leadership. She is also a mother, grandmother, writer and feminist with a life-long interest in women's health and well-being. Throughout her career her focus has always been on providing individualised evidence-based care through relationships. She has worked clinically in hospital settings, community midwifery and independent practice. She completed her PhD research on *Women's Lived Experience of Compassionate Midwifery* at Coventry University (UK) in 2018.

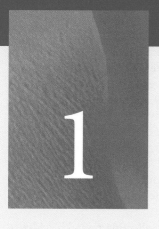

1

MIDWIFERY, RESEARCH AND EVIDENCE-BASED PRACTICE

The principal philosophy of health care in the UK, as with other 'more economically developed countries' (MEDCs) in the world, is evidence-based practice (EBP) (Schneider et al., 2014). In midwifery, this means a focus on clinical outcomes for women and their babies that are based on clear evidence of their effectiveness (Homer et al., 2019; Nursing and Midwifery Council (NMC, 2019); Renfrew et al., 2014). Although this philosophy is well matched with the philosophy of midwifery, it does demand supporting and enhancing the research skills of the midwife. These include information searching, gathering and synthesising skills and those of critical analysis. In particular, it is important that midwives, in common with other health practitioners, are research literate (i.e. they have an understanding of the principles of research and how it can be evaluated) (NMC, 2019; Spencer and Yuill, 2018). For some, it also means contributing to the generation of knowledge through research activity, and many trusts and health boards in the UK and across the globe now employ research midwives (Rowland and Jones, 2013). This first chapter prepares the way for the remainder of the book by exploring the context of research in modern midwifery and identifies some essential skills for the individual midwife.

Although this is a book on research, it cannot start without firstly discussing what is evidence and how it contributes to EBP. This is because the goals and expectations of health care from a national right down to an individual level are shaped by the demands of research and EBP. Its relevance to midwifery care has been emphasised by Bick (2011), who believes EBP is an important component to the provision of contemporary woman–centred maternity care. Implementing EBP into maternity care will improve the quality of midwifery care (Renfrew et al., 2014) and has the power to reduce maternal morbidity and mortality (Horton and Astudillo, 2014).

Furthermore, in the UK it is now an essential midwifery skill according to the NMC Standards of Proficiency for Midwives (SPM) (NMC, 2019: 29) which states:

At the point of registration, the midwife will be able to:
- **5.16** *demonstrate knowledge and understanding of the importance of current and ongoing local, national*

1

and international research and scholarship in midwifery and related fields, and how to use this knowledge to keep updated, to inform decision-making, and to develop practice

- **5.17** *demonstrate knowledge and understanding of the importance of midwives' contribution to the knowledge base for practice and policy through research, audit and service evaluation, engagement and consultation.*

Clearly, this is a powerful concept that every midwife needs to understand because it dominates so much of the thinking in maternity care (Bick, 2011). This first chapter, then, traces the development and meaning of EBP and its implications for an understanding of research within midwifery.

WHAT IS EVIDENCE?

One of the most frequently asked questions about EBP, according to Gebb et al. (2013), is, '*What counts as evidence?*' This is because there can be many sources of information used by midwives on a daily basis, all of them potentially legitimate sources of evidence. The answer for medicine is that research findings, particularly from quantitative studies, are the main form of evidence.

READER ACTIVITY

Student midwife: when you are next in practice, ask your practice supervisor (PS) what influences their decision-making. What sources of evidence do they use?

Registered midwife: when you are next on duty, ask yourself what influences your decision-making. What sources of evidence do you use?

COLLECTING RESEARCH EVIDENCE

In general, evidence is organised into a hierarchy where evidence that is regarded as higher quality is placed at the top while lesser-quality evidence is placed lower down (Fig. 1.1). While higher-quality evidence originates from studies that are considered to have more rigour and validity (e.g. systematic reviews and meta analyses), evidence towards the bottom of the hierarchy would include case-controlled studies, with randomised controlled trials (RCTs) placed in the

middle of the hierarchy. There is much criticism of the hierarchy, with debates that highlight the unique strengths and perspectives of all research methods (Vere and Gibson, 2020; Greenhalgh, Thorne and Malterud, 2018). Midwives have also argued that there should be a broader definition of what counts as legitimate evidence. Sources of evidence can include anecdotes and personal experience, findings from qualitative research, intuition and ancient wisdom, which can also contribute important perspectives to inform clinical practice.

So are all methods of collecting research evidence equally up to standard? This is important because not all methods of collecting information are equally convincing or accurate. Because of this, the 'hierarchy' of evidence would remind users that different forms of evidence should have a different weight attached to them, depending on the extent to which they demonstrate the elements that made them trustworthy or fit the criteria of sound evidence (see Fig. 1.1). At the top of the hierarchy are systematic literature reviews and meta-analyses. A systematic review is a very careful assessment of only high-quality research and, where possible, the findings of such research are combined together to overcome the difficulties found in individual research studies, such as a small sample size. At a similar level as systematic reviews on the hierarchy of evidence are meta-analyses. Meta-analyses utilise the statistical data from specific studies into a systematic review and then recalculate the statistical tests to provide further evidence of the topic (Gebb et al., 2013).

Meta-analyses are based on systematic reviews, but not all systematic reviews become meta-analyses **(Gebb et al., 2013: 5).**

Systematic reviews and meta-analyses of the literature are followed in the hierarchy of evidence by high-quality single RCTs that clearly demonstrated the qualities of well-produced research. In an RCT, patients as research subjects are randomly allocated to either receive the new treatment or care, while another group will serve as a control. The research subjects are assigned randomly, and other variables are reduced; any statistical results between the two groups can be credited to the intervention. Further down the hierarchy are less 'scientific' forms of research, including qualitative studies ending with

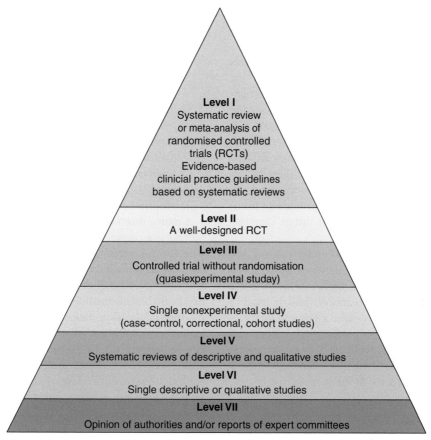

Fig. 1.1 ■ Hierarchy of evidence. (LoBiondo-Wood and Haber, 2014).

alternatives such as professional opinion or experience. Again, there has been much opposition to such hierarchies in both nursing and midwifery, where it has been argued that the emphasis on clinical trials and measurable outcomes are not the only relevant factors in care but that experience, including that found in qualitative methods, is just as important (Lützén, 2017).

Although qualitative studies are ranked towards the bottom of many of the hierarchies of evidence, it is important to acknowledge that this may have been in regard to questions of measurement and researcher objectivity in the research process. As will be discussed in Chapter 4, qualitative research does follow clearly defendable processes to support the truthfulness of findings, although it cannot claim to be generalisable in the same way that quantitative research may. Therefore in qualitative research the aim is not generalisability but instead *transferability* to other areas or *fittingness* for other groups of people.

Nevertheless, such studies have a special role to play in midwifery research because of the concern not only with clinical outcomes but also with the quality of the journey through pregnancy and birth, where there are other criteria than simply measurable outcomes. For example, the lived maternal and family experiences of midwifery continuity of care schemes or having a premature infant in a neonatal unit are examples of aspects that can inform 'best practice'. For these kinds of life events, qualitative data are important, are more appropriate and can inform both midwifery practice and policy. However, such research still needs to be rigorously conducted and so meet the criteria of sound evidence.

Only relying on evidence from the higher levels of the hierarchy of evidence may only provide one aspect of the focus of any 'problem' under investigation. Focusing just on clinical outcomes misses the patient perspective, and it cannot be assumed that findings from studies are always applicable to individuals (Smythe, 2011). Quantitative studies are also not particularly good at explaining complex issues, which is where qualitative research has the potential to explain complex phenomena and provide an innovative and novel ways of looking at things (Smythe, 2011).

This book will help develop an understanding and skills to consider the type of qualitative evidence developed from the social sciences, alongside quantitative research from the medical sciences. Midwifery, like nursing, is concerned with a wider scope and interpretation of science relevant to professional practice and so the interpretation of 'evidence' will be somewhat different from traditional medical thinking when it comes to what is judged as 'fit for purpose'.

EVIDENCE-BASED MIDWIFERY CARE

There is a clear interrelationship that exists between midwifery, EBP and research. The goal of midwifery care and practice is to provide support and management to women and their families to ensure best outcomes, whether these are physical, emotional or social (NMC, 2019). In addition, the key principle in achieving this goal is that care should be woman centred and support physiological processes.

The relationship between a mother and midwife can take many forms, as indicated in the following statement from **The International Confederation of Midwives (2017)**:

Midwifery is the profession of midwives: only midwives practice midwifery. It has a unique body of knowledge, skills and professional attitudes drawn from disciplines shared by other health professions such as science and sociology, but practiced by midwives within a professional framework of autonomy, partnership, ethics and accountability.

Midwifery is an approach to care of women and their newborn infants whereby midwives:
- *optimise the normal biological, psychological, social and cultural processes of childbirth and early life of the newborn;*
- *work in partnership with women, respecting the individual circumstances and views of each woman*
- *promote women's personal capabilities to care for themselves and their families*
- *collaborate with midwives and other health professionals as necessary to provide holistic care that meets each woman's individual needs*

(Definition of a Midwife; Adopted at Toronto Council meeting 2017).

This is a complex and extensive remit for the midwife and midwifery practice. To achieve a high standard of safe midwifery care throughout these activities and settings, clinical decisions must be based on the best available information. EBP therefore is a problem-solving and decision-making system, based on the collection, evaluation and synthesis of sound evidence to ensure best practice by midwives. This process should always be combined with professional judgement and the individual needs and desires of those receiving services and is seen as much more than research-based evidence (Menage, 2016a).

The dominance of EBP in health care has led to it being regarded as a 'movement' that has swept through so many countries and adopted as the preferred way of decision-making. Basing care on evidence has been made easier through the improved availability and accessibility of research carried out in health care. This has created an increase in midwifery knowledge based on research carried out by midwives, obstetricians and social scientists. The result has the potential to create high standards of decision-making in maternity care and improving safety across the maternity services, thus promoting positive outcomes for the mother and infant. The philosophy and practice of EBP provide the energy that encourages the use of research knowledge.

This is illustrated in the formation of guidelines such as those produced by the National Institute for Health and Care Excellence (NICE). NICE produces evidence-based guidance and advice for health, public health and social care practitioners. Their guidance is widely used to develop health policies and shape the activities of health organisations across the National Health Service (NHS) and social care systems.

Therefore it can be acknowledged that research is of fundamental importance in the promotion and development of EBP. Undertaking good-quality research and being able to read and critique research is therefore vitally important for the midwife. This is reflected in the NMC's SPM (2019), for example:

> Outcome 3.25: 'At the point of registration, the midwife will be able to use evidence-based, best practice approaches and work in partnership with the woman to provide care for the woman and the newborn infant across the continuum that optimises normal processes, manages common symptoms and problems, and anticipates and prevents complications, drawing on the findings of assessment, screening and care planning (NMC, 2019: 24).

EVIDENCE-BASED RESEARCH

Research, as defined by the Oxford UK Dictionary, is:

> The systematic investigation into and study of materials and sources in order to establish facts and reach new conclusions.

The result should be knowledge that increases understanding of a topic or problem and which can be checked for accuracy. It should be possible to apply this knowledge to a range of settings, not simply the one in which a study took place. Generalisability is one way in which quantitative research is judged: it should be capable of producing results that can be applied more generally, although this is not always useful when applied to health care settings (Futoma et al., 2020). In the case of qualitative research (which cannot usually be considered generalisable), it should be considered for its applicability or transferability to other groups or settings (see Chapter 4).

EBP and evidence-based research are not the same and should not be confused. EBP focuses on the use or application of knowledge, usually that produced by research, to produce the highest standard of care and clinical outcomes. In contrast, research is concerned with the production of knowledge that is as objective and accurate as possible. EBP is the application of this knowledge as the foundation for clinical decision-making. In this way, they can be seen as two distinct but related ingredients involved in the same process of improving midwifery care.

Bringing together EBP and evidence-based research means that EBP is not an additional or peripheral aspect of midwifery care but is part of providing care in the same way as it is accepted in nursing and other professional groups in health care.

In addition, using evidence for clinical decision-making is part of an ethical obligation for all health professionals because it demonstrates the responsibility to 'do good' as a result of professional action and 'avoids doing harm'. In the language of ethical thinking, these are known as the obligations of *beneficence* (i.e. doing good) and *nonmaleficence* (i.e. avoiding harm). It is difficult to argue that midwives are in a position to guide women in decision-making to promote positive outcomes unless they have knowledge of the research that will enable women to make sound choices throughout pregnancy and the birth of their infants. The professional duty to have up-to-date and evidence-based clinical skills and knowledge is also reinforced within The NMC Code (NMC, 2018: 9):

> 6.1 make sure that any information or advice given is evidence based including information relating to using any health and care products or services.

In summary, EBP and research are used as tools as part of the practice of midwifery, to form the optimum clinical and care outcomes for a woman and her baby, which is at the heart of midwifery practice. There are sound reasons, then, why midwifery has adopted the approach of EBP and all midwives are charged with supporting it.

USING EVIDENCE-BASED PRACTICE IN THE MATERNITY SERVICES AND MIDWIFERY PRACTICE

Midwives have increasingly been involved in developing and integrating EBP into their practice over the past few decades. Activity includes the generation of new evidence through literature reviews and primary research conducted by midwifery researchers and academics, which has influenced and changed midwifery practice. In many areas of midwifery practice, there is high-quality evidence on interventions that have been shown to improve outcomes for mothers and their babies, and midwifery practice has changed and developed through primary research (Bick, 2011).

Midwives, as undergraduate students, learn research-based skills such as database searching and critiquing skills and are encouraged to apply theory to practice within their clinical placements (NMC, 2019). The midwifery profession has also contributed to the synthesis of evidence acquiesced and knowledge transferred through systematic reviews and the development of policies and guidelines for practice, often supported by national guidance such as NICE. Midwives are also involved in audit and evaluation (Munro and Spiby, 2010) (see Chapter 2, which will explain the differences between research, audit and service evaluation).

Clinical governance is a framework through which National Health Service (NHS) trusts and organisations are accountable for continuous improvement in the quality of patient care, incorporating quality assurance, quality improvement and risk and incident management and recognises research and audit as central to this approach Public Health England (PHE, 2021).

The development and widespread use of information technology facilitate the fast dissemination of research and evidence, promoting critical appraisal and the assimilation into practice. Midwives can access information quickly through access to the internet while at work. However, the availability of guidelines has been thought to have resulted in midwives taking a more passive role in EBP, although more recently there are signs that midwives are becoming more engaged in the development of local and national guidelines (Spencer and Yuill, 2018; Munro and Spiby, 2010).

Although there have been vast improvements in care as a result of EBP, it has to be recognised that this is an ongoing endeavour, with no end, as midwifery care is constantly developing and refining. The implementation of EBP depends on several factors: timing of the proposed change, resources available, structures in place and workforce issues, all underpinned by finite resources where any change management needs to demonstrate cost-effectiveness (Scott et al., 2019; Brownson, Fielding and Green, 2018). Gaps in research coupled with a lack of application of available research can still result in variations in practice across trusts. However, Leufer and Cleary-Holdforth (2009: 35) suggest that EBP may support the allocation of finite resources available to health care:

EBP [evidence-based practice] is highly relevant in a social and healthcare environment that has to deal with consumerism, budget cuts, accountability, rapidly advancing technology, demands for ever-increasing knowledge and litigation.

However, in 2012 as part of the Health and Social Care Act, clinical commissioning groups (CCGs) replaced primary care trusts on 1 April 2013. CCGs are groups of general practitioner (GP) practices, which contract and authorise most of the hospital and community NHS services in the local areas for which they are responsible for. This has resulted in examples of 'postcode lotteries', where resources have been restricted or diverted to other priorities, despite the evidence-based research supporting implementation and change.

The introduction of EBP in midwifery was seen as a powerful tool to question and examine obstetric-led decision-making in maternity services (Munro and Spiby, 2010). There has been a steady and incremental transformation away from midwifery care based on rituals and routines, and a move towards evidence-based midwifery practices. Midwives as role models for students through their practice assessor (PA) and practice supervisor role (NMC, 2018) supported by approved education institutions (AEIs) and academic assessors (AAs) (NMC, 2018) are ensuring midwives of the future have the skills, knowledge and attitudes to continue to drive the profession forwards (NMC, 2019).

The Evidence-Based Practice Process

Implementing EBP is a five-stage activity (Table 1.1):

The starting point is to identify an area for clinical improvement and develop a question that might guide the development of best practice. This question is frequently formed using the acronym PICO, which stands for **p**opulation-**i**ntervention-**c**omparison-**o**utcome. This was originally developed by Sackett et al. (2000), and an example of PICO would be:

*In women during pregnancy (**P**) does attendance at antenatal groups (**I**), compared to those who do not attend groups (**C**), result in a higher level of women choosing to breastfeed their baby (**O**)?*

The most important aspect of this kind of statement is that the 'outcome' must be measurable (Alla et al., 2017). So, statements such as is it 'better' or 'more effective' for women to attend antenatal groups are difficult to answer because there is no indication of how it could measure either outcome statement. In comparison, breastfeeding rate is measurable.

The various elements of the PICO statement, then, guide the search for relevant literature through the use of each key word in the PICO question. The appropriate literature is systematically examined to provide a sound answer to that question. However, the literature should be included only if it has been critically evaluated and reaches a high standard. If the result is seen as strong or 'robust' enough to be used in practice, guidelines are drawn up and implemented. After a sufficient period, the results of applying the new practice are evaluated to ensure that it should continue to be used and can be demonstrated to have had an impact on the outcome measure.

Although this is a very simplified model of the process, it does highlight some of the skills required by the midwife, such as the ability to carry out a comprehensive review of literature that includes high-quality articles capable of providing sound evidence. Midwives also need critiquing skills that will allow them to assess how well research has been carried out. A decision then has to be made on whether the evidence collected is adequate or sufficient to solve the problem in the particular local clinical area so that the decision to apply the findings can be made. Finally, there is a need to know how to evaluate clinical outcomes and ensure that they have the desired effect.

This is a considerable demand on the individual midwife. However, it is not envisaged that all midwives should be carrying out all these stages in relation to every one of their clinical activities. This is clearly not possible. It is something that should be the responsibility all those involved in a clinical area or geographical area bound by the same systems. In other words, the agreeing of standards or guidelines for practice should be a team effort and can be based

on nationally available guidelines or those developed locally. Sometimes guidelines do not always keep pace with current evidence. There is huge work involved in updating guidelines, which means that it cannot happen very frequently. Thus, while guidelines have many advantages for practitioners, this can be seen as one of the disadvantages/weaknesses.

EBP, then, is a clear step-by-step activity that seeks to provide the best clinical decisions. It is a logical process that requires skill in those applying it. In most situations, the result of this process will already exist and have been agreed by clinical areas. The individual practitioner must be satisfied that these have been based on carefully evaluated information and that they are up to date. If that is confirmed, then such guidelines have the potential to increase the quality of care available and should form part of the decision-making process for the individual midwife in partnership with individual women.

Comparison Between Sources of Evidence

One way to understand the emphasis on research as a major source of evidence is to compare it against alternative forms of decision-making, such as those suggested by Polit and Beck (2014). The list later (Table 1.2) includes some of the major alternatives to research that have influenced decision-making and provides an opportunity to consider some of the advantages and disadvantages of each source against those of research.

This is a varied list, and, although each of these has its advantages, it can be seen that they all have a number of disadvantages that limit their accuracy and transferability to other clinical situations. In reality, the midwife may use several methods of decision-making almost simultaneously, and this can provide checks and balances (Menage, 2016b), but overreliance on one method to the exclusion of others is likely to be problematic. Interestingly, although clinical experience has historically been accepted as a strong basis for decision-making, Walsh (2008) presents some clear examples to suggest that clinical experience can lead to poor decision-making. Walsh includes such dangers as 'overconfidence' when predicting the way clinical events will unfold. Clinical predictions are well known for turning out to be wrong, and Walsh (2008) comments that studies have demonstrated that clinical

---

TABLE 1.1

Implementing Evidence-based Practice

1. Identify a clinical problem and turn it into a specific question
2. Find the best available evidence that relates to the specific question, usually by systematically searching the literature
3. Appraise the evidence for its validity, usefulness and methodological rigour
4. Identify best practice, and, together with the client's preferences, apply it to the clinical situation
5. Evaluate the effect on the client and the practitioner's own performance (Moule, 2015).

	TABLE 1.2	
	Advantages and Disadvantages of Different Sources for Decision-Making	
Type	**Advantages**	**Disadvantages**
Tradition	Familiar and accepted source of making decisions, especially by those receiving care and interventions. Little thought required on best clinical approach (do as has always been done).	May have been superseded by more effective methods. Clinical solutions may not have kept pace with changing demands and circumstances. Solutions can be quite narrow and do not suggest adequate thought is given to personal circumstances or alternative more effective options. The basis for traditional approaches may have not been open to scrutiny and verification. Are there tested grounds to believe them? N.B. this method is not in line with current thinking within health care that demands decisions based on convincing evidence.
Authority	Accepted as strong guide to knowledge and decision-making.	Decisions are made by those with the power to influence procedures and practices. May not be based on evidence. May be outdated.
Clinical Experience	If a solution worked before, it may work again. Taken as a strong source of knowledge in the past where experience was seen as providing 'wisdom'.	Experience may be untypical or results may have been 'one-off' outcomes, and may not work again. A number of biases associated with professional experience and expertise have also been noted.
Trial and Error	Appears to be a systematic approach, has pseudo-scientific air of comparing approaches until a solution is found.	May stop at a workable solution although a better solution may not have been reached. Not a very professional approach to care.
Intuition	Sometimes seems uncannily accurate. Provides a starting point for action.	May be drawing on subconscious memory of legitimate information and not a sudden or spontaneous source of knowledge therefore more applicable to experienced practitioners. For this reason, it is difficult to teach new or student practitioners. Not considered as a professional basis for decision-making.
Logical Reasoning	Has potential to arrive at a correct decision. Provides rational case for action.	May be flawed logic. Depends on accuracy of information used and powers of logic. Findings in one area may not be transferable to other area.
Assembled Information	Already existing data such as caesarean section or infection rates, etc. Can provide a useful indication of trends or outcomes. Appears evidence based.	Depends on accuracy of the data gathered, the method used to gather the data and the age of the data.
Research	Highly regarded as a source of knowledge. Well-conducted research reduces personal bias and controls for other influences and explanations. High level of transferability.	Can be poorly conducted. Too high a level of control of other influencing factors in the study setting might reduce the transferability of the information to other situations. May be inbuilt biases in situations. Can be overwhelming 'threats' to validity where results can be explained by other factors.

predictions are often wildly inaccurate. He also refers to 'base-rate neglect', where clinicians can overestimate the prevalence or risk of something developing that is far from the actual level or frequency. Having a long clinical experience or being in a senior position, then, does not necessarily result in a superior source of evidence. In this situation, well-conducted research is more valuable compared with other forms of decision-making.

Its main assets include the careful and closely controlled approaches to gathering evidence and the scrutiny it undergoes to ensure its accuracy. Although no midwife should have complete faith in every single study, the way research is presented allows the reader to inspect how the information was collected and processed so that they can match their own interpretations of the results to those of the author. This level of scrutiny and transparency of processes is rarely available in other forms of decision-making.

Research also has its disadvantages, and one should not feel that research is always the answer or that poor research is better than no research; it really depends on the quality of the study in question. Overall, if midwives are to make use of evidence in support of the principle of EBP they must closely examine the source and quality of that evidence to ensure it stands up to scrutiny. In this respect, there are more systematic methods the midwife can use to judge the quality of research information compared with alternatives that make it the preferred option for decision-making.

Having set the scene for the book, the next chapter will consider some of the essential concepts midwives need in applying research to practice. This will help with some of the language of research and key ideas that underpin research thinking. Later chapters will describe and discuss some essential skills such as critiquing research articles (see Chapter 5) and reviewing the literature (see Chapter 6).

Each chapter ends in a similar way, applying the content of each chapter to (1) conducting research and (2) critiquing research. It will also have some reader activities dotted within each chapter and a suggested reflective prompt at the end of each chapter. Throughout, important research terms will be *italicised* and appear in the glossary at the end of this book.

Conducting Research

This book concentrates on applied research (i.e. research designed to improve professional practice and clinical outcomes). Therefore midwifery researchers, when designing new projects, should consider the relevance of their study for practice. Will midwives and women in contact with services benefit from such a study? This is neatly summed up by the challenges *'who cares'* and *'so what'*? Therefore the decision to carry out a study should be clearly justified and its quality equally apparent.

Critiquing Research

Student midwives during their preregistration degree programme are encouraged to regularly read research articles and use research findings to support debate and

discussion within summative assessments. Curricula are designed to embed research awareness skills as a developing theme throughout the programme (NMC, 2019; Spencer and Yuill, 2018).

Chapter 5 focuses on how to read and critique research. It is concerned with recognising how the researcher has carried out the study and having an opinion about the quality of the research. The problem is what a reader of research needs to know before they can adequately express an informed opinion. One indicator might be the extent to which the findings may help improve practice. Can the results help midwives in their clinical activities? Will it help to provide the evidence to influence clinical decisions? Can the results be transferred to other settings and geographical locations? Do they appear accurate and genuine? Here midwives must be mindful that it is not only the results, but the researcher's interpretation of those results, that need to be considered. Researchers who strongly believe in a particular clinical process or technique may interpret their results in a way that only sees the outcome they hoped for. In other words, the researchers must convince the reader that they were objective and had an open mind in the way in which they conducted the study. It is these kinds of questions that will be developed through subsequent chapters.

REFLECTION PROMPTS

Why should midwives use evidence and research to underpin their practice as a midwife?

What types of evidence have you seen used in practice?

What is the role of experience and intuition in midwifery practice?

KEY POINTS

- Maternity services should provide midwifery care within the context of EBP, where knowledge, skills and practice are derived from research.
- This means that midwives must ensure that clear and acceptable evidence supports their professional practice and therefore guarantees the best use of available resources.

- EBP is compatible with midwifery philosophy because it seeks to provide the highest quality and safest levels of care. It is an ethically and professionally defendable concept.
- Working within a culture of EBP demands that each midwife can demonstrate a range of research-based skills, including an understanding of key research concepts and principles, as well as skills in searching the literature, critiquing articles and synthesising research into clinical guidelines.
- This book will provide an introduction to the knowledge and skills midwives need to understand research and play an appropriate role in the generation and application of research evidence to benefit those in contact with midwifery services.

REFERENCES

Alla, K., Hall, W.D., Whiteford, H.A., Head, B.W., Meurk, C.S., 2017. How do we define the policy impact of public health research? A systematic review. Health Res. Policy Sys. 15, 84. https://doi.org/10.1186/s12961-017-0247-z

Bick, D., 2011. Evidence-based midwifery practice: take care to 'mind the gap'. Midwifery 27, 569–570.

Brownson, R.C., Fielding, J.E., Green, L.W., 2018. Building capacity for evidence-based public health: reconciling the pulls of practice and the push of research. Ann.l Rev. Public Health. 39, 27–53. https://doi.org/10.1146/annurev-publhealth-040617-014746

Futoma, J., Simons, M., Panch, T., Doshi-Velez, F., Celi, L.A., 2020. The myth of generalisability in clinical research and machine learning in health care. Lancet Digit. Health 2 (9), e489–e492. https://doi.org/10.1016/S2589-7500(20)30186-2. ISSN 2589-7500

Gebb, B.A., Young, Z.G., Anderson, B.A., 2013. Evaluating and using the evidence Best Practices in Midwifery: Using the Evidence to Implement Change. Springer Publishing Company, New York, (Chapter 1).

Greenhalgh, T., Thorne, S., Malterud, K., 2018. Time to challenge the spurious hierarchy of systematic over narrative reviews? Eur. J. Clin. Invest. 48 (6), e12931. https://doi.org/10.1111/eci.12931

Homer, C., Leap, N., Brodie, P., Sandall, J., 2019. Midwifery Continuity of Care: A Practical Guide. Elsevier, Australia.

Horton, R., Astudillo, O., 2014. The power of midwifery. Lancet 384 (9948), 1075–1076. https://doi.org/10.1016/s0140-6736(14)60855-2. PMID: 24965820

International Confederation of Midwives, 2017. Definition of the midwife. https://www.internationalmidwives.org/assets/files/definitions-files/2018/06/eng-definition_of_the_midwife-2017.pdf

Leufer T., Cleary-Holdforth J., 2009. Evidence-based practice: improving patient outcomes. Nursing Standard. 23 (32), 35–39.

LoBiondo-Wood, G., Haber, J., 2014. Nursing research: methods and critical appraisal for evidence-based practice. Mosby Elsevier, St Louis.

Lützén, K., 2017. The value of qualitative methods in prioritised healthcare research. Nordic J. Nurs. Res. 37 (4), 175–176. https://doi.org/10.1177/2057158517745474

Menage, D., 2016a. Part 1: a model for evidence-based decision-making in midwifery care. Br. J. Midwifery 24 (1), 41–49.

Menage, D., 2016b. Part 2: a model for evidence-based decision-making in midwifery care. Br. J. Midwifery 24 (2), 137–143.

Moule, P., 2015. Making Sense of Research in Nursing, Health and Social Care, fifth ed. SAGE Publications, London.

Munro, J., Spiby, H., 2010. The nature and use of evidence in midwifery care. In: Spiby, H., Munro, J. (Eds.), Evidence-Based Midwifery: Applications in Context. Wiley-Blackwell, Chichester.

NMC, 2018. The Code: professional standards of practice and behaviour for nurses, midwives and nursing associates. https://www.nmc.org.uk/standards/code/

NMC, 2019. Standards of proficiency for midwives. https://www.nmc.org.uk/globalassets/sitedocuments/standards/standards-of-proficiency-for-midwives.pdf

Oxford UK Dictionary. What is research. https://www.lexico.com/uk-english

PHE, 2021. Clinical Governance. https://www.gov.uk/government/publications/newborn-hearing-screening-programme-nhsp-operational-guidance/4-clinical-governance

Polit, D., Beck, C., 2014. Essentials of Nursing Research: Appraising Evidence for Nursing Practice, eighth ed. Lippincott Williams and Wilkins, Philadelphia.

Renfrew, M.J., McFadden, A., Bastos, M.H., Campbell, J., Channon, A.A., Cheung, N.F., et al., 2014. Midwifery and quality care: findings from a new evidence-informed framework for maternal and newborn care. Lancet 384 (9948), 1129–1145.

Rowland, L., Jones, C., 2013. Research midwives: importance and practicalities. Br. J. Midwifery 21 (1), 60–64.

Sackett, D.L., Strauss, S.E., Richardson, W.S., Rosenberg, W., Haynes, R.B., 2000. Evidence-Based Medicine: How to Practice and Teach EBM, second ed. Churchill Livingstone, Edinburgh.

Schneider, Z., Whitehead, D., LoBiondo-Wood, G., Haber, J., 2014. Nursing and midwifery research; methods and appraisal for evidence-based practice, fifth ed. Elsevier, Marrickville, Sydney.

Scott, P.A., Harvey, C., Felzmann, H., Suhonen, R., Habermann, M., Halvorsen, K., et al., 2019. Resource allocation and rationing in nursing care: a discussion paper. Nurs. Ethics 26 (5), 1528–1539.

Smythe, E., 2011. From beginning to end: how to do hermeneutic interpretive phenomenology. In: Thomson, G., Dykes, F., Downe, S. (Eds.), Qualitative Research in Midwifery and Childbirth; Phenomenological Perspectives. Routledge Press, Oxon.

Spencer, R., Yuill, O., 2018. Embedding evidence-based practice within the pre-registration midwifery curriculum. Br. J. Midwifery 26 (5), 338–342. https://doi.org/10.12968/bjm.2018.26.5.338

Vere, J., Gibson, B., 2020. Variation amongst hierarchies of evidence. J. Eval. Clin. Pract. 27 (3), 624–630. https://doi.org/10.1111/jep.13404

Walsh, D., 2008. Research evidence and clinical expertise. Br. J. Nurs. 16 (8), 498.

2

KEY CONCEPTS IN RESEARCH

This chapter will examine some of the important concepts used by researchers and simplify the language by helping you to understand its meaning. The language of research can appear to be composed of 'jargon' (i.e. unhelpful and meaningless words). This can form a barrier to understanding research because people resent the use of words they do not understand, particularly if they feel they are just being used for effect. However, in reality, the words are a shorthand for complex ideas, and once the most commonly used words are understood, research can take on a completely different level of understanding. The chapter will also cover some of the important issues that researchers face when demonstrating that their research is accurate and carried out to a high standard. These are called 'methodological issues'. An important starting point is to recognise that research takes many different forms; in this book, we will focus specifically on research examining midwifery issues, carried out on the whole by midwives.

THE DIFFERENCE BETWEEN RESEARCH, AUDIT AND SERVICE EVALUATION

Research can be defined as:

the systematic collection of information using carefully designed and controlled methods that answer a specific question objectively and as accurately as possible.

However, *audit* and *service evaluation* have similarities to research. All three look for information (or data) to answer a question or questions (Twycross and Shorten, 2014). The basic difference is that the key role of research is to generate *new* knowledge and understanding of a particular topic or issue. The new knowledge can then lead to generalisations or new insights, which, in turn, can be used to make decisions about the information we can give to women and the way that we provide midwifery care.

Research conclusions are usually placed within a context of existing knowledge. That is, they are usually compared with previous research that has examined the same topic, to confirm existing knowledge or help to clarify or extend it. The purpose is always to enrich our understanding of the topic so that we can better use it. In contrast, *audit* is usually concerned with how a service is performing against a predetermined standard, and *service evaluation* is concerned with how the service is experienced and evaluated by those who use that service. Both audit and service evaluation are very different in their design when compared with research. Only research is designed to generate knowledge which can be applied generally, rather than the specific location to which audit and service evaluation data apply. Put another way, we could think of research as a process that starts with the question: 'What should we be doing?' whereas audit asks, 'Are we actually doing what we decided to do?' In contrast, service evaluation asks, 'How do the service users experience and perceive this?' For example, a number of good research studies have found that mother and baby skin-to-skin contact at birth is beneficial for breastfeeding initiation (Moore et al., 2016), and this knowledge has influenced global, national and local, evidence-based, clinical guidelines. Locally, maternity units may audit this activity either by observing in real time or collecting data from the records to find out whether early skin-to-skin contact is actually happening in accordance with their guidelines. Some units may wish to conduct a service evaluation by collecting data on the parent's experiences and views on skin-to-skin with their baby or babies following birth. Sometimes such evaluations may even seek the experiences of other stakeholders, such as the staff. This can be a vital part of the whole picture, and it may be particularly useful when trying to find out the reasons why evidence-based care is not happening.

One problem in trying to define research is that it is not a single entity. It has many different forms. This means that once we decide to study it, we have to learn something about the many forms it can take. At this stage, it is useful to think of research as a process that will follow a number of principles that will change depending on the type or category of research considered. In this book, we will focus on midwifery research (i.e. research that explores the problems and issues of direct concern to the midwife and that has implications for the work of the midwife more than any other discipline).

QUANTITATIVE AND QUALITATIVE RESEARCH

These two concepts are an ideal starting point for learning about research because they categorise very different approaches to research and each has its own underpinning ideas or *philosophy*. This is important because it explains why some studies look very different from others. If we know why they differ, we can make the best use of both types. Although Chapter 4 explores some of the differences in more detail, here we outline the key ideas associated with them and the implications these have for midwifery research and knowledge.

Historically, research has been synonymous with the word 'scientific', often associated with words like 'objective' or 'accurate', because these are two key characteristics that 'good' research is presumed to possess. Gerrish and Lathlean (2015: 9) see a scientific approach to research as indicating '*a rigorous approach to a systematic form of enquiry*'. The philosophy or belief on which this approach is based is that the natural or 'real' world does not depend on an individual's experience of it to exist and that it is open to study and quantification. In other words, it can be measured in some way independent of the person doing the measuring. This type of research can be characterised as '*quantitative*' research as it attempts to quantify (or measure) concepts, such as blood pressure, family size and even pain, in the form of a numeric value. These numbers can be summarised and allow the use of a range of statistical techniques to give the results greater usefulness and meaning (see Chapter 13). The purpose of quantitative research is seen as the search for relationships between things in the world so that we can understand the way they act and relate together. The ultimate aim of this understanding is to be able to control the elements in our world that impact on human existence. In midwifery, one example is the identification and measurement of the relationship between midwife-led continuity models of care and labour and birth outcomes. Once this relationship could be described and measured through a number of high-quality research studies (Sandall et al., 2016), this knowledge could be used to make decisions about commissioning, organising and delivering midwifery care.

This scientific view or *positivist paradigm* is one way of looking at things in research. It is the view traditionally embraced by medical research as the 'right' and 'proper' approach for a profession that is concerned with clinical outcomes. These words have been put in inverted commas to show that there is no longer agreement on this statement, and the scientific paradigm may not be the most appropriate for all circumstances (Rapport and Braithwaite, 2018). We must remember that this is only one approach to research. Although it is an indispensable approach in all health care, including midwifery, there are other, equally legitimate ways of conducting a study in addition to counting or measuring something that can also extend midwifery knowledge and practice.

Qualitative research has a different underpinning philosophy and therefore a different view of the characteristics of knowledge and the best way of conducting research to advance knowledge (Williamson and Johanson, 2017: 17–18). Qualitative researchers believe that the real world can be understood through our personal experience of it, and everything depends on how we experience and interpret that experience. This explains why some people are afraid of spiders or going to the dentist. It is a product of how people experience them, or the associations they hold for the individual. It does not mean that spiders or dentists themselves are frightening, but it does mean that they have different thoughts and feelings about them. Qualitative researchers (sometimes called naturalistic researchers) believe that if we are to understand a topic we need to look at it through the eyes of those who experience it and try to understand it from their point of view (Howitt, 2019: 8). Seeking the individual's perspective creates a different understanding of reality and the type of research we need to capture it accurately. This kind of research produces qualitative data, often in the form of verbal or written statements and dialogue, or extensive descriptions of observed human activity and behaviour. It uses methods such as interviews or observations, and information taken from documents such as diaries and journals that capture perceptions, interpretations, experiences or understanding.

One of the guiding principles of qualitative research is that it tries to capture people's thoughts and feelings in their own words. So, surveys or questionnaires with *fixed-choice options* would not be classed as qualitative research even though they may have tried to see things from the individual's point of view. This is because the list of alternative answers is limited and does not allow individuals to express ideas and answers in their own words, only in those of the researchers who have decided what they think are relevant alternatives. Fixed-choice options (e.g. a Likert scale in which five or seven possible responses, representing how much a person agrees/disagrees with a statement) are usually converted into numerical data for analysis.

An important visual distinction between quantitative and qualitative research is the presentation of data. Quantitative research will use numerical or visual forms of data presentation such as tables, bar charts and histograms (more of these in Chapter 13 on statistics). This form of data presentation is not a main feature of qualitative research, although some studies may present a table showing details of the study participants, such as age or number of children. This helps us to understand the participants' characteristics. In general, qualitative results (or findings) avoid numbers and instead present broad theme headings and discuss the type of comments made, often illustrated with examples of direct quotations or dialogue. As will be seen in Chapter 4, these two forms of research are so different they are almost two different entities. The importance of this is that we must avoid criticising qualitative research using the criteria of a quantitative research.

READER ACTIVITY

Consider quantitative and qualitative research in relation to midwifery research.
Which of these two approaches do you think is best suited to midwifery research?
Give reasons for your answers.

You may have thought about both approaches and feel that one is more useful than the other or perhaps you can see the advantages of both for different situations. The approach that is best is *the one that is most appropriate to the question posed*. If the midwifery question is one of quantity, or frequency, particularly in regard to clinical outcomes, then a quantitative approach will be appropriate; if the question is one of perceptions, understanding and interpretations, then the best approach will be qualitative.

Mixed methods research uses both approaches, within the same study, to increase knowledge on different aspects of a problem or issue. As health care becomes more complex, there has been an increase in the use of mixed methods (Shorten and Smith, 2017); however, there are both advantages and drawbacks. Given the differences in the underpinning philosophies of quantitative and qualitative research, it may seem obvious that a mixed methods approach poses some problems in this area. However, there are also clear benefits in being able to use both methods within one study to develop a more all-round understanding of the issue or problem (Shorten and Smith, 2017). For example, Brizuela et al. (2019) carried out an international mixed methods study to find out about health care providers' knowledge of and perceptions around maternal sepsis. Quantitative surveys measured the level of participant's knowledge on this subject, and qualitative interviews explored their perceptions regarding the environmental and professional barriers to identifying and managing maternal sepsis.

This section has introduced quantitative, qualitative and mixed methods approaches. No approach, in itself, is better than any other. It is always the *research question or aim* that will dictate the most appropriate approach.

LEVELS OF QUESTIONS IN RESEARCH

There is no shortage of questions that need to be answered through midwifery research. From the research point of view, it is the question posed by the researcher that results in the aim of the research. The aim usually begins with the word 'to' as in:

To explore first-time pregnant women's expectations and factors influencing their choice of birthplace (Borrelli, Walsh and Spiby, 2017).

Research questions will differ in their complexity, and this will have implications for the way a study is designed. Wood and Ross-Kerr (2011) make a useful distinction between what they call the three levels of research question. These levels are influenced by how much is known about a particular subject or how much theory exists in relation to it (Table 2.1). The advantage of this system is that it allows you to predict the way

TABLE 2.1		
Levels of Research Questions		
Level of Question	**Description**	**Type of Research**
Level 1 series	Examines one variable (or a series of variables) but without looking for patterns between variables. Exploratory situation where little is known about the topic.	Quantitative descriptive, (e.g. survey) Qualitative study: all types are level 1.
Level 2	Looks for a statistical relationship between variables that are present in the form of a pattern or association.	Correlation survey where variables frequently seem to be present together, (e.g. social class and likelihood to breastfeed).
Level 3	Looks for the presence of a statistical relationship between variables that indicate a cause and effect relationship (i.e. an intervention always has an influence on an outcome)	Randomised controlled trial where the effect of an intervention is measured in terms of a clinical outcome.

a study should be structured to answer a question at each of the levels.

- *Level-one questions* form the most basic level where very little is known about the topic. The purpose of this type of research is to describe a situation. The work of Wessberg, Lungren and Elben (2019) is one example of this, where the purpose was to describe women's experiences of late-term pregnancy (≥41 gestational weeks) to gain knowledge which could inform midwifery care and support. Although pregnancy beyond 41 weeks is thought to be a worrying time for women, little was known about what life is really like for women living through this. The researchers used semistructured interviews to gather the data, and analysis of the data led to the development of themes which represent a description of the experience from the perspective of the women participants.

- *Level-two questions* are those where some basic information is known about a topic, and there is an attempt to look for a possible statistical relationship between two or more factors. An example is the study by Carlisle, Seed and Gillman (2019) that sought to build on existing knowledge about poor seasonal influenza vaccine uptake in pregnant women receiving maternity care within one UK hospital. They wanted to determine whether any common characteristics could be identified as predictors of the vaccine uptake in a cohort of women receiving maternity care at one UK hospital. The researchers used existing anonymised computer records to retrospectively determine the characteristics of women who did take up the influenza vaccine and those who did not. They found that ethnic origin, age at booking, planned pregnancy, parity and booking in the first trimester were statistically significant predictors for receiving the seasonal influenza vaccination. This knowledge can be useful for identifying which women may benefit most from public health initiatives which inform women about the benefits of being vaccinated against seasonal influenza.

- *Level-three questions* are used to test hypotheses based on already established theories about a topic. A study by Daley et al. (2019) provides one example of this. Many well-established weight management programmes use target setting and regular weighing. However, there was a lack of evidence about whether this strategy could help women to avoid excessive weight gain in pregnancy. In this study, a randomised controlled trial evaluated the effectiveness of a brief behavioural intervention based on routine antenatal weighing and feedback from community midwives to assess whether it had an effect on excessive gestational weight gain in pregnancy; 656 women from four maternity centres in England were recruited and randomised to be in either the intervention group or receive usual care (control group). The study found no evidence that the intervention decreased excessive gestational weight gain and concluded that the intervention did not prevent excessive gestational weight gain.

These three levels form an important distinction because they influence the type of approach the researcher must use to gather the data. Level-one questions require a descriptive approach, perhaps using survey methods or a qualitative approach. Level-two questions require more sophistication in the method of analysis, to suggest that relationships between variables may exist. Finally, level-three questions require the use of an experimental approach that will test whether a hypothesis based on a theory can be supported by research evidence.

VARIABLES

So far, we have already been using some of the concepts that form the basic building blocks of research. Once we are familiar with their meaning in more detail, we should find our ability to analyse research has increased.

All studies are concerned with examining topics of interest to the researcher, such as level of pain in childbirth, intention to breastfeed and suturing skills. The term 'variable' is used to describe these characteristics as they differ or vary in some way. For example, length of labour, attitude towards natural childbirth methods, social class, temperature and level of pain in labour will vary from one person to another. Grove, Gray and Burns (2015: 514) state that variables are: '*Qualities, properties, or characteristics of persons, things, or situations that change or vary and are manipulated or measured in research*'. In other words, they are the 'things' that the researcher builds the study around, and so we should identify the particular variables of concern in the studies we examine.

In level-three questions involving randomised controlled trials, we can further subdivide variables into two types: *dependent variables* and *independent variables*. The variable that is the focus of concern, or sometimes the 'problem' the researcher is striving to improve or control, is the dependent variable, such as total length of time breastfeeding, or level of pain. The variable that is presumed to play a part in influencing the dependent variable is known as the independent variable. The independent variable can be thought of as the influencing factor or 'cause', and the dependent factor is the outcome consequence, or 'effect'.

An example will make this clear. Imagine a study whose aim is to examine whether women who have attended antenatal sessions or 'classes' are more assertive in seeking the type of birth they want than those who have not attended classes. The extent to which a woman is assertive in seeking the type of birth she wants would be the dependent variable; attendance at antenatal classes would be the independent variable. Experimental research, which we shall explore later in Chapter 12, revolves around the examination of cause and effect relationships, where the researcher introduces the independent variable into the experimental group and examines its effect on outcomes.

Initially, the difference between dependent and independent variables can be difficult to grasp. An easy way of sorting them out is to think of their chronological order of measurement in an experimental study, and identify which comes first and which comes last. The variable that comes first in time is the independent variable – the influence; the variable that comes last is the dependent variable – the outcome. In the previous example, attendance at antenatal classes happens before the level of assertiveness in seeking the type of birth they want, so attendance would be the independent variable, and the level of assertiveness, the dependent variable (see Table 2.2 for more examples).

One danger in many experimental design studies is that they appear to be based on the assumption that events are influenced by only one factor. Things are rarely as simple as this, and a number of other variables may influence whether a woman is assertive at the birth. Other factors in the previous example of assertiveness include influences such as personality, the quality of the relationship with their birth partner, level of education and social class. These would also be independent variables that the researcher may need to consider in the interpretation of the results. In experimental studies, then, we should identify the dependent variable and the independent variable, and ask ourselves, 'Is there anything else that could have influenced the outcome that has not been taken into account?' If we do this, then we are becoming more critical users of research.

CONCEPT DEFINITIONS AND OPERATIONAL DEFINITIONS

These two phrases explain firstly what the researcher means by the words used to describe the study variables, and secondly, how they were measured in the study. The *concept definition* is a clear statement of the sense in which the researcher is using the words describing the concept. It is similar in some ways to a dictionary definition of the word. In our example of attendance at antenatal classes and feelings of involvement, although we may feel we do not need to define the words 'antenatal classes', there are a variety of terms used to describe them in the UK, and they may well not mean the same to readers from other countries. We would also be concerned about the concept definition

TABLE 2.2		
Examples of Dependent and Independent Variables Identified From the Aim of a Study		
Aim	Dependent variable	Independent variable
To investigate an education discharge plan that included information about postnatal depression to reduce the severity of depression after childbirth (Ho et al., 2009)	Level of postpartum depression	Discharge education on postnatal depression provided by postpartum ward nurses
To evaluate the effects of an extended midwifery support (EMS) programme on the proportion of women who breastfeed fully to 6 months. (McDonald et al., 2010)	Proportion of women breastfeeding fully to 6 months	An extended midwifery support (EMS) programme
To evaluate the effect of active management of the third stage of labour on the amount of blood loss in the third and fourth stages of labour, and the duration of the third stage of labour (Kashanian et al., 2010)	1) the amount of blood loss in the third and fourth stages of labour, 2) the duration of the third stage of labour	The type of management of the third stage of labour (active versus 'expectant' or 'hands-off' approach)

of what qualifies as 'attendance at classes'. If someone attended just one or two sessions, are they referred to as having attended in the same way as those who have attended more times? The other term we would want clearly defined would be 'level of assertiveness'. What exactly does this mean? To provide an answer, criteria may be provided that specify what counts as an instance of assertiveness.

The meaning of the term *operational definition* is important from the data-gathering point of view, as it indicates how a particular concept is to be measured or '*operationalised*'. Grove, Gray and Burns (2015: 508) define the operational definition as '*an explanation of the procedures that must be performed to accurately represent the concepts*'. In other words, how we go about converting the variable into some numeric value, whether that is by means of a scale or a scoring system. So, for instance, the condition of the baby following birth may be operationalised using the Apgar score, and this converts the condition of the baby at birth into a number and will permit the condition of different babies to be compared accurately. Concepts such as pain and anxiety, are now operationalised using a scale that is regarded as a reasonably objective measure. For example, participants may be asked to mark on a 100-mm line how severe their symptoms have been for health problems they may have experienced. This calibrated line is known as a visual analogue scale (VAS) and is used to operationalise concepts that do not usually have a numeric value attached to them. The line is divided into 25-mm sections so that the location of a cross, indicated by a respondent along the line, can be given a numeric value and comparisons made between respondents.

THEORETICAL AND CONCEPTUAL FRAMEWORKS

One of the aims of research is to add to the body of knowledge on a particular subject, and to increase understanding by developing a more accurate theory about why things happen the way they do. A particular study cannot look at everything and will confine itself to a number of key factors or variables. The researcher's understanding of those variables can be expressed in terms of the theoretical framework that is adopted for the study. This provides a clear context for the study.

Grove, Gray and Burns (2015: 513) define a theory as '*an integrated set of defined concepts and existence statements, and relational statements that present a view of a phenomenon and can be used to describe, explain, predict or control that phenomenon*'. This gives the theoretical framework an important place in research as it guides the thinking of the researcher and provides the study with a specific context. So, to use skin-to-skin as an example again, the principle to provide a mother, and often the father, with skin-to-skin contact with the newborn baby is, at least partly based, on the theory of *parental attachment*. Researchers have used this to construct a *hypothesis*, for instance, that mothers and fathers who have skin-to-skin contact with their babies will show higher levels of bonding with their baby and spend more time interacting with the baby following the birth than those who do not have skin-to-skin contact. Clarity around the theories and concepts being used in research also helps to identify what information should be collected to test the theory.

The relationship between concepts is sometimes presented diagrammatically to illustrate how the author visualises the links between the dependent and independent variable(s). These diagrams are sometimes referred to as conceptual frameworks or conceptual maps, where key concepts are joined by lines and arrows to show the direction and nature of the relationships believed to exist. So a study may concentrate on the concept of breastfeeding and be concerned with some of the independent variables, which may influence the adoption of breastfeeding. A suitable conceptual framework that would illustrate the researcher's thinking may look something like Fig. 2.1.

As can be seen, conceptual frameworks provide a mental image of what the researcher sees as the influencing factors or variables that will be explored in a study. This provides the researcher with a clear picture of the topic area and should influence the design of the study, the key concepts, the elements included in the tool of data collection and the analysis and interpretation of data. In other words, they are a very powerful part of a research process. It is for this reason that a thorough review of the literature is essential to provide the theoretical and conceptual context for the study. This will then provide a clear indication of the key concepts that require concept and operational definitions.

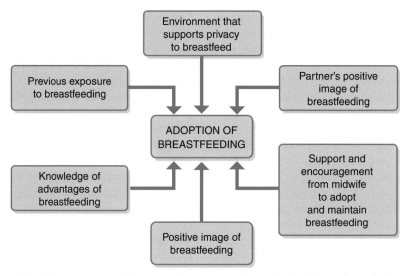

Fig. 2.1 ▪ Conceptual framework for a study exploring the decision to breastfeed.

One final word is to emphasise that the use of theories and conceptual frameworks does vary between quantitative research, which will usually start with a theory and conceptual framework, and qualitative research, which is more likely to develop one during or following data analysis. Remember, not all studies will explicitly include a theoretical or conceptual framework.

RELIABILITY, VALIDITY, BIAS AND RIGOUR

These four concepts are amongst the most valuable to use when critiquing research as they form part of the language that allows studies to be evaluated in terms of their design and way they are carried out. The words themselves may be familiar but their exact meaning may be unclear. The first two, reliability and validity, are used mainly when discussing quantitative research approaches and are concerned with the nature of measurement.

Reliability

This relates to the method of collecting data and refers to the accuracy and consistency of the measurements produced by the tool of data collection. For example, if we wanted to collect fundal height measurements from women in the third trimester of pregnancy, the use of an elastic tape measure would make us distrust the reliability

of the method of collecting the measurements. Reliability, then, relates to the *consistency and accuracy* of the measurement tool. If a study involved weighing babies as part of data collection, we would want to ensure any weighing scales used were tested for accuracy. Where a number of different scales were used, we would want to ensure that each one gave an accurate reading; otherwise, the reliability of the results would be open to question.

Validity

This relates to what is being measured and is an attempt to ensure that the measurement tool is really measuring what the researcher intended to measure. So, for instance, we could think we were looking at the satisfaction of women with the clinical skills of their midwife, when we were really measuring the influence of the midwife's personality that may influence how women felt about the care they received. Although reliability is usually amenable to checking and may become apparent in a pilot study, validity is far more difficult to confirm.

Bias

The degree of accuracy in the results of a study will be influenced by the amount of *bias* contained in the research. Bias has been defined by Polit and Beck (2018) as '*an influence that produces a distortion or error in the study results*' (p. 197). This can take a number of different forms, as we shall see in later sections. Here, we will concentrate on bias within the sample that may make them untypical or unrepresentative of the group they represent (see Chapter 14). This can happen through the method of sample selection.

In describing the sample, the researcher frequently mentions the *inclusion and exclusion criteria* used to select those in the study. These terms relate to the characteristics of those felt to be typical of the study group – the inclusion criteria, and those characteristics that were felt may either put them at clinical risk, or that would introduce bias into the group – the exclusion criteria. It is important to examine these closely and assess whether you feel the researcher has attempted to *control* for bias in the way the sample was selected. Look, too, for any changes in the size of the groups as a result of people not completing a study once they had started. This may make comparisons between groups difficult, as they may no longer be similar in composition once a number of people have dropped out of the study. The results will be distorted by the fact that, although the two groups may have been comparable at the start, they are not at the end, when a number from one of the groups did not complete the study.

Rigour

This is the final of the four major concepts used to assess studies and relates to the overall planning and implementation of the research design. It examines whether the researcher has carried out the study in a logical, systematic way and paid attention to factors that may influence the accuracy of the results. Grove, Gray and Burns (2015: 511) suggest that rigour is the '*striving for excellence in research and involves discipline, scrupulous adherence to detail, and strict accuracy*'. They argue that a rigorously conducted study has precise measurement tools, a representative sample and a tightly controlled study design. They also make the point that rigour applies just as much to qualitative research as to quantitative, where poorly developed methods, inadequate time spent gathering and analysing the data can all negatively affect the quality of the research, as discussed in Chapter 4.

Having examined these key concepts, it is evident that midwifery has a body of knowledge that draws on both quantitative and qualitative research

approaches. The issues and problems faced in research relate both to the worlds of quantification found in the scientific approach, and the naturalistic world as experienced by those who come into contact with midwifery services, including midwives themselves. This book is concerned with this wide spectrum of research approaches. Through understanding the principles of research, you will be able to identify and make use of studies which can inform evidence-based practice.

CONDUCTING RESEARCH

The key research concepts included in this chapter are essential to the researcher at the planning stage of a project. Understanding these concepts and the relationships between them will enable researchers to plan their study in such a way that it will stand up to scrutiny. Together, they provide a basic vocabulary not only to plan a study but also provide the researcher with possible ways of reducing the inevitable problems that are part of any study.

CRITIQUING RESEARCH

Research articles can appear to be written in a foreign language unless the reader has a basic understanding of the concepts introduced in this chapter. Once these have been absorbed, the reader will not only understand far more but will become more appreciative of good research and sensitive to weak research.

Knowing the distinction between quantitative and qualitative research will help anticipate the appropriate research approach and the type of data collected. There are different approaches to critiquing a research paper or article, depending on whether it is quantitative or qualitative in design, and Chapter 5 will explore the different ways of critiquing research in a lot more depth.

An ability to identify the level of the research question will allow the reader to make certain assumptions about the research and the form it takes. Knowledge of the levels also provides a way of critically examining the study to ensure that the researcher has considered the implications of the different levels and has not introduced something that is inappropriate to that level.

In reading a research report, a reader should quickly establish the variables under scrutiny. The clarity of the concept and operational definitions will ensure the reader knows exactly what the researcher is examining and how it is measured. Where the question is level three, the reader should identify the dependent and independent variables, to follow the outcome measure that forms the dependent variable, and what the researcher introduces in the form of the independent variable.

The underlying theoretical or conceptual framework will also allow the reader to understand why the particular elements have been linked and the underlying assumptions made by the researcher. In identifying the theoretical or conceptual framework, the reader should ensure that the tool of data collection and the discussion of the findings reflect the theoretical or conceptual framework.

Critiquing is about assessing how well the researcher has designed and carried out the study to address the stated research question or aim and how well they have presented their research. It is an assessment of both the strengths and weaknesses. To provide a fair assessment, the reader must always keep the concepts of reliability, validity, bias and rigour in mind. These concepts provide an informed approach to assessing, firstly, the quality of the research, and secondly, the degree of excellence achieved by the researcher.

REFLECTIVE PROMPTS

After reading this chapter, do you feel more confident to read a research paper in a journal?
Would you be able to find the research question or aim?
Would you be able to identify the approach?
Would you be able to make some assessment of the reliability, validity, bias and rigour of the study?

KEY POINTS

- Research is a lot easier to appreciate through an understanding of some of the concepts covered in this chapter.
- Quantitative and qualitative approaches to research relate to the different research designs and are based on philosophical beliefs about the nature of empirical evidence (i.e. evidence collected in the real world through the senses).
- Quantitative research is based on the belief that the truth of a situation exists in an objective state outside the personal views or perceptions of the individual. It emphasises accuracy and produces numerical data.
- Qualitative researchers believe that the truth of a situation is produced by our subjective experience and that we need to look at things from an individual's point of view. Midwifery is concerned with issues that draw on both beliefs.
- Research questions can relate to three levels of exploration. Level-one questions relate to describing one variable, usually about which little is known or that has rarely been the subject of research. Level-two questions look for relationships between variables but where little theory exists. Level-three questions relate to questions where theory exists and the aim is to test hypotheses based on the theory.
- Variables are the elements in which the researcher is interested. In level-three questions, there will be a dependent variable that is the outcome or effect, and one or more independent variables that are presumed to influence or cause the dependent variable.
- Concept definitions relate to how the researcher defines the topic in which they are interested. This can be thought of as a dictionary definition or alternative word for the topic of interest.
- Operational definitions refer to the way in which a concept is measured. They reduce the vagueness of such words as comfort, pain and benefit by producing a clear specification of how the researcher will make them visible in a specific study.
- Theoretical and conceptual frameworks provide the context and meaning for the ideas and concepts contained in a study.
- Reliability, validity, bias and rigour relate first to the extent to which the tool of data collection is accurate and consistent between different measurements, or different researchers. Validity relates to whether the method does measure what the researcher intends it to measure. Bias is the extent to which the findings are distorted either by the choice of subjects or the method of measurement. Rigour is the extent to which the

researcher has attempted to conduct the study to ensure accuracy and high-quality research.

REFERENCES

Borrelli, S.E., Walsh, D., Spiby, H., 2017. First-time Mothers' choice of birthplace: influencing factors, expectations of the midwife's role and perceived safety. J. Adv. Nurs. 73 (8), 1937–1946.

Brizuela, V., Bonet, M., Souza, J.P., Tunçalp, Ö., Viswanath, K., Langer, A., 2019. Factors influencing awareness of healthcare providers on maternal sepsis: a mixed-methods approach. BMC Public Health 19 (1) 683–683.

Carlisle, N., Seed, P.T., Gillman, L., 2019. Can common characteristics be identified as predictors for seasonal influenza vaccine uptake in pregnancy? A retrospective cohort study from a South London hospital [online]. Available from http://www.sciencedirect.com.proxy.library.dmu.ac.uk/science/article/pii/S0266613819300397

Daley, A., Jolly, K., Jebb, S.A., Roalfe, A., Mackilllop, L., Lewis, A., et al., 2019. Effectiveness of a behavioural intervention involving regular weighing and feedback by community midwives within routine antenatal care to prevent excessive gestational weight gain: POPS2 randomised controlled trial. BMJ Open 9, e030174. https://doi.org/10.1136/bmjopen-2019-030174

Gerrish, K., Lathlean, J. (Eds.), 2015. Research Process in Nursing, seventh ed. Wiley Blackwell, Oxford.

Grove, S.K., Gray, J., Burns, N., 2015. Understanding Nursing Research: Building an Evidence-Based Practice, sixth ed. Elsevier, Missouri.

Ho, S., Hey, S., Jevitt, C., Huang, L., Fu, Y., Wang, L., 2009. Effectiveness of a discharge education program in reducing the severity of postpartum depression: A randomized controlled evaluation study. Patient Educ. Couns. 77 (1), 68–71.

Howitt, D., 2019. Introduction to Qualitative Research Methods in Psychology: Putting Theory into Practice, fourth ed. Pearson Education, Harlow.

Kashanian, M., Fekrat, M., Masoomi, Z., Ansari, N., 2010. Comparison of active and expectant management on the duration of the third stage of labour and the amount of blood loss during the third and fourth stages of labour: a randomised controlled trial. Midwifery 26 (2), 241–245.

McDonald, S., Henderson, J., Faulkner, S., Evans, S., Hagan, R., 2010. Effect of an extended midwifery postnatal support programme on the duration of breastfeeding: A randomised controlled trial. Midwifery 26 (1), 88–100.

Moore, E.R., Bergman, N., Anderson, G.C., Medley, N., 2016. Early skin-to-skin contact for mothers and their healthy newborn infants. Cochrane Database of Systematic Reviews 2016 (11).

Polit, D.F., Beck, C.T., 2018. Essentials of Nursing Research: Appraising Evidence for Nursing Practice, ninth ed. Lippincott Williams & Wilkins, Philadelphia.

Rapport, F., Braithwaite, J., 2018. Are we on the cusp of a fourth research paradigm? predicting the future for a new approach to methods-use in medical and health services research. BMC Med. Res. Methodol. 18 (1), 131. https://doi.org/10.1186/s12874-018-0597-4

Sandall, J., Soltani, H., Gates, S., Shennan, A., Devane, D., 2016. Midwife-led continuity models versus other models of care for childbearing women. Cochrane Database Syst Rev. 4, CD004667. https://doi.org/10.1002/14651858.CD004667.pub5 2016 Apr 28, PMID: 27121907.

Shorten, A., Smith, J., 2017. Mixed methods research: expanding the evidence base. Evid. Based Nurs. 20 (3), 74–75.

Twycross, A., Shorten, A., 2014. Service evaluation, audit and research: what is the difference? Evid. Based Nurs. 17 (3), 65–66.

Wessberg, A., Lundgren, I., Elden, H., 2019. Late-term pregnancy: navigating in unknown waters – a hermeneutic study. Women Birth 33 (3), 265–272. https://doi.org/10.1016/j.wombi.2019.03.011

Williamson, K., Johanson, G., 2017. Research Methods: Information, Systems and Contexts, second ed. Chandos Publishing, Oxford.

Wood, M.J., Ross-Kerr, C., 2011. Basic Steps in Planning Nursing Research: From Question to Proposal, seventh ed. Jones and Bartlett, Sudbury, MA.

3

THE BASIC FRAMEWORK OF RESEARCH

An understanding of the basic framework of research projects is imperative, whether an individual is carrying out research or reading research articles. This chapter outlines the stages involved in designing and carrying out research. The framework used here applies mainly to quantitative research projects. Although qualitative research follows similar steps, the order of the stages may be different. The next chapter provides more detail on the distinction between these two approaches.

READER ACTIVITY

Where do you think ideas for research come from? When you think of any topics for research – what shaped and influenced your ideas?

How does a researcher carry out a research study? The answer to this question provides a roadmap to understanding the way the many stages in research all fit together. Before looking at the detail, the journey through the research process begins by looking at the broad phases of any research project, as suggested by Thomas (2017):

- Thinking About the Question: this is the beginning of any research; it is where the researcher develops the idea for the research and undertakes a literature review, finally deciding on the research question
- Design and Planning: the literature review will have refined the research question. In this phase, decisions on the research approach, research framework and the data collection tools are decided
- Data Collection: the activity part, involving the collection of information, also includes the pilot study, which tests the method
- Data Analysis: here, the data are analysed and a report written

- Dissemination: finally, the research report is communicated in the form of a report, article, blog, tweet, conference poster or presentation so that practice can benefit from this new knowledge

These phases can be simplified even further to a sandwich of:

THINKING – DOING – THINKING

It can be seen from this that research is based on thinking things through and interpreting the consequences of the information that has been collected. This has very close parallels with clinical work where midwives think about how to provide the best care to meet the needs of the individual, action the plan and then assess how successful it has been. Research and clinical thinking, then, are not that far apart (Menage, 2016).

The next stage is to break down the broad phases outlined above and concentrate on each of the sub-stages within them. The overall structure of the research process is summarised in Table 3.1.

STAGE ONE: THE RESEARCH QUESTION

Research begins when the researcher decides to examine a topic or answer an important question. Where do ideas for research come from? Perhaps one of the

TABLE 3.1
Stages in the Research Process

1. Develop the research question.
2. Critically evaluate the relevant literature.
3. Plan the method of investigation to include:
   a. The broad approach (i.e. quantitative or qualitative),
   b. The sample, sample size, and sampling strategy,
   c. The information to be gathered,
   d. The tool of data collection,
   e. The method of data analysis and presentation,
   f. The ethical issues to be addressed,
   g. Apply for funding and ethical approval.
4. Carry out a pilot study (if quantitative).
5. Collect the data.
6. Analyse the results.
7. Develop conclusions and recommendations.
8. Communicate the study.

most common sources is a known problem in the practice area. The researcher's first task is to take the problem and write the research question, or 'terms of reference'. This is a clear statement of the aim of the project. White (2017) emphasises that the role of the research question is absolutely central to the development of successful research, and so a great deal of effort is placed on getting it right. At the preliminary stage, the researcher may think in terms of a question that they want to answer that begins with 'why', 'what', 'when' or 'how'. Examples would be: 'what are the factors that influence women to give up breastfeeding?' or 'who is likely to decide on a home birth?'

These questions are then converted into the research aim by removing the 'why', 'what', 'when' and replacing it with 'to identify', 'to compare', 'to determine' or a similar phrase. So, for instance, it could say the aim of the study was 'to identify the factors that influence women to give up breastfeeding', or 'to determine the characteristics of women who are likely to decide on a home birth'.

In experimental and some correlation studies, the researcher will usually state a *hypothesis*, or even more than one. A hypothesis is different from a research question as the hypothesis is 'precisely testable' (Thomas, 2017: 16). In more simple terms, it is the 'hunch' that the researcher has about the outcome of the study. In experimental studies, the aim is to predict the nature of the relationship between the independent and dependent variables (for more details, see Chapter 12).

Although a hypothesis is not required in descriptive research, as the purpose is not to test the relationship between variables, it is sometimes helpful for the researcher to consider what assumptions they have about influencing factors. These can be used in deciding what information to gather. So, in describing what attracts some women to a home birth and not others, the researcher might hypothesise that factors such as social class, age and parity may be influential. These would then be included as questions in the tool of data collection.

An important consideration at this stage is whether the question is researchable. This relates first to the practical aspect of the study in terms of whether it is the kind of question that could be tackled by research reasonably easily (White, 2017). Second, it is important to realise that not all questions are amenable to investigation. Philosophical questions, or ethical issues, cannot be answered through research. Such questions as 'should midwives wear a uniform' or 'should midwives reserve the right to strike' belong in this category and are really the subjects of debate, not research.

The first stage of research is complex. The type and nature of the question are important, not only from the professional point of view of whether it is necessary to know the answer, but also in relation to the research method. Many of the other stages in the research process will be influenced by the way the aim is written (Thomas, 2017). So, for instance, the broad approach, the method of data collection, the sample and method of data analysis should all be implicitly influenced by the aim of the study.

STAGE TWO: REVIEWING THE LITERATURE

Studies are not undertaken in isolation from previous research; therefore, the second stage of the research process consists of a critical review of current literature on the topic. The purpose of this is to gain more information about the topic being examined. The literature also helps to clarify the research question and possible ways of answering it (see Chapter 7). It also confirms whether there is a need for such a study and focuses on how further study could enhance the understanding of a topic. As Lacey (2010) points out, there is no point in carrying out research if the question has already been competently answered. All researchers regard reviewing the literature as an important part of clarifying ideas and as a necessary early stage in the research process, particularly in identifying a gap in the literature and therefore justifying the need for such a study.

The literature review is important not only to provide information on the topic but also to provide guidance on the approach and methods used by those who have studied a particular topic previously. The 'methods' section of research articles provides useful guidance on the way data can be gathered in a study and any possible pitfalls that might be attached to some methods. Most researchers are expected to provide some details of problems encountered and comment on what they would have done differently with hindsight. All these are valuable to the researcher planning a study.

Once this stage is reached, it is worth the researcher stopping and asking the following three questions:

- Does it need to be done, or should practice be based on the research evidence already available?
- What use will be made of the results? Are the results likely to influence practice?
- Can I do it? Do I have the resources, skills and time for this to be carried out rigorously?

Unless the answers to these questions are in the positive, there may be little point in moving on to the next stage of planning the study.

STAGE THREE: PLANNING THE STUDY

Once the first two stages are complete, the researcher is ready to plan the study from beginning to end. The quality of the research is influenced by the amount of preparation and planning that have been invested in the process. *Rigour* is an important aspect in research and is dependent on this thinking phase. As has been seen in Chapter 2, rigour involves the researcher attempting to produce the highest-quality study. This is achieved by considering possible problems that may be encountered and planning to reduce them as far as possible. Table 3.1 lists the considerations that should be included in this planning stage.

The Research Design

This is the outline of the process the researcher will follow and is influenced by the purpose of the research. There are three types of research questions:

1. **Descriptive:** this is where the study is designed essentially to describe what is occurring or what happens
2. **Predictive (or Relational):** this is where the study is intended to look at the relationships between two or more variables
3. **Causal:** this is where the study is planned to determine whether one or more variables causes or influences one or more outcome variables.

If the researcher aims to establish causal relationships, then the research approach would be experimental. If the purpose is to describe a situation, as in a descriptive question, then a descriptive approach would be appropriate, perhaps using a survey method. A survey may also be used where the researcher wishes to identify if certain variables are related, as in a predictive (or relational) question that looks at correlation (Kamper, 2020) (see Chapter 9).

There are other approaches, such as *action research*, where the action researcher is seen as the facilitator and evaluator of change (Meyer, 2010). There are few clear examples of its use in midwifery (Crozier et al. 2012; Shallow et al. 2018). Its emphasis on change makes it appealing to those who want to develop clinical practice, and the involvement of those working in the areas involved in change in its design and implementation is a strong feature. This level of local involvement avoids the introduction of change for its own sake and ensures that any developments demonstrate benefits over the current situation. Meyer (2010) does highlight that it differs from other research approaches in that there is a blurring of the boundaries between education, practice and research. To be truly a research approach, it should provide an original contribution to increasing midwifery understanding or have the potential to be 'theory generating', adding to the existing body of knowledge, which is what distinguishes it from other forms of change strategies, audit and evidence-based practice (Cate et al. 2017) (see Chapter 4 for more discussion on action research).

Historic research is another method that has had only limited application within midwifery, despite the potential for providing a sense of development within the profession. It relies on the use of historical records and accounts, such as diaries, to chart the course of a particular issue or problem. The work of Langtree et al. (2019) provides some guidelines for conducting this type of research and the dangers of misinterpreting the past.

Mixed methods is a strategy increasingly used in healthcare research design. The aim of using this approach is to achieve a more encompassing understanding of often complex healthcare issues (McBride et al. 2018). Using this methodology, the research question is studied using both qualitative and quantitative data collected simultaneously or sequentially (in any order), often through a multiphase project. Lukasse et al. (2017) researched Norwegian midwives' opinions of their midwifery education within a cross-sectional study, where they collected quantitative and qualitative data, which included postal questionnaires and follow up open questions.

Finally, audit should be mentioned despite not being a research approach, as the use of audit in midwifery has become so common as part of the process of evidence-based practice that it merits inclusion here. *Audit* often looks like research and certainly requires the same systematic approach and rigour found in research. However, its purpose is not to add to midwifery knowledge, nor can the results of one audit be applied elsewhere; yet, it does answer important questions that are very similar to level-one research questions in terms of the level of performance within a maternity service against a standard (Mansfield, 2018) (see Chapter 2 for more discussion on the role and use of audit).

The Sample

The sample is the term used to describe the people, items, or events included in a study (see Chapter 14). In the planning stage, the researcher must consider the characteristics that make individuals eligible for selection and those that would make them unsuitable or even put them at risk or at a disadvantage. These considerations form the *inclusion and exclusion criteria* of a study. The researcher should also attempt to estimate the intended size of the sample when drawing up the research proposal for an ethics committee or funding body, as the sample size will both affect the credibility of the study and have consequences for funding. Comparisons with previous research may provide some clue as to optimum size, as well as helping with the sampling method. Increasingly, participants are being recruited through social media and online platforms.

Deciding on the Data to be Collected

In any study, it is important to avoid collecting information simply for the sake of it, in the belief that everything is relevant and should be included. This will result in information overload and make it difficult to do anything with the findings, as well as increasing costs related to processing the information. The researcher should consider each item of information to be included and ask two questions:

- Is this relevant to my research aim?
- What use am I going to make of this information?

Unless both can be clearly answered, the information should not be included.

The Method of Data Collection

There are several alternative tools of data collection that can be used to gather information. Those most frequently used include:

- questionnaires,
- interviews,
- observation,
- documentary methods,
- clinical measurements (scales, physiological measures related to clinical outcomes)

Each one will have its advantages and disadvantages, so how does a researcher know which one to choose? One of the main considerations in selecting the data collection tool is the research aim (Thomas, 2017). If the research question is related to staff or women's experiences, views and opinions and they are in the best position to provide an answer, then questionnaires or interviews will be appropriate. Where the researcher is interested in behaviour or techniques, such as methods of conducting antenatal classes, then observation will be a more reliable method. This is true of any question where researchers are concerned with what people do rather than with what people say they do. Remember, too, that much of an individual's behaviour and actions are carried out at a subconscious level, so they may find it difficult to accurately describe. For everyday quantitative data, midwifery notes or the medical record may be the best source of information. Finally, when researchers are carrying out a causal study where they want to establish the possible existence of cause-and-effect relationships, they would use clinical measurements, including physiological measurements or scales that will accurately quantify the outcome they are examining.

It is possible to use more than one method of collecting data in a single study to cross-check the accuracy of the information gathered, and this is one form of *triangulation*. The term is used to describe the combination of alternative elements in research to examine the same variable. Here researchers are using it to describe combining information from different tools of data collection examining the same variable, but triangulation can describe the combination of two or more theories, methods, sources of data, researchers or analysis methods in a single study (Noble and Heale, 2019). Each of these is used for the same purpose, which is to overcome the limitations of a single method of collecting data and so increase the validity of the results or its interpretation. As part of triangulation related to data collection, researchers might interview midwives on how they discuss smoking in pregnancy with mothers and then observe interactions to provide a completer and more accurate picture of what goes on.

The Method of Data Analysis and Presentation

Whichever tool is selected to gather the data, the method of analysis should be considered at the design stage, not after the data are collected. If the analysis will involve the use of statistical methods, then the researcher must decide which ones would be most appropriate and the form in which the data would need to be collected (see Chapter 13). Frequently, the researcher would consult a statistician or someone who can provide appropriate advice. At this stage, it is also important to think about how the numeric results will be presented, for example, in tables, graphs, or another form of display. This will also include thinking about how different variables in the study may be combined in the form of cross-tabulation where one variable is subdivided by another variable. An example would be where the method of infant feeding is to be presented by parity. The method of analysis will also influence the form in which the information is collected. For example, if the researcher wants to provide an analysis of the average length of time babies were breastfed, it would be necessary to ask women for the time in weeks and not ask them to tick a box that related to a spread of weeks, for example, 3 to 6 or 7 to 10 weeks, as averages are calculated using specific numbers and not a broad range.

Ethical Issues

Just as the midwife is bound by a Professional Code of Conduct (NMC, 2018), so the researcher is bound by an ethical code in conducting research. Ethics in research relate to several issues concerned with the correct behaviour and processes followed by the researcher and include the following:

- informed consent,
- confidentiality,
- the avoidance of harm or exposure to risk,
- the avoidance of raising expectations that it may not be possible to meet,
- the approval of a research ethics committee (REC) as part of research governance.

All of these issues are covered in more detail in Chapter 8. At the planning stage, the researcher must consider the implications of the study for each of these issues and plan for how they will be addressed during the study. These details are then highlighted when applying for ethical approval.

Once the planning stage is complete the researcher will be required to produce a research proposal. This is a written outline of the study and includes the justification for the study, the aim and many of the details developed in the planning phase. It will also contain a cost for the whole study and an estimation of the time scale and numbers of staff to complete the study. The research proposal may be used to gain permission to undertake the study and apply for funding or submitted to the ethics committee, if appropriate, to gain ethical approval or to a scientific scrutiny panel to consider the methods being proposed. The importance of gaining this kind of permission and support means that the researcher must demonstrate the ability to complete the work involved. The proposal also allows the researcher to assess how well all the aspects of the study will fit together. This may reveal some aspects of the study that had not been previously considered.

STAGE FOUR: PILOT

Before the study is carried out, the researcher must ensure that there are few unanticipated problems in gaining access to the data and that the method used to collect the data will work. This is the role of the *pilot study*. Eldridge et al. (2016) consider a pilot study as a pre-run of a full study with the aim to test whether the components of the main study can all work together. This is different from a feasibility study that occurs earlier in the research process and assesses whether something can be done and if it should proceed and if so, how. Although the main purpose of a pilot usually relates to assessing the accuracy of the data collection tool, it should be used to consider a range of factors. These include the whole study design including resources, time, availability of subjects, their willingness to participate and the support required from others to facilitate data collection. All these need to be assessed before a total and perhaps expensive commitment to the study is made.

The results gathered in any pilot should also be analysed to test the way they will be processed in the main study. The major outcome of the pilot will be the assessment of the reliability of the data collection tool and the opportunity to practice using it. Refinements can then be made that will allow the main study to progress as efficiently as possible. In this respect, the pilot study is very much like a dress rehearsal that allows all the elements in the study to be tested and adjustments made before the opening night.

STAGE FIVE: DATA COLLECTION

Once the pilot had been completed, the researcher is ready to start data collection. As can be seen, this comes quite some way into the total process. Despite attempts to reduce problems, unexpected things do go wrong. For example, problems with Wi-Fi coverage may hinder online interviews, sickness and absence reduce the number of people available for interview, and social media, newspapers and television influence respondents by suddenly promoting the very topic being examined in the study. All this is inevitable and a normal part of the research process.

STAGE SIX: DATA ANALYSIS

This is the stage in the research process that, according to Lacey (2010), is the most demanding from an intellectual point of view as it relates to first grouping the data so that they can be examined and second to interpreting the data in a way that is sound and logical. Data analysis takes place when the data have been collected. Descriptive statistics may be used to present a picture of the results using techniques such as averages that can take the form of the 'mean', 'mode' or 'median' (Thomas, 2017). Terms such as these are explained in Chapter 13. Statistical tests or correlation may be used to establish if there are any statistical associations present. In qualitative research, the vast amount of information collected is analysed to establish themes and categories. These are then compared with the literature to achieve greater validity of the findings and to help in theory construction. The process is very complex but, as with statistical analysis, follows a systematic approach (Adams and Lawrence 2018; Thomas, 2017). The exact form of analysis varies with the type of qualitative design used. In many instances, computer-generated online programmes (e.g. ATLAS and SPSS) are available to examine some aspects of the data, although a great deal of the analysis and interpretation is carried out by the researcher. Once the data have been 'ordered' in some way, the researcher must then to interpret it so that an answer to the research question can be established.

STAGE SEVEN: CONCLUSIONS AND RECOMMENDATIONS

The data analysis should lead to conclusions. These should be based on and supported by the results. The conclusion should also provide an answer to the aim of the study and, where appropriate, say whether the study hypothesis has been accepted or rejected. Please note: researchers do not say proved or disproved because there is always a margin of error. The implications of the findings are then discussed and will result in recommendations both for further research and for changes in practice where appropriate.

STAGE EIGHT: COMMUNICATION OF FINDINGS

Research will only be useful if it is communicated. The last stage in the research process consists of the production of a report, article or verbal presentation where the author will provide the following details:

- what they set out to do (aim),
- why they did it (rationale),

- how they did it (methodology),
- what they found (results),
- what it all means (discussion and recommendations).

How midwives can now use this knowledge of the research process will be discussed in Chapter 5, which covers critiquing research. Further chapters will look at some of the topics and issues covered in this chapter in more detail.

CONDUCTING RESEARCH

This chapter has presented the basic framework the researcher follows in carrying out research. This framework is very methodical and has an internal consistency where every stage has implications for further stages. Although it is presented here as a series of steps, it should be acknowledged that some of these are carried out in parallel, or the researcher may go back to certain stages and carry out further work on them. It is not necessarily as neat as it appears.

The essence of good research is planning, and the researcher will increase the chances of a successful project the more time that is spent on this stage. The importance of the review of the literature is not only to provide a context for the study but also to guide the way the study will be conducted. This includes influencing the questions included in the data collection tool. Above all, the researcher should not be tempted to economise by neglecting a pilot study, as so many unanticipated problems can be revealed at this stage (Byars-Winston et al. 2018).

The practical feasibility of the study should be carefully considered, and two important elements at the planning stage are, first, to think about permission to conduct the study, and second, to design the method of data analysis, whether this involves statistics or qualitative data analysis. It is important to determine if ethical approval is required as soon as possible as ethical applications can take some time to complete and a delay in this can seriously delay the study (see Chapter 8 for details on this). A research proposal, which is the outline of the intended research, will have to be submitted to these various groups, so get advice from someone who has experience in this. Similarly, at this stage, advice should be sought from someone who has an understanding of statistics or the analysis of qualitative data. The method of data analysis will have a profound effect on the type and format of the information included in the data collection tool. A mistake at this point could mean that a large part of the information collected is unusable because it has not been collected in the right format.

Although researchers can spend a great deal of time on planning, and even on piloting the study, inevitably things do not always run smoothly, and the unexpected might well happen to you. Research is a skill acquired through experience over time. However, do not give up when things go wrong – adjust the plan and move on. Seek support from an experienced researcher or mentor, dissertation supervisor or doctoral supervisor team at every stage.

CRITIQUING RESEARCH

The research process framework provided in this chapter gives a useful structure to use in evaluating or critiquing published research. As the reader reviews a study, there should be clear evidence that the stages in the research process have been followed, and the issues outlined in this section addressed. If they have not, then questioning the rigour of the study is justified. Remember, however, that qualitative research has a different structure and will look different in comparison to quantitative research reports. More details on this appear in the next chapter. Once a reader is familiar with the stages of research, they will see the structure clearly evident in all the reports they read.

REFLECTION PROMPTS

The important question when critiquing a study is: *'has the researcher followed a sensible plan of action given the nature of the research question?'*
The next question should be: *'does each decision fit with the previous decision made in the process?'*

KEY POINTS

- Research projects are structured according to a number of stages that provide the researcher with a path to follow.

- The aim of this framework is to increase the objectivity, reliability, validity and rigour of the research.
- The exact sequence of steps will vary depending on the broad research design, i.e. qualitative research is different in structure and process from quantitative research.
- Knowing these steps enables the reader of a research project to assess whether the correct stages have been followed.

REFERENCES

Adams, K., Lawrence, E., 2018. Research Methods, Statistics and Applications, second ed. Sage Publications, California.

Byars-Winston, A., Womack, V., Butz, A., McGee, R., Quinn, S., Utzerath, E., et al., 2018. Pilot study of an intervention to increase cultural awareness in research mentoring: implications for diversifying the scientific workforce. J. Clin. Transl. Sci. 2 (2), 86–94. https://doi.org/10.1017/cts.2018.25

Cate, O., Derese, A., Durning, S.J., O'Sullivan, P., 2017. Excellence in PhD dissertations in health professions education: toward standards and expectations. Med. Teach. 39 (9), 926–930. https://doi.org/10.1080/0142159X.2017.1302573

Crozier, K., Moore, J., Kite, K., 2012. Innovations and action research to develop research skills for nursing and midwifery practice: the innovation in nursing and midwifery practice project study. J. Clin. Nurs. 21 (11–12), 1716–1725.

Eldridge, S.M., Lancaster, G.A., Campbell, M.J., Thabane, L., Hopewell, S., Coleman, C.L., et al., 2016. Defining feasibility and pilot studies in preparation for randomised controlled trials: development of a conceptual framework. PloS One 11 (3), e0150205. https://doi.org/10.1371/journal.pone.0150205

Kamper, S., 2020. Types of research questions: descriptive, predictive, or causal. J. Orthop. Sports Phys. Ther. 50 (8), 413–469. https://doi.org/10.2519/jospt.2020.0703

Lacey, A., 2010. The research process. In: Gerrish, K., Lacey, A. (Eds.), The Research Process in Nursing, sixth ed. Wiley-Blackwell, Chichester.

Langtree, T., Birks, M., Biedermann, N., 2019. Separating 'fact' from fiction: strategies to improve rigour in historical research. Forum Qual. Soc. Res. 20 (2). ISSN 1438-5627. https://doi.org/10.17169/fqs-20.2.3196

Lukasse, M., Lilleengen, A.M., Fylkesnes, A.M., Henriksen, L., et al., 2017. Norwegian midwives' opinion of their midwifery education – a mixed methods study. BMC Med. Edu. 17 (1), 80. https://doi.org/10.1186/s12909-017-0917-0

Mansfield, J., 2018. Improving practice and reducing significant postpartum haemorrhage through audit. Br. J. Midwifery. 26 (1). https://doi.org/10.12968/bjom.2018.26.1.35

McBride, K.A., MacMillan, F., George, E.S., Steiner, G.Z., 2018. The use of mixed methods in research. In: Liamputtong, P. (Eds.), Handbook of Research Methods in Health Social Sciences.

Springer, Singapore. pp. 1–19. https://doi.org/10.1007/978-981-10-2779-6_97-1

Menage, D., 2016. Part 1: a model for evidence-based decision-making in midwifery care. BJM. 24 (1), 41–49.

Meyer, J., 2010. Action research. In: Gerrish, K., Lacey, A. (Eds.), The Research Process in Nursing, sixth ed. Wiley-Blackwell, Chichester.

NMC, 2018. The code: professional standards of practice and behaviour for nurses. Midwives and Nursing Associates. https://www.nmc.org.uk/standards/code/

Noble, H., Heale, R., 2019. Triangulation in research, with examples. Evid. Based Nurs. 22 (3), 67–68.

Shallow, H., Deery, R., Kirkham, M., 2018. Exploring midwives' interactions with mothers when labour begins: a study using participatory action research. Midwifery. 58, 64–70. https://doi.org/10.1016/j.midw.2017.10.017

Thomas, G., 2017. How to Do Your Research Project. A Guide for Students, third ed. Sage Publications Ltd, London.

White, P., 2017. Developing Research Questions, second ed. Palgrave and Macmillan Education, UK.

4 QUALITATIVE RESEARCH APPROACHES

Research comes in many shapes, sizes and 'brands'. As indicated in Chapter 2, one common broad categorisation is the distinction between *quantitative* and *qualitative* research approaches. These terms are associated with the types of data produced by each category; however, a more fundamental difference is the researcher's beliefs concerning the nature of research, and the principles they should follow in completing it.

As the majority of research used in evidence-based practice is quantitative, the aim of this chapter is to provide a balance between these two approaches by concentrating on qualitative research. It will extend the discussion on these two approaches in Chapter 2 by examining some of the main differences between quantitative and qualitative research, and describe some of the major types of qualitative design. The importance of feminist approaches to midwifery will also be emphasised and its relationship to qualitative approaches outlined.

The development of health care knowledge has traditionally been associated with the 'scientific' image of research. This is particularly true of research used in evidence-based practice, which, in the past, has focused largely on quantitative research, frequently in the form of randomised control trials (RCTs). This leaves qualitative research with many challenges, as it has taken time to develop a strong position in health service decision-making. In the past, the distinction between 'hard' and 'soft' data, and talk of a quantitative/qualitative 'divide', has exacerbated the view that qualitative research is not objective and therefore in some way inferior to quantitative. In reality, it is far better to see these as two distinct research approaches or 'research paradigms'. A *paradigm* is a world view with a set of philosophical principles about the nature of something, that shapes how people see and understand things related to that concept. In research, it has been thought to influence the different ways researchers who adopt either a quantitative or qualitative paradigm see the nature of research, its purpose and the role of the researcher. However, it is worth considering whether this divide is always a useful one. Arguably, the idea that researchers have fixed paradigms that limit them to one approach or another may be old-fashioned and does not reflect the complexity of modern health care. Particularly in midwifery, there are many questions where best practice can be informed by research that focuses on understandings, interpretations and experiences, requiring a qualitative approach. There is growing recognition that it is not just **what** we do, but **how** we do it that matters. In childbirth, outcomes matter a lot but so does experience. Midwives seek to improve both outcomes **and** experiences. As Downe has so clearly pointed out, women want **both** safety **and** well-being (Downe and Byrom, 2019).

How does qualitative research differ from quantitative research? The key difference is that qualitative research does not concentrate on the measurement of clinical outcomes; instead, it explores human experiences and processes (including those of midwives) and our understanding of health and illness issues from the perspective of those involved. Examples include women diagnosed with post-traumatic stress disorder (PTSD) post-childbirth describing their experiences of care (Patterson et al., 2019) and midwives' experiences of caring for women who make unconventional birth choices (Feeley et al., 2019). Is this knowledge important to us? How can it not be? We need to understand how people experience health care if we are to provide a meaningful, sensitive and appropriate response to health needs. Pregnancy, birth and childcare are all extremely personal experiences, so any research approach that values human experience will be compatible with a profession that emphasises individuality and an empowering approach to care. Qualitative research, then, is an appropriate choice in exploring some of the important issues facing midwifery.

The conclusion to be drawn from this is that all midwives need to be familiar with both quantitative and qualitative approaches to research if they are to demonstrate evidence-based practice. Qualitative approaches balance the narrow focus of quantitative research by examining the bigger picture and the more human side of service provision, and help to determine the needs

and preferences of those receiving health care. The following section examines some of the major differences between the two major approaches of quantitative and qualitative methods.

THE CONTRAST BETWEEN QUANTITATIVE AND QUALITATIVE RESEARCH

Qualitative research is a broad term covering a number of different but related approaches to research. Denny and Weckesser (2019) describe it as research that:

considers why individuals think or behave the way that they do and how they come to understand these complex thoughts and actions within their lives. It also allows the voice of patients and carers to be included in research.

Like quantitative research, it is carried out in an organised and methodical way, but whereas quantitative research can tell you *what* happened, qualitative research explores the human experience and particularly the way in which people make sense of the things that happen to them. For this reason, qualitative research is sometimes referred to as *interpretivist* or *constructivist* research, as it is based on the belief that how we see things 'constructs' how we experience our reality or world through subjective interpretations (Harvey and Land, 2021). Researchers using this approach analyse the words used by the participants to describe their experiences and to build understanding around the meaning they attach to those experiences (Gray, 2019: 59). Polit and Beck (2008) elaborated on this by outlining some of the key characteristics of qualitative approaches (Box 4.1).

As these characteristics are important in understanding the differences between quantitative and qualitative research, they require further elaboration, as their meaning is not always clear. One way of simplifying matters is by demonstrating how the two approaches differ in the following three phases:

- Planning,
- Data collection, including the role of the researcher and the nature of their relationship with the participants, and
- Analysis and interpretation of the results.

BOX 4.1
CHARACTERISTICS OF QUALITATIVE APPROACHES TO RESEARCH

Qualitative design:

Often involves a merging together of various data collection strategies (i.e. triangulation);

Is flexible and elastic, capable of adjusting to what is being learned during the course of data collection;

Tends to be holistic, striving for an understanding of the whole;

Requires the researcher to become intensely involved, usually remaining in the field for lengthy periods of time;

Requires the researcher to become the research instrument; and

Requires ongoing analysis of the data to formulate subsequent strategies and to determine when field-work is done.

Polit, D., Beck C., 2008. Nursing Research: Generating and Assessing Evidence for Nursing Practice, eighth ed. Lippincott Williams and Wilkins, Philadelphia.

Planning

Perhaps the most important characteristic of qualitative research is the holistic approach that attempts to provide a total picture of individuals or groups and their life experiences and beliefs. This is in contrast to isolating a single biophysical entity, such as heart rate or blood pressure. This holistic approach of qualitative research is necessary if it is to discover how people interpret life events and give them meaning within their life. To achieve this, the researcher's exploration takes into account a broad outline of people's lives and cultural influences that may affect behaviour and beliefs and so allow the researcher to contextualise the topic and their findings (Holloway and Galvin, 2016). As a consequence, the research question will be broader than that found in quantitative research so that it can capture the bigger picture. The research process followed in qualitative research is also less structured and more flexible to adapt to new ideas and insights as they grow and develop throughout the study.

These features have considerable implications for the planning process, which tends to be shorter than in quantitative research. For example, in some qualitative methodologies, less time is devoted to a comprehensive literature review. The researcher should always search the literature to ensure that study has not already been undertaken, and consulting the literature will provide a broad understanding of concepts that may be related to the study (Holloway and Galvin, 2016). However, the literature should not 'direct' or 'influence' the path of the research. In qualitative research, the literature can be seen as part of data analysis, where it is used as a way of confirming the credibility of the researcher's interpretations and descriptions of behaviour.

A further planning stage distinction is that the qualitative researcher does not develop a structured tool of data collection based on the literature review or use a tool that has been validated in previous research. This is because the researcher attempts to keep an open mind on what may be important within the study. The implication of this is that a pilot study is not needed in the same way as in quantitative research, as there is no highly structured research tool to test for consistency and accuracy. Data is often collected through interviews, but many others forms of data collection can be used (e.g. observation, photographs, journals and social media posts). Each interview (or other data collection method) will be different and not standardised as in quantitative research, which seeks to ensure consistency. However, small pilots can still be useful in qualitative studies and may be used as a means of picking up unforeseen practical problems and refining interview questions.

Data Collection

Whatever data collection tool is used, one of the clearest differences between the two research approaches is the way the researcher forms a relationship with the participants during data collection. As the aim of the research is to gain an understanding and insight into human behaviour, there is a social closeness in the relationship between the researcher and the participants. This mainly develops over a sustained time period not characterised by the quick interview or the faceless questionnaire approach. Traditionally, in quantitative research, there was a belief that the researcher should keep a social distance from the subjects of the research to avoid undue influence on the results. The question of power in the researcher/participant relationship is an import consideration. This is a particularly important aspect of feminist research, which emphasises the need to recognise and minimise inequalities in power, the aim of feminist research being to amplify women's voices and empower them (Holloway and Galvin, 2016).

This means that the researcher must have a great deal of personal awareness of the relationship with subjects where this may have influenced the findings. This is referred to as *reflexivity*, where the researcher considers and takes responsibility for their own position within the research and the effect that it may have on those being studied, the data being gathered and its interpretation (Dodgson, 2019). The impact of the researcher on data gathering is so important that researchers in qualitative research are sometimes thought of as the *tool* of data collection, or research *instrument*, because the researcher makes decisions on what should be highlighted through the analysis and presentation of findings.

Another consideration is the concept of the researcher as *insider*. Burns et al. (2012) explored the advantages and disadvantages of being midwife/researchers in an observational study carried out within a maternity unit well-known to the researcher. In these circumstances there can be advantages around access, acceptance and blending-in, which is of course valuable in an observational study. Another advantage was having prior understanding of the workplace culture and systems. However, disadvantages included feelings of role conflict and ethical dilemmas, for example, when the ward was busy and women needed assistance. It is not that it is wrong or right to be an 'insider' researcher. What is important is that the qualitative researcher engages in *reflexivity* around their role and engages in critical reflection of themselves and their relationships in the research setting. This should become part of the research process. Reflexivity is revisited in relation to qualitative interviewing in Chapter 10.

Data Analysis and Interpretation

Visually, one of the clearest differences between quantitative and qualitative research is the form of data presentation; the former is presented using numbers and analysed statistically, and the latter uses words in the form of direct quotations and descriptions of activities and is analysed through the researcher's interpretation of emerging themes. Extracting themes from the data requires a great deal of attention to the data, whether it be interview transcripts, journals or observational field notes. This is often done by hand and involves the researcher immersing themselves in the data, although computer software packages can also assist in this process.

The sequence of events between data gathering and analysis is also different. Unlike quantitative research where the process of analysis starts once data collection has finished, in qualitative research data gathering and data analysis can be carried out at the same time. Fieldwork may stop when the researcher feels that no new themes or elements are emerging and *data saturation* has been reached, that is, when further data collection would be redundant.

Analysis in qualitative research is characterised by an *inductive* approach rather than a *deductive* one. This means that the researcher takes the individual elements emerging from the analysis and gradually builds up a picture to provide a broad explanation of what may be happening. In contrast, the quantitative researcher starts with general principles, often in the form of a theory or hypothesis, and examines the individual units of data to either confirm or reject that theory or hypothesis.

The two approaches of quantitative and qualitative are very different, and Table 4.1 illustrates some of the major differences. The following section examines some of the more popular qualitative approaches.

QUALITATIVE RESEARCH DESIGNS

Although qualitative research can take many different forms, there are three main traditions that dominate nursing and midwifery research, all of which seek an *emic* view: that is from the perspective of the participant or *insider*. This is in contrast to the *etic* view: from the perspective of the outsider, and in research that would mean the researcher (Hennink et al., 2020: 15). However, as touched upon earlier in the chapter, while researchers seek data from participants, they may also influence the data in some way.

The three main traditions are:

- Ethnography
- Phenomenology
- Grounded theory

TABLE 4.1 Summary of Differences Between Quantitative and Qualitative Approaches		
Characteristic	**Quantitative**	**Qualitative**
Focus	Narrow and specific	Holistic and general
Research question	Precisely worded	Broadly worded
Type of evidence	Objective	Subjective
Belief about reality and research activity	The social world is similar to other 'sciences' and open to measurement by the researcher Reality is 'out there' and objective	The social world can only be known through an individual's experience and understanding of it Reality is inside all of us
Researcher's relationship to subjects	Detached to ensure it does not influence subjects, although rapport sought	More equal and reciprocal relationship characterised by social warmth
Review of the literature	Critical to the development of the process	Can be used to provide a broad picture, but often used to support findings It is included as part of written report.
Planning	Carried out in depth	High level of planning avoided so as to reduce preconceived ideas about the nature of the topic
Tool of data collection	Emphasis on accuracy and consistency, to ensure reliability and validity	As the tool is used flexibly and continually developing, a pilot may not be appropriate
Sample size	Emphasis on large numbers to reduce bias and to allow statistical procedures	Small numbers but appropriate experience explored
Sample referred to as	Subjects	'Participants' or 'informants' to avoid dehumanising
Analytical approach	Deductive	Inductive
Data	Numeric	Words
Data gathering	Extensive to gain maximum coverage	Intensive to gain maximum depth and rich, 'thick' data
Product of data analysis	Referred to as 'results'	Referred to as 'findings', although some publications use the term 'results'
Generalisability	Major concern to achieve this to a high level	Not generalisable but transferability considered
Ethical concerns	High, particularly where an intervention is invasive	High, harm is concerned with psychological and social elements and the protection of human dignity
Methodological concerns	Reliability, validity and bias	Trustworthiness, in the form of credibility, dependability, confirmability and transferability
Emphasis on rigour	High	High
Application to evidence-based practice	Highly rated, notably in the form of RCTs	Increasing emphasis on user views and experiences is increasing the acceptability
Applicability to midwifery practice	High	High

RCTs, Randomised control trials.

These traditional approaches are certainly not the only approaches to qualitative research. Qualitative approaches and methodologies are constantly being developed in different ways, and hybrid approaches are being recognised, published and critiqued. In this way, qualitative research has its methodological roots in traditional approaches, and yet it is also a dynamic, evolving phenomenon.

The next section will outline the three main, traditional approaches as well as some contemporary methodologies or approaches.

Ethnography

The holistic approach taken by the qualitative researcher is clearly illustrated in the work of the ethnographer. Grove et al. (2019) explore ethnography as a discovery of the interrelated parts of a particular culture to create a clear picture of the culture as a whole. Holloway and Galvin (2016) see it as a way of studying human behaviour in the context of cultural rules and norms. It is not surprising then, to find that this approach has its roots in anthropology, where the objective of the anthropologist was to describe and interpret human activities within a culture or cultural subgroup. The earliest ethnographic studies were with isolated indigenous communities or tribes where the researcher attempted to learn something about the people and the society as a whole.

The use of this approach is now applied to everyday social groups or cultures, but still with the purpose of understanding the rituals and beliefs that people hold and that influence their behaviour. The underlying assumption of ethnographic research, according to Polit and Beck (2008: 224), is that every human group evolves a culture that guides the members' view of the world and the way they structure their experiences. The aim of the ethnographer is to learn from (rather than to study, as in a laboratory) members of a cultural group. This again gives clues as to the way qualitative researchers think and the values they hold about research.

The anthropologist's techniques of observation, interviews, participation and immersion in the culture have all been adopted to various extents by the ethnographic researcher in health care. Like the original anthropologists, the ethnographer is described as carrying out *fieldwork* (i.e., a study in the natural environment or field in which those involved in the study are usually found). This usually lasts for sustained periods of time in order to observe a particular group under a range of circumstances. This does hold dangers, as the longer the period of observation, the more likely a close and familiar relationship develops between the observer and the observed. This can lead to what anthropologists have called *going native* (Madden, 2010). This phrase refers to the researcher who no longer sees the group's activities through the eyes of an enquiring stranger, but rather as another member of the group with *tacit* knowledge, or knowledge taken for granted. To overcome this, the researcher attempts to use the technique of 'cultural strangeness'. This means trying to see things 'with the eye of an outsider' (Holloway and Galvin, 2016), so that they can question the purpose and meaning of behaviours those within the group see as unremarkable. This is perhaps one of the difficulties facing the midwife ethnographer, in that it is very difficult to see things as culturally strange once socialised into the midwife role.

There are also practical difficulties facing the midwife ethnographer, particularly the investment of sufficient time to carry out the fieldwork. Ethnographic research takes time. The researcher needs time to gain trust, acceptance, and a clearly identified role within the group. It is a very intimate relationship where those in the study are prepared to share deep feelings and shared understandings that they may not want to reveal to strangers. This can make for a potentially expensive study in terms of time required.

Anthropologists are typically concerned with what people do and say, how it is said, the objects they make or use and how they use them. This helps us understand the approach of such studies and the focus of attention. The methods of data collection to achieve these aims typically consist of observation and interviews, both of which tend to be flexible and intense; that is, they are carried out over a long period of time in the field. Other forms of data collection can also be used to shed light on the situation, such as written accounts, including health records or diaries. The approach of ethnography is very similar to making a 'fly-on-the-wall' documentary. The purpose is not to manipulate a situation, but rather to record it and try and make sense of it. Instead of a camera, ethnographic researchers keep a 'fieldwork diary' in which they capture the details of their observations, interviews and personal interpretations and understandings. In presenting results, reference may be made to a fieldwork diary or field notes to add detail and support the accuracy of the observations and interviews.

Examples of ethnography in midwifery research include a study by Arnold et al. (2019) which sought to understand some of the factors surrounding poor quality care, reported by women in Afghanistan. Arnold and colleagues observed and examined the everyday lives of the maternal healthcare providers working in a maternity hospital in Kabul, Afghanistan. The aim was to understand their notions of care, varying levels of commitment, and the obstacles and dilemmas that affected standards of care.

Another study by Goodwin et al. (2018) looked at the nature of the midwife-woman relationship in a South Wales community by observing midwives and women at antenatal appointments. In addition to observation, this study collected data using semi-structured interviews, media, and field notes as a way of enhancing the *thickness* or denseness of the data and therefore its ability to provide rich, detailed descriptions. Many ethnographic studies use observation alongside other data collection methods for this reason. Sosa et al.'s (2018) ethnographic study involved observing women and midwives to learn about the culture of midwife-led birth environments that were providing one-to-one labour support. Interviews at a later date added to the thickness of the data.

Phenomenology

The origins of phenomenology are in the discipline of philosophy. Phenomenology attempts to understand the essential nature of people's experiences and interpretations of key features in their life so that the core *essence* of a concept can be revealed. 'Essence', according to Polit and Beck (2008: 227), is *'what makes a phenomenon what it is, and without which it would not be what it is.'* This is clearly useful for the midwifery researcher who wants to understand the essence of the experiences that women encounter during pregnancy, birth and motherhood, so that the experiences can be understood by midwives.

As a research method, phenomenology can be defined as a method of gaining the *lived experience* of

a particular phenomenon as seen through the eyes of those involved so that its essence can be discovered. The phrase *lived experience* is often found in the title of such studies. As with other qualitative approaches, there is not one 'method' that produces a phenomenological study, but several variations. Many researchers who claim to follow this approach credit the influence of one of two key German philosophers, Edmund Husserl (1859–1938), and one of his students, Martin Heidegger (1889–1976), who developed Husserl's ideas in a different direction. However, the philosophy of phenomenology has also been influenced by French thinkers, such as Maurice Merleau-Ponty (1908–1961) and Paul Ricoeur (1913–2005). These influential figures were not researchers, but their philosophical ideas have influenced the way that phenomenological researchers think about the purpose of their research and how people experience the world.

Phenomenological research is often, although not always, conducted by means of in-depth interviews. The approach will differ depending on whose work has influenced the study. For example, if the main influence comes from Husserl, the emphasis will be on a descriptive approach to the lived experience. Here, the researcher is encouraged to put aside (or *bracket*) their personal understandings, values and preconceptions so as not to influence data collection and interpretation. Those following Heidegger do not attempt to bracket; the focus is on the interpretation of what it is like for those in the study. Prior understanding of the topic or situation is not suppressed as such but is instead seen as a necessary part of the researcher's interpretation. A great deal of controversy exists in the literature over the process of bracketing, particularly in regard to whether it is possible to suspend what we already know (Gelling, 2010), and what the researcher should do when attempting to 'bracket' (Hamill and Sinclair, 2010).

Phenomenology has a great deal to offer midwifery, as it provides the perspective of those receiving services and so may open up understandings that would not be available through other methods. Samples tend to be small, but studies can produce rich and very detailed data. One example of this approach is a study conducted by Barros et al. (2020) to understand the health care experiences of homeless pregnant women. In this study, in-depth interviews with 10 women were conducted, and analysis of these led to rich insights into the participants' experiences of discrimination, violence, prejudice, racism and vulnerability.

Another interesting example of this approach was the work by Dibley in 2009. Dibley undertook a study of 10 lesbian parents' experiences of health care in the UK, focusing on interactions with midwives. She adopted a Heideggerian phenomenological approach for the study as she wanted to use her own experiences as a lesbian mother and nurse to interpret the findings without 'bracketing' her own connectedness with the topic of the study. There are two ways of looking at this. Some would argue that it creates potential for bias. Others argue that the researchers' personal insights and experiences in this area aid rapport with participants and enhance interpretation of the data and thus the quality of the study. The study provides stark information on the way some lesbian mothers were treated by midwives at that time and their published paper gave recommendations on improvements that needed to be made to increase the quality of experience for this group of women.

Interpretive Phenomenological Analysis

Interpretive phenomenological analysis (IPA) has been an important methodological development, and particularly over the last decade there has been an increase in studies using an IPA approach. As the name suggests, IPA has its roots in phenomenology, yet it can be seen as a more modern and flexible methodology. First described by Smith in 1996, it was initially popular in psychology research because it is especially good at examining concepts which are complex, ambiguous and emotion-laden (Smith and Osborn, 2015). IPA also has an *idiographic* focus; that is, a focus on the unique experience for the individual (Smith et al., 2009). It is now used in a wide range of healthcare disciplines and is seen as very suitable for qualitative midwifery research which seeks to gain in-depth, rich understandings of women's (and midwives') experiences (Roberts, 2013).

The controversy in phenomenology about whether the researcher should 'bracket' off their own experiences and knowledge (as Husserl thought) or acknowledge and embrace these (as Heidegger believed) is not debated in IPA. In IPA, the researcher is acknowledged as a part of the process of interpretation of

the data. Therefore, reflexivity (as discussed earlier in this chapter) is important, and researchers may make reflexive notes or keep a journal as part of the research process (Smith et al., 2009). Examples of IPA approaches used in midwifery research include a study to understand women's lived experience of receiving compassionate care from midwives (Menage et al., 2020) and a study by Norris et al. (2020) which studied women with high body mass index (BMI) to try to understand their perceptions of their risk during their childbirth journey.

Grounded Theory

This research approach was developed in the 1960s by two American sociologists, Glaser and Strauss, to explore hospital staff's behaviour towards dying patients. Although the approach may look similar to either a phenomenological study or an ethnographic study, the crucial difference is in its purpose. The purpose of grounded theory is not only to describe and build understanding, but also to try to explain, through a proposition, why things might take the forms they do. These propositions can be said to form a theoretical explanation that is 'grounded' in the data collected; hence the term *grounded theory* (De Chesnay, 2014: 6).

In grounded theory, data collection and analysis are carried out in parallel, and they stop once no new categories arise from the data. This is called 'saturation'. The analysis also consists of '*the constant comparison method*' where new data and emerging categories from the analysis are compared with previous data and categories to ensure consistency and the possible development of links between the categories.

Grounded theory uses methods such as observation alone or with other methods, such as interviews or focus groups. These are similar to the previous qualitative approaches in being very flexible in design. An important source is also the fieldwork diary in which researchers keep a running commentary on the way events unfold and their own reflections and developing understanding of the situation. The main emphasis in the findings section of a grounded theory study is the presentation of a model or theory that explains the data collected. It is through these theoretical models that midwifery theory can be expanded and practice developed in line with the experiences and perceptions of both midwives and those for whom they care. One excellent example of grounded theory in midwifery research is a study by Borrelli et al. (2016) which set out to conceptualise first-time mothers' expectations and experiences of a good midwife during childbirth. Participants were interviewed both before and after giving birth, and data was constantly compared with interviews for the same person and also with other participants' interviews. In this way, the interviews' components were put into context and grounded in the whole data to eventually build a theoretical model of the 'good midwife'.

REFLECTIVE PROMPT

Do you think that you could briefly describe to a colleague the key features of ethnography, phenomenology and grounded theory and the sort of research questions they are used to answer?

Narrative Methodologies

Narrative approaches focus on the stories that people tell about themselves and their experiences. In this form of research, data collection is through participant's narratives, which are usually analysed through a technique called narrative analysis. Nolan et al. (2018) used narrative inquiry to study adolescent mothers' use of social media.

Discourse Analysis

Discourse analysis is not one specific methodology but a family of approaches for studying the way that people talk and write to examine its broad meaning or the cultural discourses upon which it draws (Willig, 2008). The important distinction here is that the focus is on the purpose and effects of the language used. It is not just the structure and vocabulary in the language used, it is the meaning and intent within and the way it is used to influence, control or manage. For these reasons it is surprising that it has not been used more in midwifery and maternity research. However, there are some useful examples in the literature. An Australian study by Ferndale et al. (2017) studied the ways in which midwives negotiate the conflict between medical and midwifery philosophies of care during midwifery consultations. They collected recorded data of the real conversations between pregnant women and midwives during their antenatal appointments. Analysis of their discourse revealed that midwives occupied a complex and sometimes conflicted position as they negotiated the medicalisation of childbirth and a risk discourse while also trying to foster women's trust in their bodies.

Discourse analysis also lends itself to analysis of legal documents, polices and guidelines. For example, Amodu et al. (2018) carried out a study on Nigerian Government policies aimed at eradicating obstetric fistula. Obstetric fistula is a severe, long-term complication of prolonged, obstructed labour, with the highest prevalence in low-resourced sub-Saharan African and Asian countries, with Nigeria accounting for around half of all cases (USAID, 2016). Systematic study of the policy documents using discourse analysis techniques found that the policy revealed no inherent commitment to eradication of obstetric fistula and did not live up to its title. The value of this evidence is that it assists in holding policy makers to account and, in this case, it strengthens arguments to go beyond the well-intentioned rhetoric and actually link policy to improved reproductive rights and maternal health.

Studies may also use discourse analysis on data such as leaflets, books, newspapers, websites, social media posts and text messages. Studies that use photographs and pictures can also use a discourse analysis approach or similar methods, such as *content analysis* or *image analysis*. For example, Bowden et al. (2016) used discourse analysis and image analysis to examine internet images of birth rooms in developed countries to understand what messages and norms were being communicated through images. They concluded that messages reinforced the idea that bed was the most appropriate place to birth, and that medical equipment is intrinsically involved in the process of birth.

Action Research

Action research comes under the broad heading of practice-based research (McNiff, 2013: 23) and encompasses a number of similar but distinct methods. Action research in healthcare settings blends action, often in the form of seeking to improve care and implement changes, with processes which increase understanding and help to refine and focus the action. In this way it is very different to other types of research, as the research and the implementation are going on simultaneously, and it could be argued that it is more of a change theory than a research theory. An alternative view is that it is research which relates to implementation process. One important feature is that the participants and the researchers are the same people; hence, it is often called *participatory action research* or PAR. It is a methodology that Kurt Lewin saw as creating knowledge through problem-solving in real-life situations (Herr and Anderson, 2015). Reflection on action is an important part of the process, and action research aligns closely with a reflective learning cycle. In maternity settings it can be a really valuable tool for implementing evidence-informed practices in context, while simultaneously gathering information and reflecting on actions to gain new, deeper understandings. For example, much is now known about the extent of disrespect and abuse of women in childbirth settings around the world through a large number of quantitative and qualitative studies, as well as systematic reviews (Bohren et al., 2015; Bohren et al., 2019; Kassa et al., 2020). Now that this is known, an obvious question might be: how do maternity settings, where disrespectful care is entrenched, implement respectful care? Sando et al. (2016) used an action research study to select, implement and evaluate a package of interventions designed to prevent and reduce disrespect and abuse in a large urban hospital in Tanzania. Open days for women and respectful care workshops for staff were implemented and all levels of staff were involved, and senior managers and leaders played an important part in modeling behaviour and encouraging dialogue on respectful care. This is just one area which lends itself to action research, but there are many others.

READER ACTIVITY

Can you think of evidence about a best practice that you would like to see implemented in your area of practice?

Do you think that an action research project could be used to guide this?

Co-operative Methods

Co-operative research methods go hand-in-hand with action research approaches in that they are about conducting research **with** people rather than **on** people. Co-operative enquiry or collaborative enquiry is a type of action research which involves working with other people who have similar positions or interests in order to understand and make sense of a situation or concept and to develop new and creative ways of examining it (Heron and Reason, 2006: 144–154). In co-operative research, as with other action research approaches, boundaries between the researcher and participants do not really exist, and therefore it is associated with being a much more equitable process with less potential for power dynamics to influence the process or the findings. From a midwifery perspective it can be particularly useful when bringing together interested parties to identify the meaning and relevance of a topic or concept in the context of maternity care. This is exactly what Crowther et al. (2021) did when they conducted an international collaborative inquiry in which a group of people, experienced in the field of birth care or birth room design, explored ways that spirituality could be honoured in 21st century maternity care settings. What added to this study was the fact that the participants were based in different countries and the study was conducted entirely using online platforms. The study is a reminder of how the internet has opened up many different types of research to people who would not usually be able to participate face-to-face, due to a variety of barriers, including some hard-to-reach groups.

QUALITATIVE RESEARCH WITHIN MIDWIFERY

The previous sections have indicated how each approach has been applied within midwifery research, and some examples of these are illustrated in Table 4.2. However, as qualitative research takes so many diverse approaches, not all midwifery research falls neatly into one of these categories. Indeed, some researchers may simply state that they have broadly followed a qualitative approach and not specify a particular category. In these instances, they may have followed some of the basic principles of a qualitative approach in valuing the individual's views, experiences or perceptions, or have followed some of the principles of qualitative data analysis to make sense of the findings. The depth of analysis will also vary from article to article. Studies can be of practical value even if they do not always follow the criteria applied to a specific qualitative approach, like those described above. However, the researcher should provide in-depth 'backstage' information on how the study was carried out and the analysis achieved.

Sometimes, researchers will use a very descriptive approach to present the study and summarise the main points made under various headings or themes. A tried and tested method of looking for themes in the data is *thematic analysis* (Braun and Clarke, 2006). Here, the attempt is to paint a picture of the situation from the individual's perspective without attempting to provide analytical comment. Occasionally, a study is described as a *thematic analysis*, although this can be confusing because it is really a versatile method of qualitative data analysis and not a complete research methodology like phenomenology or ethnography.

MIXED-METHODS RESEARCH

Mixed-methods research are studies which use quantitative and qualitative methods as already seen in Chapters 2 and 3. This can provide a deeper understanding of people and their behaviour and the meaning behind it (Wurtz, 2015). Mixed-methods studies integrate both quantitative and qualitative data to develop a more comprehensive understanding than if either had been used alone (Creswell and Plano Clark, 2017). Typically, they are asking the *what* and the *why*. The *what* will be best answered using quantitative data, and the *why* requires qualitative data. In mixed-methods studies, the data will be quite different and require different methods of analysis, but the findings are combined to provide more detail than one method could on its own. A mixed-methods study by Agwu Kalu et al. (2018) looked at the issue of midwives' confidence to support bereaved parents in Ireland. The researchers used a quantitative method, a survey, to measure confidence levels using a validated tool. However, they also wanted to understand why confidence might be high in some midwives and low in others, and for this they needed qualitative methods, collecting data from midwives in focus groups (see Table 4.2).

FEMINIST RESEARCH

Qualitative researchers will often state that they have drawn on a particular approach such as a phenomenology or grounded theory as a part of the methodology section of a research article. This helps the reader anticipate the way the material has been analysed and also the concepts and theories behind that analysis. This can be thought of as the researcher's *theoretical lens* through which one sees the world and, because of this, the way one sees the research findings.

The aim of this section is to consider what is meant by feminist research and its relevance to midwifery knowledge. The starting point is to place feminist research within the context of feminism. Feminism is based on the belief that gender is a fundamental organiser of society. In other words, many of the things that happen (or do not happen) to women are because of the way society is set up to favour men, and this impacts all aspects of life to the detriment and disadvantage of women. A major goal of feminism is to raise the profile of women and give them a legitimate voice by redressing the imbalance of power in society. A further goal is the acceptance and legitimisation of a female social agenda and the development of an action plan for the issues raised by it. This is accepted as a long struggle, as it is felt that the negative position of women in society has existed for so long that many women themselves no longer question the disadvantages they face and have come to see them as 'normal'.

Women's health can be seen as a particular area in which women are vulnerable and do not always have the power to control the process in which they are involved. Throughout the life cycle, women's reproductive and general health becomes controlled by medicine. The history of obstetric care is a good example of how a predominantly male obstetric profession has dominated the ideas and discussion on what constitutes a desirable form of care for women during pregnancy and birth. This has led to some clearly oppressive situations for women in the name of safety and convenience. The quality of the birth experience and subsequent relationship with their baby have also been influenced by obstetric values and practices. Midwives' position in all of this is problematic. This was illustrated by the feminist analysis in Keating and Fleming's (2009) study, which identified the difficulties midwives faced in trying to facilitate a normal birth in an obstetric-led unit in Ireland. The conclusions of this study of births in three units found that midwives were impeded in their attempts to support normal birth practices by the culture of the birth

TABLE 4.2

Examples of Qualitative Approaches Used in Midwifery Research

Author and Year of Publication	Aim	Approach	Sample Size	Sampling	Data Collection Tool	Method of Data Analysis
Borelli et al. (2016)	To conceptualise first-time mothers' expectations and experiences of a good midwife during childbirth in the context of different birthplaces	Grounded theory	14	Purposive	Semi-structured interviews before and after birth	Coding, conceptualising and constant comparison
Häggsgård et al. (2021)	To explore experiences of the second stage of labour in women with spontaneous vaginal birth.	Phenomenology	21	Purposive	Semi-structured interviews	Thematic analysis based on descriptive phenomenology using NVvivo software
Norris et al. (2020)	To explore childbearing women with a high BMI (>35 kg/m²)	Interpretive phenomenological analysis	7	Purposive	Semi-structured interviews ×3 for each	IPA approach according to Smith et al. (2009)
Sosa et al. (2018)	To explore midwifery one-to-one support in labour in a real-world context of midwife-led birth environments	Ethnography	29 women 30 midwives	Purposive	Direct observation and semi-structured interviews	Data ordered and categorised into themes using NVivo software
Crowther et al. (2021)	To collaboratively and through consensus explore ways that spirituality could be honoured in 21st century maternity care.	Action research/ Co-operative enquiry	17, 9 & 7 (Phases 1, 2 & 3)	Convenience	Workshop, online group meetings, asynchronous online discussion boards and shared Dropbox folder	Themes slowly distilled with, and by, participants through discussion and reflection
Ajayi et al. (2021)	To describe and understand pregnant and new mothers' lived experiences during the COVID-19 pandemic using authentic birth stories	Narrative Analysis	83 YouTube video birth stories	Purposive	Narrative content and other details extracted onto Excel spreadsheets	Manually coded into themes using a coding strategy that the researchers had developed
Agwu Kalu et al. (2018)	To explore within an Irish context, the psychosocial factors that impact on midwives' confidence to provide bereavement support to parents who have experienced a perinatal loss.	Mixed methods Quantitative used to identify midwives' confidence in providing support Qualitative used to explain and clarify the reasons for the different levels of confidence	277 (survey) 11 (focus groups)	Convenience Purposive	Survey and Focus groups	(SPSS statistical package for quantitative data) Qualitative content analysis

BMI, Body mass index; *IPA,* interpretive phenomenological analysis.

setting, and the hierarchy of health staff who supported a medical philosophy of birth. Ten years later, a study by Keedle et al. (2019) explored the experiences of women planning a vaginal birth after caesarean (VBAC) in Australia. They concluded that women's confidence and sense of control is undermined in paternalistic and patriarchal maternity systems in which women's subordination and lack of control is part of the system of care.

Feminist research developed in response to the dissatisfaction felt by some researchers that the definition of research and the way it was conducted was overly influenced by the dominance of a male approach to research, which was often characterised by a distant and disengaged relationship with those who were its 'subjects'. Moreover, it was seen as a relationship in which the researchers held the power (Naples and Gurr, 2014: 19–20). It was felt that the quantitative research agenda neglected many of the questions that would benefit women, and feminist research was developed to form a more appropriate approach to addressing issues that were seen as woman-centred and ignored by the current research agenda. It sought to ensure that the relationship between a female researcher and the women taking part in the study was not exploitative, but more equal and based on a sharing of information and knowledge. Therefore, data collection in feminist research is often, but not always, through interviews which are much more like conversations, with a greater social balance between the two individuals involved. Attempts are made to ensure that the women participants have some control over the production of written or audio narratives. For example, feminist research is more likely to favour techniques like *member checking* or *respondent validation* where the process of sending transcripts back to participants for checking and agreement is carried out (see section below on critiquing qualitative research). This can be a method of increasing the trustworthiness of the data and therefore the validity or credibility of research, and it invites participants to be actively involved in the research process (Iivari, 2018).

There are many different branches of feminism with different theories or standpoints which emphasise different social issues and different approaches to research. These are continually being debated, explored and expanded upon by feminist researchers

(Naples and Gurr, 2014: 35), and this adds complexity when trying to understand what feminist research is as a whole. While there is no one unified definition, Gray et al. (2015) have cut through some of the complexities and contradictions within different branches of feminist research by highlighting three guiding principles on which all feminist theorists are likely to agree, which are:

- Understanding women's experiences
- Seeking to improve women's lives
- Addressing the balance of power in the relationship between the researcher and the researched.

The importance of the research question or aim cannot be underestimated. However, when the research question relates to the disadvantage of women during a vulnerable period of their lives, or highlights the disadvantages faced by women in general, and the intention is to highlight and possibly reduce this problem, then a feminist approach is usually relevant. Yet, given the tradition of supporting and empowering women in the midwifery profession, there are a surprisingly small number of midwifery studies that follow a feminist research tradition. The reason for this underrepresentation is not clear. However, there are signs that this is a changing picture and that feminist research is now gaining ground in midwifery. This section emphasises the way in which research is not just simply a process that is totally objective, but a process that can make a statement concerning a group as a whole, such as women in society. Although the tools employed are similar to those used elsewhere, it is the philosophy or values underpinning the way the study was conducted and interpreted that holds the key. Here it is argued that feminist research has much to offer midwifery research, and that, until recently, it has been underutilised as a legitimate methodological approach within the profession.

CONDUCTING RESEARCH

Once the researcher has decided that a qualitative approach is appropriate, a particular category of qualitative method has to be selected. The wording of the research question and purposes of the research will need to guide this. Questions that ask, 'What it is like to have a certain experience, such as elective Caesarean section, or twins?' may require more of a phenomenological approach that uncovers the 'lived experience' of individuals. If the question is concerned with behaviour or the structure of activities of an identified group or 'culture', such as midwives or breastfeeding women, then a more ethnographic approach will be appropriate. If the approach sets out to provide an explanation for a particular activity or belief, such as why some women feel that birth in a midwifery-led unit is the preferred option, then a grounded theory approach should be adopted.

Although these different qualitative forms of research originally followed strict principles, variations, adaptations and hybrids have arisen through use and changing ideas. The flexibility of these approaches has sometimes made it difficult to find consensual guidelines for those wanting to carry out this type of research. There is also a lack of learning opportunities to study and practice the techniques of data collection and analysis required by these approaches. For this reason, it is more usually thought of as being 'informed by' a particular approach or tradition rather than following it to the letter.

In the same way that quantitative researchers must ensure that they fully understand the process of quantitative data collection and analysis, so qualitative researchers must ensure that their work is carried out ethically and rigorously. A number of helpful texts exist that provide some guidance on the conduct of qualitative research (Silverman, 2017, Green and Thorogood, 2018), and how it should be written up (Hennink et al., 2020: 292–317). It is advised that potential qualitative researchers study these texts and participate in courses that specialise in this form of research. The novice qualitative researcher should also read as many examples of this type of research as possible in order to get a feel for the way it is conducted and presented.

This is not an easy choice of approach, particularly with phenomenology, because of its history and underpinning with philosophy. Where possible, try to read articles that describe the researcher's experiences in conducting qualitative research. Hunt and Symond's (1995) work remains a classic and very readable account of a qualitative study that includes many 'backstage' details. The book describes in great detail many of the problems, pitfalls and dilemmas Hunt encountered in carrying out her research in a midwifery unit.

Ethical considerations are just as important with this type of research as with quantitative approaches. One added difficulty, however, is that ethics committees may not be totally familiar with the approach of qualitative research in comparison to quantitative approaches. Some researchers have, therefore, found it useful to attach brief extracts or explanations of techniques or procedures from research texts as part of a submission.

In carrying out qualitative research, one ethical dilemma is the emotional closeness established between midwifery researcher and participant. This can lead to details of behaviour or descriptions of events being revealed that might oblige the researcher to break the confidentiality between the researcher and participant. An example might be a confession regarding conduct towards a child that might suggest the child is at risk. Under the professional code of conduct, a midwifery researcher would have to report that confession or detail. When outlining the nature of the researcher's role, participants should be told that if certain information is revealed to them, the researcher might have an obligation to inform others. Similarly, if participants seem close to revealing information that might lead to this, they should be reminded of the midwife researcher's professional duty to break confidences in certain circumstances (see Chapter 8 on ethics).

It should also be remembered that the nature of qualitative research is very intensive and emotionally challenging. Support from supervisors and personal support can be important in managing the emotional demands that arise.

CRITIQUING RESEARCH

As qualitative research is so different from quantitative research, the same approach to critiquing cannot be used. More details of this will be given in the next chapter on critiquing.

The first stage is to confirm that a study is qualitative in nature and then to identify which type of approach has been used. Although articles will usually indicate their qualitative nature in the title, or at least in the methods section, some authors go no further than stating that their research is qualitative in nature. This means that the method of critiquing can only be broad, and the specific criteria associated with the various approaches cannot be used. However, it is important to satisfy yourself that the common elements that unite qualitative approaches are present.

As with quantitative research, the important question in reading qualitative research is, 'Can I trust it?' In quantitative research, the key concepts are reliability and validity. It is also important to establish if the research is generalisable. However, in qualitative research, the emphasis is different, as will be discussed in more detail in the next chapter. The methods of undertaking research follow different principles. In qualitative research, we consider *credibility and auditability* when assessing the quality of a study. We do not talk of *generalisability* but instead we consider the *transferability* or *fittingness* (Byrne, 2001).

Credibility is concerned with the trustworthiness of the findings. Are they accurate descriptions of what was said or done? This is sometimes confirmed either by checking written accounts with those who participated in the research that they are a true record of the interview or observation; this is called a '*member's check*'. Alternatively, or sometimes in addition, the researcher checks with peers to establish whether others would come to the same conclusions or categories.

Auditability is concerned with the extent to which the researcher illustrates the progress from individual comments or observations to themes. It illustrates how researchers developed their analysis in order to show that it is based on an inductive process. Usually, in the methods section there will be details on the procedure followed to analyse the findings.

Transferability or fittingness is concerned with the extent to which the basic principles can be applied to other situations. Although this may appear similar to generalisability in quantitative research, it is not the same. Qualitative research findings are never generalisable but they may be applicable to some other settings.

Although many people find statistical presentations of results in quantitative research intimidating, the unfamiliar terminology and thinking behind qualitative research can also be challenging. As qualitative research has a great deal to offer midwifery knowledge,

do not be inhibited by unfamiliar terminology or ideas; instead, try to identify the underlying messages that can be applied to practice. You should find that qualitative research can be more engaging and interesting than the presentation of many quantitative studies because of its emphasis on the spoken words and feelings of those involved in midwifery care.

KEY POINTS

- Qualitative and quantitative research approaches do different jobs and answer different types of questions. One is not superior to the other; it is the research question or aim that should determine the approach.

- Qualitative research is concerned with illuminating the interpretations and meanings people give to features in their life, including those relating to pregnancy, birth and parenthood. This leads to a more holistic and person-centred approach to generating knowledge than quantitative research could achieve.

- Three major categories or traditions within qualitative research are ethnography, phenomenology and grounded theory. However, many other different approaches exist, including narrative and discourse analysis and cooperative approaches. All attempt to present situations through the eyes of those involved.

- Qualitative research is frequently characterised by a close relationship between the researcher and those participating in the study. To some extent, the researcher is the tool of data collection in qualitative research whose social skills are paramount to effective data collection.

- Issues relating to rigour and ethical considerations are just as important in this type of research as in quantitative research.

- Mixed-methods studies integrate both quantitative and qualitative data to develop a more comprehensive understanding of the research topic.

- Feminist approaches to research contain many of the characteristics of qualitative methods. Feminist research seeks to improve the situation of women disempowered by their position as women within health care arenas and society as a whole.

- Criteria used for critiquing qualitative research are different to that used for quantitative research. Knowledge of the principles of qualitative research is fundamental to a critique of such studies.
- Midwives need an understanding of both types of research in order to take a balanced approach to evidence-based practice.

REFERENCES

Agwu Kalu, F., Coughlan, B., Larkin, P., 2018. A mixed methods sequential explanatory study of the psychosocial factors that impact on midwives' confidence to provide bereavement support to parents who have experienced a perinatal loss. Midwifery 64, 69–76. https://doi.org/10.1016/j.midw.2018.06.011

Ajayi, K.V., Harvey, I.S., Panjwani, S., Uwak, I., Garney, W., Page, R.L., 2021. Narrative analysis of childbearing experiences during the COVID-19 pandemic. MCN 46 (5), 284–292.

Amodu, O.C., Salami, B.O., Richter, M.S., 2018. Obstetric fistula policy in Nigeria: a critical discourse analysis. BMC Pregnancy Childbirth 18 (1), 269. https://doi.org/10.1186/s12884-018-1907-x

Arnold, R., van Teijlingen, E., Ryan, K., Holloway, I., 2019. Villains or victims? An ethnography of Afghan maternity staff and the challenge of high quality respectful care. BMC Pregnancy Childbirth 19 (1), 307–307.

Barros, K.C.C., de Cássia Rocha Moreira, R., Leal, M.S., Ferreira Bispo, T.C., Azevedo, R.F., 2020. Healthcare experiences of homeless pregnant women. Rev. RENE 21, e43686. https://doi.org/10.15253/2175-6783.20202143686

Bohren, M.A., Vogel, J.P., Hunter, E.C., Lutsiv, O., Makh, S.K., Souza, J.P., et al., 2015. The mistreatment of women during childbirth in health facilities globally: a mixed-methods systematic review. PloS Med 12 (6), e1001847.

Bohren, M.A., Mehrtash, H., Fawole, B., Maung, T.M., Balde, M.D., Maya, E., et al., 2019. How women are treated during facility-based childbirth in four countries: a cross-sectional study with labour observations and community-based surveys. Lancet (British edition) 394 (10210), 1750–1763.

Borrelli, S.E., Spiby, H., Walsh, D., 2016. The kaleidoscopic midwife: a conceptual metaphor illustrating first-time mothers' perspectives of a good midwife during childbirth. A grounded theory study. Midwifery 39, 103–111.

Bowden, C., Sheehan, A., Foureur, M., 2016. Birth room images: what they tell us about childbirth. A discourse analysis of birth rooms in developed countries. Midwifery 35, 71–77. https://doi.org/10.1016/j.midw.2016.02.003

Braun, V., Clarke, V., 2006. Using thematic analysis in psychology. Qual. Res. Psychol. 3, 77–101. https://doi.org/10.1191/1478088706qp063oa

Burns, E., Fenwick, J., Schmied, V., Sheehan, A., 2012. Reflexivity in midwifery research: I insider/outsider debate. Midwifery 28 (1), 52–60.

Byrne, M.M., 2001. Evaluating the findings of qualitative research. AORN Online Retrieved from http://www.aorn.org/journal/2001/marrc.htm. [PubMed].

Creswell, J.W., Plano Clark, V.L., 2017. Designing and Conducting Mixed Methods Research, third ed. Sage Publications, Washington, D.C.

Crowther, S.A., Hall, J., Balabanoff, D., Baranowska, B., Kay, L., Menage, D., Fry, J, 2021. Spirituality and childbirth: an international virtual co-operative inquiry. Women Birth 34 (2), e135–e145.

De Chesnay, M., 2014. Nursing Research Using Grounded Theory: Qualitative Designs and Methods in Nursing. Springer Publishing Company, New York.

Denny, E., Weckesser, A., 2019. Qualitative research: what it is and what it is not: study design: qualitative research. BJOG 126 (3), 369–369.

Dibley, L., 2009. Experiences of lesbian parents in the UK: interactions with midwives. Evid. Based Midwifery 7 (3), 94–100.

Dodgson, J.E., 2019. Reflexivity in qualitative research. J. Human Lact. 35 (2), 220–222. https://doi.org/10.1177/0890334419830990

Downe, S., Byrom, S., 2019. Normal Birth: What's Going on? From the Northern Midwifery and Maternity Festival UK. Available at: https://www.youtube.com/watch?v=Qy5RTDuHdvs (accessed 14 May 2021).

Feeley, C., Thomson, G., Downe, S., 2019. Caring for women making unconventional birth choices: a meta-ethnography exploring the views, attitudes, and experiences of midwives. Midwifery 72, 50–59.

Ferndale, D., Meuter, R.F.I., Watson, B., Gallois, C., 2017. 'You don't know what's going on in there': a discursive analysis of midwifery hospital consultations. Health Risk & Soc. 19 (7–8), 411–431.

Gelling, L., 2010. Phenomenology: the methodological minefield. Nurs. Res. 17 (2), 4–6.

Goodwin, L., Hunter, B., Jones, A., 2018. The midwife–woman relationship in a South Wales community: experiences of midwives and migrant Pakistani women in early pregnancy. Health Expect 21 (1), 347–357. https://doi.org/10.1111/hex.12629

Gray, J., 2019. Introduction to qualitative research: Chapter 3. In: Grove, S.K., Gray, J. (Eds.), Understanding Nursing Research: Building an Evidence-based Practice, seventh ed. Elsevier, St. Louis.

Gray, M., Agllias, K., Schubert, L., Boddy, J., 2015. Doctoral research from a feminist perspective: acknowledging, advancing and aligning women's experience. Qual. Soc. Work 14 (6), 758–775.

Green, J., Thorogood, N., 2018. Qualitative Methods for Health Research, fourth ed. SAGE, London.

Grove, S.K., Gray, J., Burns, N., 2019. Understanding Nursing Research: Building an Evidence-based Practice, seventh ed. Elsevier, St. Louis.

Häggsgård, C., Nilsson, C., Teleman, P., Rubertsson, C., Edqvist, M., 2021. Women's experiences of the second stage of labour. Women and Birth: Journal of the Australian College of Midwives. https://doi.org/10.1016/j.wombi.2021.11.005

Hamill, C., Sinclair, H., 2010. Bracketing – practical considerations in Husserlian phenomenological research. Nurse Res. 17 (2), 16–24.

Harvey, M., Land, L., 2021. Research Methods for Nurses and Midwives: Theory and Practice, second ed. SAGE, London.

Hennink, M.M., Hutter, I., Bailey, A., 2020. Qualitative Research Methods. SAGE Publications Ltd, London.

Heron, J., Reason, P., 2006. The practice of co-operative inquiry: research 'with' rather than 'on' people. In: Reason, P., Bradbury, H. (Eds.), Handbook of Action Research.pp. 144–154.

Herr, K., Anderson, G.L., 2015. The Action Research Dissertation: A Guide for Students and Faculty, second ed. SAGE, California.

Holloway, I., Galvin, K., 2016. Qualitative Research in Nursing and Healthcare, fourth ed. John Wiley & Sons, Incorporated, Hoboken.

Hunt, S., Symonds, A., 1995. The Social Meaning of Midwifery. Macmillan, Houndmills.

Iivari, N., 2018. Using member checking in interpretive research practice. Info. Tech. People (West Linn, OR) 31 (1), 111–133. https://doi.org/10.1108/ITP-07-2016-0168

Kassa, Z.Y., Tsegaye, B., Abeje, A., 2020. Disrespect and abuse of women during the process of childbirth at health facilities in sub-Saharan Africa: a systematic review and meta-analysis. BMC Int. Health Hum. Rights 20 (1),23–23. https://doi.org/10.1186/s12914-020-00242-y

Keating, A., Fleming, V.E.M., 2009. Midwives' experiences of facilitating normal birth in an obstetric-led unit: a feminist perspective. Midwifery 25 (5), 518–527.

Keedle, H., Schmied, V., Burns, E., Dahlen, H.G., 2019. A narrative analysis of women's experiences of planning a vaginal birth after caesarean (VBAC) in Australia using critical feminist theory. BMC Pregnancy Childbirth 19 (1), 142–142.

Madden, R., 2010. Being Ethnographic: A Guide to the Theory and Practice of Ethnography. SAGE, London, England.

McNiff, J., 2013. Action Research: Principles and Practice, third ed. Routledge, Abingdon.

Menage, D., Bailey, E., Lees, S., Coad, J., 2020. Women's lived experience of compassionate midwifery: human and professional. Midwifery 85, 102662.

Naples, A., Gurr, B., 2014. Chapter 2. Feminist empiricism and standpoint theory: approaches to understanding the social world. In: Hesse-Biber, S.N. (Ed.), Feminist Research Practice: A Primer, second ed. SAGE.

Nolan, S., Hendricks, J., Williamson, M., Ferguson, S., 2018. Using narrative inquiry to listen to the voices of adolescent mothers in relation to their use of social networking sites (SNS). J. Adv. Nurs. 74 (3), 743–751.

Norris, G., Martin, C.J.H., Dickson, A., 2020. An exploratory interpretative phenomenological analysis (IPA) of childbearing women's perceptions of risk associated with having a high body mass index (BMI). Midwifery 89, 102789.

Patterson, J., Hollins Martin, C.J., Karatzias, T., 2019. Disempowered midwives and traumatised women: exploring the parallel processes of care provider interaction that contribute to women developing Post Traumatic Stress Disorder (PTSD) post childbirth. Midwifery 76, 21–35.

Polit, D., Beck, C., 2008. Nursing Research: Generating and Assessing Evidence for Nursing Practice, eighth ed. Lippincott Williams and Wilkins, Philadelphia.

Roberts, T., 2013. Understanding the research methodology of interpretative phenomenological analysis. Br. J. Midwifery 21 (3), 215–218.

Sando, D., Ratcliffe, H., McDonald, K., Spiegelman, D., Lyatuu, G., Mwanyika-Sando, M., et al., 2016. The prevalence of disrespect and abuse during facility-based childbirth in urban Tanzania. BMC Pregnancy Childbirth 16 (1), 236–236.

Silverman, D., 2017. Doing Qualitative Research, fifth ed. SAGE Publications Ltd, London.

Smith, J., 1996. Beyond the divide between cognition and discourse: using interpretive phenomenological analysis in health psychology. Psychol. Health 11, 261–271.

Smith, J.A., Flowers, P., Larkin, M., 2009. Interpretative Phenomenological Analysis: Theory, Method and Research. Sage, London.

Smith, J.A., Osborn, M., 2015. Interpretative phenomenological analysis as a useful methodology for research on the lived experience of pain. Br. J. Pain 9 (1), 41–42. https://doi.org/10.1177/2049463714541642

Sosa, G.A., Crozier, K.E., Stockl, A., 2018. Midwifery one-to-one support in labour: More than a ratio. Midwifery 62, 230–239. https://doi.org/10.1016/j.midw.2018.04.016

USAID., 2016. Repairing Obstetric Fistula in Nigeria. https://www.usaid.gov/sites/default/files/success/files/fp_nga_fistulapdf

Willig, C., 2008. Introducing Qualitative Methods in Psychology: Adventures in Theory and Method. McGraw-Hill, Maidenhead.

Wurtz, K., 2015. Using Mixed methods Research to Analyse Surveys. Retrieved from http://www.chaffey.edu/research/ir_pdf_files/presentations/other/0809-mixedmethods.pdf (accessed April 2016).

5

CRITIQUING RESEARCH ARTICLES

The main purpose of midwifery research is to increase the quality of care through the application of evidence-based knowledge gained from systematic data collection and analysis. There is a problem, however, and that is research does vary in quality. The perfect research project is almost impossible to achieve as researchers seldom have ideal conditions in which to carry out their work and so find themselves making the best of a challenging situation. So how does the midwife reading research assess the quality of the literature? Developing critiquing skills is part of the answer. This chapter clarifies the meaning and purpose of critiquing. The skill of critiquing is illustrated with the aid of two critiquing frameworks: one for qualitative research articles and the other for qualitative research. Some of the details within both frameworks are based on information in later chapters. This means that the reader may need to look at these for more details on certain points. This chapter appears at this point in the

book as critiquing is a skill that should be developed early in gaining an understanding of research.

READER ACTIVITY

How do you approach the literature when reading research papers?

How do you as the midwife or student midwife reading research distinguish between the good, the misleading and the dangerous?

There are some research skills that all midwives need to develop, and critiquing is one of them. This is because, as Lavender (2010) emphasises, it is no good relying on others to critique research, as they may have a different agenda and interpret studies differently. According to Halcomb and Newton (2017: 137), '*determining best available evidence requires nurses* (and midwives) *to be able to effectively critically evaluate research*' which by critiquing, or critical appraisal, means the systematic, unbiased careful examination of all aspects of a study in order to judge the merits, limitations, meaning and relevance to practice. Although the word critique sounds like the word 'criticise', it is meant to be a constructive evaluation and should be objective, unbiased and impartial. It should take a balanced view of both the content and process of research as followed by an author. It is a way of using critical skills to reflect on not only the whole process in which the research was undertaken but also the thinking and assumptions on which the research was based.

Critiquing is a skill that requires practice, so read this chapter alongside a research article that is not too complex. This will help readers become familiar with applying the critique framework. The first section reviews quantitative studies, where the results are presented in the form of numbers, and in the second part, a qualitative study where dialogue, quotes or descriptions of events is used.

APPLYING A CRITIQUING FRAMEWORK

Before starting to critique, it is useful to consider if an individual paper is worth reading. How to tell? The first of two criteria that will help is to limit any effort to peer-reviewed articles. This will indicate it is from a reliable source, such as a well-known professional journal that first gets experts to review and confirm that the study is worthy of publication.

Secondly, consider the title and its relevance to the topic under exploration by reading the abstract. An abstract is an outline or summary of the paper or the research and should be succinct and brief. It is subdivided into an introduction, main findings, discussion and conclusion, with the aim of highlighting the key points of the research. Readers often peruse the abstract of a research paper before deciding on whether they should take the time to read the complete paper. Sanganyado (2019) identifies a good abstract as '*like a traffic sign on the edge of a busy highway; easy to see even in the chaos of a rush hour, easy to understand, and accurate*' (p. 1).

Once an article has been chosen, three questions need to be answered:

- What does it say?
- Can I trust it?
- Will it contribute to practice?

The first question relates to comprehension and is a description of what the authors examined. How did they justify the need for the study? How did they carry out the study? What did they find? What did they conclude? The second question relates to an assessment of the rigour applied to the research process – how well was it thought through, and what steps were taken to reduce problems of bias, reliability and validity. This second question requires knowledge of some of the kinds of issues and techniques of research covered throughout this book. The third question relates to an evaluation of the study's contribution to professional practice – does it provide clear evidence for continuing, adapting or challenging practice. Who might benefit from the study, and in what way?

Reading research articles requires an active, analytical and reflective approach. To help improve active reading and analytical skills, first of all, it is necessary to separate a research article into its components. This illustrates the overall outline of the research and shows how all the pieces fit together. Second, to be an active reader, there are questions to be critically considered when reviewing a research paper. To help the reader appraise a research paper, there are several frameworks for critiquing research that act as an aide memoire. The Critical Skills Appraisal Programme (CASP) frameworks help readers check different types of health research for trustworthiness, results and relevance (https://casp-uk.net/casp-tools-checklists/). (For examples of frameworks, see Boxes 5.1 and 5.2). The following sections add detail to the use of a framework.

FOCUS

The first thing a reader needs to identify is the broad topic the research covers so they can put it in the context of existing knowledge. This should be stated in a few words that include the key concepts or variables covered in the article. These might be found in the title and most certainly in the aim. Ask what is the basic theme of this article? The answer might be 'making informed choices', 'care of the perineum', or 'breastfeeding support'. Notice that these are not questions, nor are they long or detailed. At this stage, the reader is looking at the broad canvas of which this study forms a part.

BACKGROUND

The opening to an article should provide a convincing justification for choosing the topic area. Here, the reader should expect a clear argument or evidence as to why the topic is a problem, the nature and implications of that problem, and how it has been examined in the literature. A study should start with the identification of a problem.

The author may use the subheading '*Review of the literature*' (or '*Literature review*') in which previous studies are examined. Some articles may contain only a summary or synopsis of previous work. Where

---

BOX 5.1
FRAMEWORK FOR CRITIQUING QUANTITATIVE RESEARCH

Do not expect to get answers to every question in each section, as what is important will vary from study to study. The questions provided here are to give some guidance.

1. **Focus:** In broad terms, what is the theme of the article? What are the key words to file this article under? Is the title a clue to the focus? How important is this for the profession/practice?

2. **Background:** What argument or evidence does the researcher provide to suggest this topic is worth exploring? Is there a review of previous literature on the subject, or reference to government or professional reports that illustrate its importance? Are gaps in the literature or inadequacies with previous methods highlighted? Are local problems or changes that justify the study presented? Is there a trigger that answers the question 'why did they do it then?' Is there a theoretical or conceptual framework that helps us to see how all the elements in the study may be related?

3. **Research Question:** What is the research question or aim? The research aim will usually start with the word 'to' (e.g. the aim of this research was '*to examine/ determine/compare/establish/etc*'). If relevant, is there a hypothesis? If there is, what are the dependent and independent variables? Are there concept and operational definitions for the key concepts?

4. **Study Design:** What is the broad research approach? Is it quantitative or qualitative? Is the design experimental, descriptive or correlation? Is the study design appropriate to the aim?

5. **Data Collection Method:** Which tool of data collection has been used? Has a single method been used or triangulation? Has the author addressed the issues of reliability and validity? Has a pilot study been conducted or tool used from previous studies? Have any limitations of the tool been recognised?

6. **Ethical Considerations:** Were the issues of informed consent, confidentiality, addressed? Was any harm or discomfort to individuals balanced against any benefits? Did an ethics committee approve the study?

7. **Sample:** Who or what makes up the sample? Are there clear inclusion and exclusion criteria? What method of sampling was used? Are those in the sample typical and representative of the larger group, or are there any obvious elements of bias? On how many people/things/events are the results based?

8. **Data Presentation:** In what form are the results presented: tables, bar graphs, pie charts, raw figures, or percentages? Does the author explain and comment on these? Has the author used correlation to establish whether certain variables are associated with each other? Have tests of significance been used to establish to what extent any differences between groups/variables could have happened by chance? What sense can be made of the way the results have been presented, or could the author have provided more explanation?

9. **Main Findings:** Which are the most important results that relate to the aim? (Think of this as putting the results in priority order; which is the most important result followed by the next most important result, etc. There may only be a small number of these.)

10. **Conclusion and Recommendations:** Using the author's own words, what is the answer to the aim? If relevant, is the hypothesis accepted or rejected? Are the conclusions based on, and supported by, the results? What recommendations are made for practice? Are these relevant, specific and feasible?

11. **Readability:** How readable is it? Is it written in a clear, interesting style, or is it heavy going? Does it assume a lot of technical knowledge about the subject and/or research procedures (i.e. is there much unexplained jargon?).

12. **Practice Implications:** post-review, what is the answer to the question: the 'so what'? Was it worth doing and publishing? How could it be related to practice? Who might find it relevant and in what way? What questions does it raise for practice and further study?

BOX 5.2
FRAMEWORK FOR CRITIQUING QUALITATIVE RESEARCH

Do not expect to get answers to every question in each section, as what is important will vary from study to study. The questions provided here are to give some guidance.

1. **Focus:** What is the key issue, concept or problem the work examines? What are the key words to file this article under? Are there clues to the focus in title? How important is this for practice and the profession? Is the type of qualitative design included in the title?

2. **Background:** What argument or evidence does the researcher provide for exploring this issue, concept or problem? Is there a review of previous literature on the subject or reference to government or professional reports that illustrate its importance? Are gaps in the literature or inadequacies with previous methods highlighted? Does the literature review examine the concepts or issues that form the focus? Is there an attempt to justify the study within the context of a qualitative research design? If this is grounded theory, there may not be a comprehensive review of the literature at this point, although some reference to previous work may be included as an illustration of its importance. There should be some argument or background information to justify looking at this particular subject.

3. **Aim:** What is the stated aim of the research? This will usually start with the word 'to'. There will not be a hypothesis or the identification of dependent and independent variables, as qualitative research answers a level-one question. There may be an attempt to provide a concept definition for the concept that forms the focus of the study. On the whole, the aim will be very broad and general and not as detailed as in quantitative research.

4. **Study Design:** There may be an acknowledgement that the study is qualitative in design and then the type of method specified. The main alternatives are (1) *phenomenological*, which explores what it is like to have a certain experience such as a birth, a pregnancy or threatened miscarriage, and how people interpret that experience; (2) *ethnographic*, where the researcher enters and participates in the world of the subject by listening, observing and asking questions in order to understand their view of the world; or (3) *grounded theory*, which identifies concepts that arise from the analysis of the data collected and may also suggest a theory or hypothesis that explains or predicts some of the behaviour that has emerged in the study. It is important that the philosophy behind the method suits the intentions of the research.

5. **Tool of Data Collection:** Here focus not only in the technique used to collect the information, but the amount of detail there is on the circumstances under which the data were collected. This contributes to the credibility of the study. This should include details of the environment in which the data were collected, over what period of time data collection took place, and any other details that allow us to visualise the conduct of data collection. Did the researcher spend sufficient time, either in observing the life and behaviour of the subjects, or in interviewing subjects, to produce sufficient depth to the data? Because of the flexible way that data are gathered, and the way the method will change during data collection, a pilot study will not usually be employed. The researcher should, however, include detail of how they have attempted to achieve procedural rigour in the way the study was conducted. Did the researcher check with those in the study that the information collected was accurate (member's check)?

6. **Ethical Considerations:** As with qualitative studies, it is important that the researcher has protected the participant from harm, and has gained informed consent from those taking part in the study. It should not be possible to identify individuals or places where the study took place where this might affect anonymity. The researcher should illustrate ethical rigour

7. **Sample:** Who forms the sample and what are their basic characteristics? The sample size may be quite small, even down to 3 or 4, but more usually about 10–15. This may be dictated by theoretical saturation, that is, data collection stops once no new themes or categories emerge from the analysis. In qualitative research, it is important to assess whether the participants possess the relevant knowledge or carry out the activity in which the researcher is interested. Has the researcher demonstrated that the participants are able to provide relevant information and are not open to any kind of bias? The reader must consider to what extent the findings, theory or conceptual categories may apply to other settings. This contributes to its *fittingness* to be applied elsewhere.

8. **Data Presentation:** The data will be presented in the form of description, dialogue or comments from participants. Is this 'thick' and 'rich' description? Is there sufficient detail for us to almost feel that the reader is there? Do the quotes from participants clearly illustrate the concepts they are being used to illustrate? Is there overdependence on comments from a small number of the participants in the sample? Have the researchers detailed how they ensured that the data were accurately recorded and representative of the data gathered? Is there anything about the circumstances in which the data were collected that could have threatened the accuracy of the data? Is it possible to discover the *'decision trail'* used by the researcher to determine how the raw data was processed into

BOX 5.2
FRAMEWORK FOR CRITIQUING QUALITATIVE RESEARCH—Cont'd

the categories presented in the results section? This contributes to its *auditability*. Given the same data, it should be possible, following the decision trail, to arrive at similar categories and conclusions. Does the researcher present the findings in the participant's own words rather than reinterpreting what was said or done?

9. **Main Findings:** What are the key concepts or categories developed from the data? Do the concepts and categories presented cover all the data gathered? Were the findings checked either by the participants (member's check) or examined by other experts in the field (*peer review*)? Are the main findings credible, that is, have attempts been made to support the accuracy of the results through rigour in the way in which the study was conducted? Does the researcher discuss the findings and relate these to the literature, or do they leave the quotes to speak for themselves?

10. **Conclusion:** Is there a clear answer to the question or aim? Does the researcher propose a relationship between the concepts and categories developed in the analysis to form a clear conceptual or theoretical framework? Does the conceptual or theoretical framework reflect the data? Has the conclusion been arrived at inductively (built up from the findings)?

11. **Readability:** Does the researcher present the description of the social circumstances described in the research in sufficient detail that one can almost imagine being there, and hear the participants talking and carrying out the activities described? Is it possible to recognise the concepts described as related to practical experience? Is the report written in a simple and understandable way? Is there a clear 'story line' emerging from the research?

12. **Relevance to Practice:** Are the findings relevant to practice or professional knowledge? Is it an important area related to current concerns and issues within the profession? Does the research satisfy the criteria of *transferability*, that is, can the findings in the form of the theory, concepts or categories developed through the study be applied to other situations, or are they only applicable to the place and the people where the study took place? How has the research highlighted practice issues or provided further insight? Has it confirmed views that might have been already held?

---

possible, however, an author should provide a critical review of the literature. This should draw attention to both strengths and weaknesses of individual studies and the literature overall. In this section, the author may explicitly or implicitly draw together the theoretical or conceptual framework of the study. This will answer the question, 'which concepts or variables are seen as linked for the purpose of this study'? The review of the literature section should open with some indication of how the search for appropriate literature was conducted, for example, the databases, key words and time frame used (see Chapter 6). These will help identify if a comprehensive review was conducted.

AIM (TERMS OF REFERENCE)

The background should prepare the way for the aim or 'terms of reference', which is the question the data will be collected to answer. There are two places where the aim can usually be found. The first is in the abstract, sometimes found underneath the title. The second place is just before the subheading, 'method'. Although the aim usually begins with the word '*to*', sometimes

because of the grammatical construction of the sentence, the reader might have to insert it themselves (e.g. if it says 'this study examines the problem, etc.' it may help to rephrase it as '*to* examine the problem, etc.'). If the work is experimental, there might also be a *hypothesis* or assumption the researcher is testing. The author's stated aim and hypothesis will help us identify if these were achieved or answered.

With the aim, and the hypothesis if present, it should be possible to identify which of the three levels of research question has been used (see Chapter 2). The study variable(s) should also be clear at this stage. Where the research question is level three, there will be dependent and independent variables, and the researchers should provide a concept and operational definitions for the variables. It may be helpful to return briefly to Chapter 2 for a reminder of these terms and their meaning.

In writing or producing a critique, it helps to use the author's own words, rather than paraphrase them, to avoid changing their meaning. Try to both describe under each heading in the critique framework and also say how well the author has accomplished each aspect.

In other words, it is not simply what they said but how well they said it. This results in a critical analysis of the article.

METHODOLOGY

This section identifies the research design of the project and matches its suitability to the research question. The first stage is to classify it under one of the following:

- experimental design with an experiment and control group
- correlation, where the researcher searches for patterns or associations between variables
- a survey where the purpose is description
- a qualitative design where the purpose is to gain insights into people's perceptions, beliefs or behaviour.

Is there a match between the design and the aim? Within the broad research approach, can it be identified which tool of data collection has been used. What are some of the strengths and weaknesses of the tool of data collection that makes it appropriately chosen here? Are the limitations of that tool recognised? Has triangulation been used, where the author has used more than one method of data collection to look at the same variable? Has the researcher attempted to strengthen the accuracy or 'reliability' of the tool? For instance, has the researcher used a pilot study to check the consistency of the tool of data collection?

The critique considers the ethical issues related to the tool of data collection. Here, consider the principles of research ethics and governance, such as informed consent, confidentiality, and an evaluation of the possible negative consequences of taking part in the study. Has the researcher gained approval from an ethics committee or is it not appropriate in this case? In an increasing number of research publications, there may only be a comment that ethical approval has been given by an appropriate ethics committee. As these committees are very careful in giving permission to carry out a study, it can be assumed that all the other elements were therefore present; otherwise, permission would not have been granted (see Chapter 8 for more detailed discussion on ethical considerations and processes).

Examine the sample of people, events or objects involved in the study. Are there clear inclusion and exclusion criteria that will help us to consider if they were appropriate for the study (for more detail, see Chapter 14)? Identify the total numbers on whom the results are based. Here, it is important to be careful, as large numbers could be initially involved or targeted but, through a poor response rate, individuals dropping out, or being eliminated from analysis for one reason or another, the final numbers could be quite small. The main concern with the sample is whether it is typical of the group it represents. It is not only sample size, but also geographical variations and characteristics of the sample that need consideration. Could there be cultural patterns related to the country or part of the country, or social class, that might also influence the results? What was the name of the method used to draw people into the study, and does this have particular strengths or limitations? The wrong or inappropriate sampling strategy might seriously limit the extent to which findings may be generalised.

MAIN FINDINGS

This section is concerned with the results (quantitative research) or findings (qualitative research) of the data collection. It is necessary to review these in the light of what might be an anticipated response to questions or measurements against which a comparison can be made with the findings. For example, what proportion of women would be expected to have held the baby within 5 minutes of the birth? If the expectation was in the region of 85%, and the results showed that only 48% of women held her baby within 5 minutes of the birth, would this be considered as a main finding? In any study, there may only be a small number of perhaps three or four main findings. How easy is it to pick these out?

The results section of studies can look intimidating, especially if the reader does not have a full understanding of some of the statistical terminology and symbols. However, it does not take long to learn some of these meanings, and the results section can become clearer once the reader has learnt a few of these (see Chapter 13). Although it is reasonable for authors to make some assumptions about the level of statistical knowledge readers of certain journals should possess, unfamiliar specialised terms and procedures should be clarified. If the author is interested in reaching the widest audience, these terms should be explained. The author should also highlight what is noteworthy from the tables and graphs so the reader can understand the researcher's viewpoint. Understanding the results section can take time and perseverance, but a critique cannot be made unless the reader is clear on the results of a study.

DISCUSSION, CONCLUSION AND RECOMMENDATIONS

Following the results section, the author presents the issues that have arisen from the findings in the discussion. This section may also include the author's own comments on any limitations to the study, such as the size and composition of the sample, or the limitations of the tool of data collection. These comments should be seen as positive, and a demonstration of rigour, as the researcher is seeking to help the reader form a balanced view of the results. The discussion section takes some of the issues or implications raised by the results and presents the author's interpretation of their relevance for the aim of the study. The discussion may also refer to the findings of other studies to compare or contrast with the findings in the study under review. While reading the discussion, it is important to consider the readers own view of the arguments put forward. Is this correct, or are there other possible interpretations?

The discussion should be followed by the conclusion and provide an answer to the study's aim using or 'echoing' some of the same words as those used in the research question. Be wary of a 'conclusion' section that contains only recommendations. If this happens, the 'real' conclusion may be hidden at the start of the discussion. Where the aim is made up of more than one part, question or hypothesis, each should have a clear conclusion. In the assessment, consider whether the conclusion was based on and supported by the results. Given the findings of the study, would the reader have come to the same conclusion? Is the evidence strong enough to support the conclusion, or are there alternative conclusions that the author has not considered?

The final element should be the recommendations. Sometimes these can be placed in a box or labelled as 'implications for practice'. What does the author suggest could improve the situation? Do these suggestions flow naturally from the discussion? Are the recommendations realistic and concrete or are they so vague and general that it is unlikely that improvements could be made? Do they give a clear idea of what the reader could go away and do, having read the report?

If the reader was to produce a critique of an article, there are two remaining categories to consider. The first is how to describe its readability. Although research convention dictates the structure of a research article, report or presentation, this does not mean that it has to be dull and hard going to read or listen to. Any study has the potential to be presented in an interesting way.

The reader should expect that a research article is written in a clear style, with a minimum of jargon. Complex terminology should be explained or clarified. However, the researcher should expect readers to be familiar with common research terms and to be prepared to look up unfamiliar terms known to the majority of readers.

Finally, the most important consideration is the application of the research to clinical practice. Once the reader has read the study, what is the answer to the question, 'so what'? What is the message for practice? Is there something that should happen now as a result of these findings? The reader needs to consider some of the points in the recommendations to see if there are some things that relate to their own practice or clinical area.

Once the reader has applied all the sections of a framework to an article, they should feel that they have a clear understanding of how the author carried out the study. The reader should also feel that they have not accepted the author's work uncritically. Critiquing a research article is a meeting of minds: the researcher's and the reader's. The result should be a greater understanding and consideration of the topic under study.

Critiquing a research article should not automatically result in change. It may take a synthesis of other similar studies in the form of a literature review to produce sufficient evidence to change practice. A single study, however, could make a midwife question their practice and its effectiveness. The midwife might start to think whether some of their knowledge has passed its 'sell-by-date' and whether they need to look at their knowledge and skills more critically.

If the reader has conducted the critique robustly, they should be able to evaluate research from an informed and objective standpoint and not reject it simply because it does not agree with their personal views. Midwives need to exercise the skill of critiquing for the benefit of all concerned. However, like all skills, it does need practice. As the reader works through this book, they will gain more and more knowledge to apply when critiquing. It may be really helpful if as a reader of research if a critique can be discussed with others, perhaps in the form of a journal club. Becoming familiar with a critiquing framework and using it consistently over time facilitates becoming an analytical consumer of research.

CRITIQUING QUALITATIVE RESEARCH

The aim of qualitative research, like that of quantitative research, is to increase knowledge, and so improve practice. As a number of areas important to midwifery do not lend themselves to numeric results and statistical accuracy, other methodological approaches are applicable. Qualitative research is one such alternative (see Chapter 4). It also allows midwives to identify those areas that women themselves value in relation to the care given to them by health professionals. This is now well-established as an important source of evidence that can be used to improve maternity care.

The last chapter emphasised that the differences in the way qualitative research is conducted and presented means that the use of a quantitative critiquing framework is not just difficult but in many ways inappropriate. Any attempt to use the quantitative approach to critiquing would inevitably lead to unfair criticism, as the way qualitative research is conducted appears to break many of the principles of quantitative research. These include such things as a tool of data collection that is standardised and measures consistently, a variable that is open to quantification, the use of a pilot study to check the measuring accuracy of the data collection tool, or the use of a previous measuring tool, and relatively large sample sizes – all of these are not found in qualitative research.

The reader of research needs to adapt the critiquing framework to take account of these different principles and philosophy of research. This can be a challenge, as

the reader must be open and willing to move from often in-built assumptions of the quantitative world or paradigm of research to that of the qualitative researcher. They warn that this can involve setting aside personal and sometimes strongly held views as well thinking on a more conceptual basis to follow the inductive thinking of the qualitative researcher as they interpret the accounts gathered from participants. It is also clear that a qualitative critiquing framework should include some of the unique features of the research processes involved that differ considerably from those of quantitative research (see CASP). In this section, some of these essential features are outlined and applied to a framework for critiquing qualitative studies (see Box 5.2).

Focus, Background and Aim

Qualitative research often centres on a key human or social concept, issue or theme. As with quantitative research, the researcher should provide a clear rationale as to why the study has been undertaken. This will consist of the identification of important professional issues, local problems, or key concepts relevant to the profession or clinical practice. These concepts should be clearly defined in the background of the study. In the case of some forms of qualitative research, such as grounded theory, the researcher may avoid reading too much literature in detail prior to data collection. This is in case it directs the research too much and influences what is seen as key structures in the study. Qualitative researchers should allow the issues to arise naturally by participants to highlight what is important for them. In other qualitative studies, particularly those that do not take a grounded theory approach, the researcher might present a critical review of the literature, in the same way as quantitative studies. The researcher will state an aim, but this may be deliberately broad to provide flexibility and avoid preconceived ideas. It may well simply say the intention is to examine the experience or perception of some concept or other, such as the experience of a home birth or having a baby with a cleft palate. The question will not be at level two or three as each of those require numerical measurements to answer them.

Methodology

In outlining the methodology, the researcher should be rigorous and illustrate the steps taken to make the process of data collection as accurate as possible. There is usually an attempt is made to avoid separating those taking part from the social contexts in which they function. There should be comprehensive descriptions of the setting that go beyond a surface reporting of phenomena and so uncover feelings and the meanings given to their actions. This should produce a richly visual picture of what is going on and be so detailed that the reader almost feels to be there.

As the researcher attempts to be as flexible as possible in collecting the data, there is rarely a pilot study aimed at testing the measuring accuracy of the data collection tool. However, some researchers carry out a number of 'practice' interviews to experience the response to the interviews or observations. These different approaches to data gathering raise the question of what evaluative criteria can be used to assess the quality of these studies. Whereas quantitative research is evaluated using the concepts of reliability, validity, bias and rigour, the flexibility of qualitative designs has led to a great debate as to whether any evaluative criteria can meaningfully be applied when critiquing them (Connelly, 2016). In qualitative research, the concept of trustworthiness is used and relates to the level of confidence that any reader has in the results of a study (Schmidt and Brown, 2009). The concept of trustworthiness encompasses the components of credibility, dependability, confirmability and transferability (Bryman, 2015; Connelly, 2016; Nowell et al., 2017; Schmidt and Brown, 2009), and so trustworthiness is said to have been satisfied if the following criteria can be satisfied:

- *Credibility:* This relates to whether the details of the study are believable and appear accurate. This can be helped by the amount of description researchers provide and whether they have checked their data and interpretations with any of the participants to ensure they are 'recognised' by those involved as true and accurate. This technique is called a '*member's check*', where those in the study confirm the accuracy of the researcher's transcription or interpretation. Other techniques include '*negative case analysis*' where the researcher deliberately looks at the findings for examples that do not fit their developing ideas and may then refine their categories, and keeping a '*reflective journal*' that captures ideas and

thoughts to ensure they contribute to the analysis and interpretation process

- *Dependability/Auditability:* This illustrates the researcher's decision-making process and allows the reader to see how they developed the category headings and themes from the analysis of the interviews or observations. The researcher should give examples of what was categorised under the theme headings, and the reader should have confidence in the extensive data that the researcher used to develop this analysis
- *Confirmability:* This provides support for the researcher's ideas to show they are not preconceived ideas or subjective views but can be shown to be taken from the findings of the study
- *Transferability:* Although qualitative research cannot be generalised to other situations in the same way as quantitative research, there is still a desire that the insights or interpretations may be useful in other settings
- *Reflexivity:* Evidence of researcher reflexivity may also contribute by showing how the researcher's prior knowledge and subjectivity was acknowledged and dealt with

All of these terms are abstract and therefore can seem confusing at first. However, many qualitative studies refer directly to these terms in their methods section in an attempt to demonstrate the rigour of their study.

The sample size of qualitative research tends to be much smaller than quantitative research as data collection is a more extensive for each person. In other words, the emphasis is the depth rather than breadth of data collection. The aim is not to produce a sample that is statistically similar to the larger population; the intention is to include those in a position to talk in an informed way about the concept of concern to the study. In qualitative research, the researcher is often dependent on '*participants*' who volunteer information or agree to provide an insider's view of things. There is an attempt to acknowledge and limit bias as much as possible so that a range of experiences or interpretations are covered by the sample. Decisions about sample size are discussed in Chapter 14, and there are a number of methodological processes that may influence this. One method that may be used is that once the researcher feels that subjects are revealing no new insights or themes, data collection may be ended on the grounds that '*data saturation*' has been reached and further participants would not add anything new to the study.

The issue of ethics should also be addressed, as they are equally as important as in quantitative research. Here, the researcher ensures that the individual is not put at any disadvantage as a result of being part of the study and should gain informed consent from participants. Where appropriate, the National Research Ethics Service (NRES) and local Trust Research and Development departments (if appropriate) will also be approached to give approval for the study (see Chapter 8 for more detail).

Analysis

In qualitative research, data analysis works in harmony at the same time as data collection. At this point, the researcher inductively analyses the findings for what they might reveal about the focus of the study. If the researcher is to avoid the accusation of bias and researcher subjectivity, it should be clear how decisions have been made throughout the research so that the reader can understand the thinking employed, not only in conducting the research but also in the analysis of the findings. This element of *dependability* should take the form of an '*audit trail*' for the reader to follow, showing how the raw data have systematically and consistently led to category headings that have been applied in the same way for the same elements.

The results section of qualitative research is usually referred to as the '*findings*' and differs from that of quantitative research as it will take the form of direct quotations, either from a participant or from a dialogue involving both a participant and the researcher. It may also include descriptions of places or events. In some instances, these are extracts from the researcher's '*fieldwork diary*' or notebook.

Along with the presentation of this form of data, the findings section may also draw on the literature to support the credibility of the findings and their interpretation.

Conclusion

The conclusion of the study may give both the answer to the research aim and put forward a possible explanation or interpretation of the findings. This may result in the statement of a theory or a conceptual framework that may be explored by subsequent research.

Application to Practice

The reader of qualitative research will want to apply the research to clinical and professional practice. As one of the aims of qualitative research is to sensitise the reader to the position and experiences of those in the study, the application to practice will include the extent to which new insights and awareness have been achieved through reading the study. Although the findings of qualitative research are not considered generalisable, the concept of *fittingness* suggests that there may be wider issues and principles that are transferable or applicable to other settings, providing the analysis relates to similar situations. The rigour relating to the way in which the research has been conducted will also be brought into question at this point, as the accuracy of the findings must be considered, and the extent to which any theoretical or conceptual frameworks really do fit the situation described.

This outline of the framework for qualitative research indicates that this form of research is no less rigorous than quantitative research. In the same way, the critical reader approaches the published work is no less systematic than with any other study.

CONDUCTING RESEARCH

This chapter is relevant to those undertaking research in two ways. First, the skill of critiquing is an essential part of reviewing the literature, and therefore, the researcher should approach the literature in a critical and analytical way. The frameworks in this chapter can be used by the researcher when considering the work of others. Second, researchers should remember that when they publish the results of their study, they will be subjected to the type of scrutiny suggested here. If researchers are aware of the criteria and framework that readers will use to evaluate their work, then they can ensure that these areas are addressed when writing up their study.

In the section on qualitative research, it has been emphasised how important it is for researchers to paint a very clear and vivid picture of their experience in conducting the study. This process is facilitated through the use of a fieldwork diary, or field notes (Bryman, 2015). These should contain all the essential descriptive elements relating to the fieldwork. They should also contain the major analytical processes that unfolded throughout data analysis. It is from these that the researcher can clearly demonstrate the decision trail by illuminating how the different conceptual categories arose from the mass of findings.

CRITIQUING RESEARCH

This chapter has focused on the need to question and critically analyse published research. If practice is to be evidence-based, all practitioners must develop analytical skills to allow them to assess the quality of evidence available for decision making. This should not be a purely negative activity, but should take a balanced view, identifying both the strengths and weaknesses of the work. Remember, research is a difficult activity, and it is important to identify the limitations of a study whilst recognising the constraints under which research is conducted.

It is important that the appropriate critiquing format has been used in the research. There is no use applying the quantitative critiquing framework on a qualitative article or vice versa. This chapter has attempted to provide suitable frameworks for each of these research approaches so it is possible to critique articles, and research reports, and even verbal research presentations and posters. A tip might be to photocopy the two tables into a readily accessible checklist to follow when critiquing research papers.

REFLECTION PROMPTS

Read the Hannah et al. (2000) research; now, use the critiquing tool (see Box 5.1)

Now, review the criticism of the Hannah Breech Trial (Sanders and Steele, 2014; Walker, 2012; Walker, 2013) – *what have you gleaned from this exercise about critiquing research?*

KEY POINTS

- Research is rarely conducted under perfect conditions and so weaknesses can be found in most published research. This means that just because a piece of research has been published, it is not above constructive criticism.
- Critiquing research articles should be accomplished using a systematic approach. This chapter has provided two critique frameworks: one for quantitative research articles, and the other for qualitative articles. As these two designs are based on different principles, it is important that the criteria for judging one form are not applied to the other.
- A critique should have a balance between description – what the researcher(s) did, and analysis – how well it was done.
- Undertaking a critique provides a sound basis for establishing evidence-based practice as it ensures that published research is carefully evaluated and not accepted at face value.

REFERENCES

Bryman, A., 2015. Social Research Methods, fifth ed. Oxford University Press, Oxford.

Connelly, L., 2016. Trustworthiness in qualitative research. Med. Surg. Nurs. 25 (6), 435–436.

Halcomb, E., Newton, P., 2017. Research in nursing. In: Daly, J., Speedy, S., Jackson, D. (Eds.), Contexts of Nursing: An Introduction, fifth ed. Elsevier, Australia.

Hannah, M.E., Hannah, W.J., Hewson, S.A., Hodnett, E.D., Saigal, S., Willan, A.R., 2000. Planned caesarean section versus planned vaginal birth for breech presentation at term: a randomised multicentre trial. Term Breech Trial Collaborative Group. Lancet 356 (9239), 1375–1383.

Lavender, T., 2010. Is there enough evidence to meet the expectations of a changing midwifery agenda. In: Spiby, H., Munro, J. (Eds.), Evidence-Based Midwifery: Applications in Context. Wiley-Blackwell, Chichester.

Nowell, L., Norris, J., White, D., et al., 2017. Thematic analysis: striving to meet the trustworthiness criteria. Int. J. Qual. Methods 16, 1–13.

Sanders, R., Steele, D., 2014. Re-engaging with vaginal breech birth: a philosophical discussion. Br. J. Midwifery 22 (5), 326–331.

Sanganyado, E., 2019. How to write an honest but effective abstract for scientific papers. Sci. Afr. 6, e00170.

Schmidt, N., Brown, J., 2009. Evidence-Based Practice for Nurses: Appraisal and Application of Research. Jones and Bartlett, Sudbury.

Walker, S., 2012. Breech birth: an unusual normal. Pract. Midwife 15 (3), 18–21.

Walker, S., 2013. Undiagnosed breech: towards a woman-centred approach. Br. J. Midwifery 21 (5), 316–322.

6

REVIEWING THE LITERATURE

A literature review should produce a picture of what is currently known about a problem or situation and identify what knowledge gaps may exist. A review of the literature is not simply a task carried out by researchers; it has now become an important part of evidenced-based practice as well as a familiar activity in many educational course assignments. The aim of this chapter is to provide practical advice on producing critical reviews of the literature suitable for many situations including student assignments and dissertations.

The process of reviewing the literature has changed considerably over time from a simple summary of what some of the literature says to a critical evaluation and synthesis of carefully sourced high-quality research evidence that can be used to support clinical decision-making. However, we will start with the following simple definition:

A review of the literature is the systematic and critical examination of a defined selection of published literature on a particular topic, issue or problem.

The key aspects highlighted in this definition are that reviews must be planned very carefully to provide the best-quality evidence, and that evidence should be subject to critical analysis to ensure that the findings are sound and transferable to practice. Reviews come in a number of forms, such as the following:

- *Narrative*: where the emphasis is on summarising the literature on a given topic or question,
- *Integrated*: where a critical evaluation of key studies is brought together in a systematic way,
- *Scoping review*: describes existing literature and also other sources of information on a broad topic. It is a fairly new, non-traditional approach in that it may not attempt to answer a question and it does not attempt to assess the quality of the literature, but it can be a useful way of gaining an understanding of the available information out there on a given topic.
- *Systematic review*: It is important to know that there is a difference between a *systematic review* and a literature review which used a systematic approach. This can be confusing! All good literature reviews (and certainly those that are required in a dissertation) should be carried out

in a systematic way. However, a *systematic review* is the name given to a very specific system of selecting and extracting key information and it is usually performed by teams of reviewers who ensure only the highest quality research informs evidence-based practice. The best-known systematic reviews in health care are Cochrane systematic reviews and these can be found in the Cochrane Library online. A student midwife carrying out a literature review for a dissertation cannot usually carry out a systematic review as such; instead they will usually do a literature review using a systematic approach.

- *Meta-analyses*: This is sometimes used in conjunction with a systematic review of similar types of **quantitative** studies. It is a process in which study results are combined statistically as if they were all one large study rather than several smaller ones. This overcomes the problem of small sample sizes and improves estimates of effect.

Meta-analysis is only ever possible with quantitative studies, but a comparable process which can be carried out with qualitative studies is referred to as meta-synthesis. In meta-synthesis, findings from qualitative studies on a particular topic or question are brought together to interpret meaning and create theories. In evidence-based practice the most sophisticated and highly sought source of evidence is the systematic review. This is because of the strict quality control placed on the studies included and the expertise of those who conduct them. In most academic courses and clinical settings the goal is usually a well-conducted integrated review that critically evaluates the studies. This chapter will mainly focus on the skills involved in the integrated review.

Why carry out a review? There are perhaps four main reasons for reviewing the literature, two of which are clinical and two academic:

- To search for best practice on which to base clinical decisions.
- As the basis for standards, protocols and guidelines for practice that will later lead to an audit of 'best practice' based on the review.

- As part of the research process where its purpose is to inform the researcher on the present state of knowledge on the topic they will research and to locate their current study within the context of that knowledge.
- As an integral part of a student assignment, or as the main focus of an assignment or dissertation for an educational course.

This demonstrates that reviews are not simply an academic exercise, they are an essential skill for all health professionals. The method of producing a review will be different within each of these four activities. In the educational setting, the depth of analysis will vary by the academic level of the course or programme of study. Most academic levels now encourage critical analysis and not just a summarising of content. At dissertation level, the depth of analysis will be paramount and the research knowledge of the student should be clearly demonstrated. The dissertation will also concentrate on a far greater conceptual or abstract level of analysis, often relating the literature to a theoretical or conceptual framework. In the clinical setting, the review will seek best practice for an activity or choice of intervention. In the research context, the three key reasons for carrying out a literature review are:

- To find out what is already known about the subject and identify gaps in the knowledge.
- To assist in defining the research question.
- To place the research in the context of other studies which address the topic.

THE PROCESS OF REVIEWING THE LITERATURE

The literature review is a research method in itself and the need for a systematic approach has already been explained. The planning stage is key to its success. Producing a rigorous review of the literature consists of the following three stages, each with its own demands and skills required to accomplish them:

- sourcing, or searching for and locating appropriate literature,
- evaluating the results of the search and extracting relevant detail,

■ writing the review based on the synthesis and evaluation of the material.

There are surprising similarities between conducting a review of the literature and a research project; both should start with a precise question. A statement such as: '*I want to find out about women who have twins*' is unlikely to be successful. There should be a clear question that the review is going to answer. A more suitable wording would be '*What are the main physical, psychological and social problems faced by women who have twins*?' Even this may be too ambitious for one assignment or review and just one of those three aspects may be more appropriate.

The review, when written, will consist of a number of subheadings under which 'clusters' of literature can be grouped. The key words that may help to clarify the headings under which the review will be structured are listed in Box 6.1.

Not all of these would be used for every subject. If we take the example of reviewing the literature on twins discussed above, we can see how they can be applied in practice. The process of planning the review may follow similar lines to that outlined in Box 6.2.

If at this stage, it is evident that the review is going to be large, the scope can be reduced to look at an aspect of it, such as the consequence of birthing twins in the first 6 weeks following birth. In this way, the planning stage helps to clarify the question that the review will answer.

BOX 6.1
KEY WORDS THAT MAY HELP TO IDENTIFY SUITABLE THEME HEADINGS FOR STRUCTURING A REVIEW

What (definitions of key terms or concepts)
Why (what are the causes/influences of the key term/ concept)
Who (is particularly affected/at risk/involved)
When (are there particular times when this might happen or action ought to be taken)
How (does it happen/take place/can we do something about it)
Problems
Solutions/recommendations
Advantages
Disadvantages
Implications for practice

BOX 6.2
PLANNING A REVIEW OF THE LITERATURE

Aim of the review:
   To consider the physical, psychological and social implications of the birth of twins on the mother and family, and to identify the implications of these factors for the midwife.
   Possible theme headings:
What are twins – how is this clinically defined, what variations are there?
Why do twins occur – what are the factors associated with twin pregnancies?
Who is most likely to have twins?
When should some of the implications be considered?
How do twins influence physical, psychological, social factors related to the mother and family?
Problems – what problems are associated with twins in pregnancy, birth and early months?
Solutions – how can some of the identified problems he reduced?
What are the *implications* for the midwife and maternity services?

The structure of the review may be reassessed as the material is gathered. For instance, it may be better to put some of the material, such as that which defines the terms used, in an introduction. The main body of the review may concentrate on the two headings of '*the main problems faced by the mothers of twins*' and '*ways in which problems can be reduced*'. A final heading may then be '*implications for practice*'. This would consider what the literature suggests are possible steps that need to be taken and would not be the writer's views. The review has to be located squarely in the literature and not take an 'essay' style coming mainly from the writer using some apt quotes to support the writer's arguments. Often, the main section of the review is written under several identified theme headings. As a general guide, two to five themes is usual, but that does vary.

REFLECTIVE ACTIVITY

Have you read many published midwifery literature reviews? Can you think of any examples?
Midwives: Could a literature review on a particular topic assist you to provide evidence-based care?

Student Midwives: Could a literature review on a particular topic assist you when writing assignments?

SOURCING THE LITERATURE

Once there is a clear question to answer, the next step is '*sourcing*' the literature. A review is only as good as the quality of the literature on which it is based, so this phase must be accomplished to a high standard. This is time consuming, but knowing how to make effective use of databases and search engines can reduce the time and effort required. This section will explain some of the principles in gathering relevant references quickly and making judgements on what is worth using in the review.

Reviews draw, in the main, on journal articles (sometimes called journal papers). This is because journals are usually more up to date than books and researchers will usually want to publish their study in a relevant, professional journal. The key principle is to use only the full text of articles as the basis for a review. The 'abstract' of an article is the short summary written under the title and used in databases to provide a quick overview but it is wholly insufficient for conducting a literature review. Relying on the abstract is likely to be very misleading as it is an incomplete view of the article. It is impossible to make a valid assessment of only an incomplete part of something.

In sourcing the literature, the first stage is to write a clear question to be answered through the review, and then break this down into the key words or variables that may help with searching for relevant literature. Specific methods used to develop a research question can be helpful in deciding which are the most relevant words or terms to use (see Chapter 7). It is useful, once these words are established, to write below them alternative terms to describe the same situation (synonyms) and use all the alternative words to maximise the search strategy. List any possible variations in spelling, especially with American variations such as 'labor' (US) and 'labour' (UK). The trick is to think of this as finding the door behind which the required information is kept, where each door has a variety of words used to describe its contents. The task is to discover which words will open

the maximum number of doors. For example, 'teenage' as in 'teenage pregnancies', may have synonyms such as 'adolescent', 'young people', 'young parents' and '13–18 years'. Similarly, 'antenatal education' may have synonyms such as 'parentcraft', 'childbirth education' or 'parenting education'. Some of these options may be listed automatically by some databases under 'subject' headings where a range of words used to store this information is listed. Some databases will then allow the search to be built up gradually by gradually adding the various search terms so that all the search terms are added together and the database will display articles for the combined words. By combining terms in this way, the number of articles is reduced as it excludes duplicate articles or articles that do not include the combination of words.

Another important aid to searching databases are words which apply logical commands for the search combinations called *Boolean Operators* (Aveyard, 2019). Do not be alarmed if this term is unfamiliar. It just means using the words *AND, OR* and *NOT* in an advanced search to make the search more focused. The way these are used is outlined below.

AND If you use this you will search for literature which includes both search terms. So if you search for **pregnancy AND alcohol** you will search for any literature which contains both search words.

OR If you use this, you will search for literature with includes either term (or both). So, for example, if you search for **pregnancy OR antenatal** you will search for literature which contains either word (or both of these words). **OR** broadens the search.

NOT If you use this, you will search for the first term but eliminate literature that also contains the second. It can sometimes be a way of excluding irrelevant literature. If for example you search for **postnatal depression NOT baby blues**, you will search for literature which contains the term postnatal depression but not baby blues. **NOT** narrows the search. However, it is important to be cautious when using **NOT** because even if you were only interested in literature about diagnosed postnatal depression and not baby blues, it is possible some useful articles on postnatal depression might also mention baby blues.

As there are a number of possible databases to search, decisions must be made on which ones are most appropriate to search for a particular topic or question. Topics of a clinical nature will be covered in databases such as **The Cochrane Library**, **NICE Evidence Search** and **Medical Literature Analysis and Retrieval System Online (MEDLINE)**, whereas more professional issues or woman-centred issues will be more likely in the **Cumulative Index to Nursing and Allied Health (CINAHL)** or **British Nursing Index (BNI)**. The **Applied Social Sciences Index and Abstracts (ASSIA)** may be useful if the question or aim of the review is strongly related to social factors, for example if it is about women who are pregnant and homeless. Similarly, depending on the topic area it may be useful to search databases that specifically cover psychology articles like **APA PsycINFO** or **APA PsycArticles or even Academic Search Complete**, which is a very large multidisciplinary database covering a lot of disciplines including psychology.

Do not simply search one database, as each one is designed to cover a slightly different aspect, and no database is complete. It is important to demonstrate that a comprehensive search has been undertaken by searching across those databases that are relevant to the specific research question or aim. The words or search terms used will be guided by the question or aim for the literature review and keywords or terms can be used. Additionally, *Medical Subject Headings* (MeSH) are used for indexing articles for the MEDLINE/PubMED database. Each research article and journal reference is associated with a prescribed set of MeSH terms to identify the content of the reference. There are hundreds of thousands of MeSH terms and they are continually being updated and added to. Using MeSH terms the researcher is able to enter phrases that the search engine recognises (instead of keywords) to assist with focussing the literature search more effectively. CINAHL also has a similar system of *Subject Headings* which allows researchers to build one-line simple or complex searches.

It is customary to name the databases and the key words used to find the literature, and any inclusion/exclusion criteria for articles (e.g. only UK articles, or excluding articles on babies in neonatal units), and the time frame used to search (how far back the search extends, e.g. 5 or 10 years). This section of the literature review should include the number of articles found ('hits') in various databases, and the numbers rejected for stated reasons.

The next four sections are written for the student midwife or midwife who is required to conduct a literature review as a part of an academic course or to inform clinical practice. These sections will cover guidance on searching effectively, extracting relevant details, common questions and writing the review. Ensure that you have read the first part of this chapter before reading on as it will be building on what has come before.

GUIDANCE ON SEARCHING EFFECTIVELY

It is important to accurately and meticulously record the details of searches so that you can clearly demonstrate how you arrived at the articles in your review. It will help to be systematic in your own records by building up a table for yourself where you can record the date of a search, the databases, search terms and the number of hits and references retrieved. As you build up your search of key words on a particular database, make sure that you save, screenshot or print out the search details to allow you to record this information. The search details should be like a recipe for arriving at your selected articles. It should include sufficient information for someone else to follow closely.

It is worth being clear here on the distinction between databases and search engines. Search engines, which include 'Google' and 'Google Scholar', do not keep their own lists of articles but sweep the web to locate references and sometimes locate the original article for you to download or print, while a database is a listing of articles and their abstracts, and may or may not offer a link to download the article. In academic work, the emphasis is on databases such as CINAHL, British Nursing Index and MEDLINE, as the journals they list tend to be those that have been '*peer reviewed*', that is, they have been filtered first (by those working in the same professional field) to ensure that they achieve a high quality. If practice is to be evidence-based, it must be built on high-quality articles, otherwise the wrong conclusion may be made. This is why your reviews should be based only on full '*primary references*', that is, complete articles written by the authors of a study themselves; avoid the use of '*secondary references*', that is, someone talking about or summarising another author's work, as you have thus not read the original and you are not in a position to personally judge its value.

One useful technique in searching for clues for relevant literature is '*back chaining*'. This involves finding one article relevant to your topic, either as a 'hard' paper copy or as a database search, and checking its list of references. The reference lists of these articles are then checked for further suitable articles, and so on. Once this has been completed several times, you should find the same names keep appearing. These are the references you must try to locate, as they are the ones that play a major part in our understanding of the topic.

An alternative to 'back chaining' is '*forward chaining*', where titles offered in databases offer the option, 'cited by' or 'similar references'. This means that a more recent author has mentioned the work of the author you are currently considering. Choosing this option will take you forward in time to a possibly relevant article.

At the end of this stage of searching the literature, the reviewer may be faced with one of two problems to overcome. The first is a shortage of useful articles, that is, when there are very few 'hits'. In these cases, it is worth checking that relevant or accurate search terms have been used. The problem may just be a typing or spelling error. If the word appears to be correct, then it could be that the database keeps the information under a different key word. Try an alternative word. If you have any articles on the subject, check if they list key words that the article has been listed under and try those. If this still does not produce many references, you may need to broaden the topic to include a wider subject of which your key word may form a part. Librarians are a valuable source of help when searching the literature, so do not be afraid to seek their support.

The second problem you may be faced with is the opposite of the above, where you have far too many hits, and are faced with 'information overload'. Here, you may have to limit the search in some way. One alternative is to reduce the time frame covered by the review to fewer years. You could also try to reduce the topic by taking one aspect of it rather than the whole topic. So if you are looking for literature on information giving, you may limit it to the antenatal period rather than information giving in general.

Before we leave this section, it is important to recognise that databases can be challenging. Never forget that you are dealing with a machine and not a person. The way

they 'think' and operate can take some time to work out and so lead to feelings of frustration. Remember, using these resources is a skill, and it does take some practice. It can be very helpful to ask for support from a colleague who is proficient. They may be able to demonstrate something that you are unsure of or answer specific questions.

REFLECTIVE PROMPT

How confident are you to search for literature?
Do you need to develop your skills in this area?
If so, reflect on what steps you will take and who could help you with this?

EXTRACTING RELEVANT DETAILS

At the end of the sourcing phase, you should have a reasonable number of references to articles on which to base your review. Once you physically have your articles, either as a paper copy or electronic copy, it is time to critically assess the material and extract relevant information for your review. To achieve this, you will need to examine all the articles systematically using a critiquing system such as the ones provided in Chapter 5. It is important to state that a review is not written as a series of critiques placed back to back. You need to compare and contrast different studies and comment on the importance of these for the question or aim of the review in the process of synthesis. You do not have to wait for all the articles to be collected before starting this stage. You should start evaluating the studies as you get hold of them, as this may lead you in different and productive directions.

Given the potentially large number of articles forming the basis of the review and the work required to extract the information, it is very important that a systematic process is used. It is vital to keep the research question or aim in mind during this process. When reading each paper the question to keep in mind is: does it contribute evidence that helps to answer the question or address the aim? This is what will guide your selection. During the initial stage of going through each article, one simple but still very popular system is to use a highlighter pen to mark key passages in paper copies of articles. Although these are very useful as a preliminary stage, it is not helpful at the writing stage. This is because highlighter pens can be overused and you can be left with so much highlighted text that the really important quotes and points become very difficult to relocate. Using different colours to code different ideas or topic areas can be useful. However, many people have found that using touch screen devices with a highlighter function works well or underlining text with a stylus. The stylus is particularly useful for making notes in the margins too.

To move from the highlighting/annotation stage to the writing up, a data extraction grid can be helpful. This can be in the form of a simple grid or even a spreadsheet which can be used to extract and organise relevant text, quotes and key points. Different theme headings can be used to assemble key quotes. Always ensure you record the author and page number if you combine quotes from different authors. It is useful to add your own comment underneath each one, saying what you feel about the comment or how you might use it in the review. This will allow you to build up your analysis of the literature and already be developing a critical and analytical approach as you go along.

It is worth examining some published literature articles, to see if they have used *data extraction tools or tables*. These are used to extract, summarise and organise the necessary information about study characteristics and they can sometimes be seen in the body or appendix. Each column in the table or grid (you will find landscape a better format than portrait) should contain a theme or category heading that will be useful for comparisons. Although these headings may vary depending on the themes or issues in your review, the headings used in the data extraction sheet in Fig. 6.1 will provide you with some useful ideas.

When reading an article or report it is possible to speed-read, until material relevant to one of the headings in the table is encountered. The material must then be read slowly and a decision made as to whether any, or some, of the passage should be entered in the grid. When writing the review, details and comparisons between studies can be easily seen and used as the basis for critical analysis and comment. Sections or the entire table may be used in the body of the review, or included in your appendix.

COMMON QUESTIONS

One of the most frequent questions asked by students writing a review is 'how many articles do I need for my review?' Unfortunately, there is no magic number. The advice is to obtain as many articles as you can in as short a period of time as possible. The more articles you gather, the easier it will be to see a pattern under the various columns in your summary table. If time is limited, there should be two main priorities: include as much recent material as possible, as these will contain current thinking and evidence, and secondly, include as many of the 'classics' as possible. The latter are the titles that appear in the majority of writers' work on a particular topic.

A second question is 'how far back do I need to go?' The usual guide is to go back approximately 5 years. If there is a lot of material, that may be sufficient, but if there is very little material, go back further. However, it is unwise to go further than 10 years for material unless it is classic or seminal work or unless you have a good rationale for doing so. Changes in health care and social factors mean that older information may not necessarily apply to the present.

A further question is 'do all the articles have to be research articles?' The answer is to focus on research articles as they are the result of a systematic process and therefore stronger evidence than an opinion piece. However, the review question is important in guiding you to the kind of articles that will provide answers for the questions. It is sometimes acceptable to include some descriptive reports based on individual thoughts, opinions or experiences, as well as policy documents, in your background section or when you set your findings in context in your discussion section.

A final question is 'can I use another review of the literature in my own review?' Aveyard (2019) warns that this needs to be considered carefully as if they are fairly up-to-date and have the same (or very similar) research question, they may leave you little to do. In which case how can your review be justified? However, the answer is not always 'no'. Previous reviews that differ in the question they asked compared to yours or have included more or different outcome measures to the ones in which you are interested may well be relevant. They may provide high-quality evidence but, as with any article, they will need to be carefully evaluated for their quality and relevance. There is also the issue of age, as newer articles, which you will include, may have emerged since a review was carried out.

Author (year)	Aim	Design and data collection tool	Sample number and selection method	Results	Conclusions	Recommendations	Your comments on strengths limitations
Author 1							
Author 2							
Etc.							

Fig. 6.1 ▪ Literature extraction sheet for use with research studies.

WRITING THE REVIEW

Writing a critical review of the literature is a high-level skill. It is not simply a collection of quotes 'cut out' of the literature and pasted together, nor is it a series of critiques of individual research articles. It should contain both description of the content of studies and analysis and reflection on what they contain, how well it is presented, and most importantly how it all relates to the question the review will answer. The real essence of a good review of the literature is not simply to present all the published work, it is to evaluate and synthesise it in order to address the question.

In your review, the selected articles are not just presented in turn but woven together to show what different authors say or have found on the same aspects, and includes your views of the strengths of the studies based on your understanding of research processes and issues. There should be a sense of what the chosen articles contribute **as a whole**. It is this approach to reviewing the literature that gains the marks in written assignments based on literature reviews.

In terms of style, the review should present a balanced view, looking at those studies that might support opposing views and look at the strength of evidence or argument presented. It should be written to demonstrate that you have been fair in presenting the evidence and have not let personal biases influence how the studies are presented. The review should be written under theme or topic headings and provide readers with the body of the evidence that has been examined and help them understand the relative importance of the key papers and any limitations. In this way, you should demonstrate ownership of the knowledge presented. It is not a summary of all the studies, but a careful analytical presentation of the studies you have selected. All the time you should be using the approach of:

DESCRIBE → COMPARE → CONTRAST → COMMENT

In this way, there should be a balance between description and critical evaluation. The question driving the review should be foremost throughout, so that the reader does not have to keep thinking, 'How does this study fit in?' The relevance of studies should be made clear, and their contribution to the evidence judged in the light of other studies or views.

One important caution is to avoid being overconfident on the results of studies. Since the perfect conditions in which to conduct research rarely exist, there is rarely a situation where you would say this study 'proves' something. Rather you would say the study 'presents strong evidence' or 'supports the view that' something is the case. It is worth looking closely at reviews of the literature for the range of phrases and ways of writing the review so that you build up a repertoire of useful phrases and well-chosen words.

At this stage, it is possible to suggest a systematic process to follow that takes into consideration all the above sections covered so far. This is presented in Box 6.3.

THE LITERATURE REVIEW AS PART OF CONDUCTING A RESEARCH STUDY

A thorough review of the literature increases the researcher's ability to plan research effectively and efficiently. So much can be learned from the published work of others, both in terms of content (what has already been established) and process (how others have gone about exploring this topic). Research must be set within the context of current studies, so it is important that the review is comprehensive. The researcher should ensure that the review is based on a clear and well thought out search strategy. There should be an emphasis on more recent research, as this will provide information on the latest findings, understandings and approaches. Classic or seminal work should also be included.

The researcher should consider the literature critically, and compare and contrast the views and findings of key authors. This should be considered in relation to the aim of the intended research. In particular, examine concepts with their operational definitions, and the experiences of using data collection tools. The method of data analysis and presentation should also be considered for the way in which they might guide the study.

The review of the literature plays a key role in developing the tool of data collection. The main elements or variables identified as important in the literature will be reflected in the tool of data collection. Similarly, the literature review will guide the development of a theoretical or conceptual framework for the study.

Although in some qualitative research methodologies, for example, grounded theory, there is a view that

BOX 6.3
THE PROCESS OF REVIEWING THE LITERATURE

1. Decide on a clear question you want to answer through the review.
2. Plan the structure of the review by thinking of the themes that will be applicable. Remember that the following are useful starting points: what, why, when, who, how, problems and solutions or advantages and disadvantages, implications for practice.
3. Decide on the key words you may need for the topic along with synonyms and alternative spellings.
4. Identify a search strategy by listing possible sources references. Explore key databases such as Cumulative Index to Nursing and Allied Health (CINAHL), The Midwives Information and Resource Service (MIDIRS) or The Cochrane Library. Be creative and use backward and forward chaining; use colleagues, other students, people in education and specialists in the topic.
5. If there seems too little material, broaden the topic; if there is too much, focus the topic down to one aspect.
6. Decide on a time period (frame) to be covered; initially this could be 5 years. If there is too little, go back further; where there is too much reduce the number of years but remember to include the classic (seminal) work.
7. As you locate material, whether it is articles, books or reports, ensure that all the information for a complete reference is recorded, or use a referencing computer programme.
8. Read through the material with your theme headings in mind. Scan fast until you meet with relevant material and then slow down and decide whether to extract it.
9. Enter the important material onto a grid or summary table. Don't forget your own comments on the material.
10. Examine your material for patterns by comparing and contrasting different authors.
11. Write a rough draft under the theme headings. Make sure you have both description (what the various authors say) as well as analysis (how well they say it). Make connections between the material for your reader, and relate studies and points to the purpose of the review. Keep telling the reader why the material included is relevant so they are not left thinking 'so what'.
12. When you are ready for the main draft, write a clear introduction including the question you set out to answer through the literature and describe your search strategy, which includes the databases, key words, time frame, the parameters used to select the material (the source of the material, e.g. British or British and American) and the themes used to group the literature.
13. At the end, make sure you relate the conclusion to practice. What can we say now, based on the literature? The conclusion should comment not only on the subject and what has been learnt, but also on the literature as a body of work itself. Is the available literature comprehensive, or are there gaps? Is the research of a high standard and rigorous, or does it contain weaknesses?
14. Remember, a review is not an essay that puts forward your views supported selectively by the literature. Neither is it a series of critiques. In writing the review, you should always start from the literature. What does it say?

reviewing the literature early on could influence the whole research process, generally it is considered useful and necessary when developing a research proposal. In conducting research, then, the literature review is a fundamental building block of the research process, particularly in quantitative research.

CONSIDERING THE LITERATURE REVIEW WHEN CRITIQUING RESEARCH

When critiquing a research article, the review of the literature section can provide vital information on what stimulated the researcher's thinking. The design and the nature of the research question will have been influenced by what the researchers discovered in their review. This should be clearly evident in the article.

Some of the preliminary pointers the reader should consider include the extent of the review – how much literature is included and how up to date it is. Is there any area obviously missing? In particular, the reader should consider the extent to which the writers critically review the available literature. Do they identify strengths, weaknesses and particularly gaps in the literature that will be addressed in their study?

READER ACTIVITY

Find two or three research papers from peer-reviewed journals and read the section entitled 'literature review' or 'background' and try to address the questions in the above paragraph.

The review of the literature should inform the reader and provide a clear rationale for conducting the study. The literature review at the start of an article should provide an understanding of some of the key issues on the topic and indicate some of the research that has already been undertaken in the area. It should point out what is known and what knowledge gaps still exist and therefore the rationale for the study. In this way, it should lead the reader to the specific research question or aim.

KEY POINTS

- A review of the literature is the critical analysis of good-quality relevant work on a topic.
- Carrying out a review has a great deal to offer midwives in practice to increase the standard of evidence-based practice. It is the starting point for most research projects. It is also the focus of many student assignments and theses.
- Reviewing the literature is a skill that can be developed by following the principles outlined in this chapter.
- Sourcing the literature is influenced firstly by the identification of the relevant key words that allow access to the literature through databases. A search strategy should be produced at the start of the search and a record kept of each stage of the search and the results of that search.
- It is important to be systematic in the method of retrieving information from individual books and articles.
- In writing the review, the topic should be presented under relevant themes.
- A review of the literature is not a series of critiques joined together but an examination of the body of knowledge on a stated topic following the selection criteria stated in the review.
- If a review is to be relevant to practice, it should include both description and critical analysis. It should end with clear recommendations for practice.

REFERENCES

Aveyard, H., 2019. Doing a Literature Review in Health and Social Care: A Practical Guide. McGraw-Hill Education, Maidenhead. Available from: ProQuest Ebook Central.

7

THE RESEARCH QUESTION

Midwifery has no shortage of questions that need to be answered. However, constructing a sound and researchable question is an art that takes practice, and the observation of a number of principles. Careful thought is essential, as the success of a project is measured against the question it set out to answer. The research question, then, is the gateway into the heart of the research process; the researcher must get this stage right, as so many other parts of the research process are influenced by it.

READER ACTIVITY

Where do research questions come from?
What makes a good question?

This chapter will outline their importance and address some of the issues relating to their construction. The purpose of a hypothesis will also be examined, and the different forms they take will be outlined.

THE ROLE OF THE RESEARCH QUESTION

If research is compared to setting out on a journey, then the research question is the statement of the destination, or as Thomas (2017: 324) suggests, it is '*a clear statement in the form of a question about an issue that a researcher wishes to study*'. A researcher cannot map a clear and effective route unless they know where they are going, and they certainly will not know whether they have arrived unless they know where they wanted to be at the end of their journey. In the same way, the research question allows the researcher to plan the research in the best possible way and make important decisions to ensure that the correct destination is reached.

The following are aspects of the research process that will be influenced by the research question:

- the broad research approach (design)
- the tool of data collection (the method)
- the sample
- the form of data analysis
- the ethical considerations

Research questions evolve from the choice of a particular topic area (White, 2017). This is often a topic felt to be problematic or where questions are raised on what is best practice for optimum care. The choice of topic can emerge from a desire to improve the quality of services, whilst others arise from reviewing the literature, or from searching for ways to provide clinically effective care. Often, the search for research problems is one of the easiest parts of the research process, and that is certainly true within midwifery.

Can research answer every kind of question? The answer is 'no'. Some questions demand a value judgement for their resolution and are not open to research. For example, 'Should midwives carry out some of the more technological procedures currently performed by obstetricians?' Although researchers can survey midwives' views or those of obstetricians, the answers would not indicate whether it is 'right', only what people feel about it. Similarly, some questions are ethical or philosophical questions and cannot be answered by research but need to be discussed and debated.

One important consideration before pursuing a research question is that of relevance. Does the research need to be done? Every research idea should be evaluated in terms of the contribution it will make to midwifery: 'Is there a need to know the answer to the question?' This can be characterised as the 'so what' and 'who cares' test, which ensures that thought is given to the outcome of research and its relevance to practice, the development of theory or its contribution to shaping policy.

Perhaps the most important criterion in judging the relevance of a research project is whether women, their babies and their family gain from this research. Even if the topic relates to midwives themselves, those receiving care may still benefit indirectly through an increase or change in midwives' knowledge, skills or attitudes.

Having considered the relevance of a particular study, the next issue is that of feasibility. This includes such factors as:

- availability of time
- availability of funding and resources
- ethical considerations
- researcher expertise
- participant availability and willingness to take part
- cooperation of key decision-makers such as clinicians and managers who will be affected by the data-gathering process and its possible disruptive effect and economic cost

The researcher must be able to confirm that all of these issues can be successfully addressed before the research can go any further.

TYPES OF RESEARCH QUESTIONS

Research questions are structured in a number of different ways according to the level of question (Blaikie and Priest, 2019; White, 2017) (see Chapter 2). The way the question is written or 'framed' will illustrate the level it addresses. Each level is associated with an appropriate broad research approach. For example, a level-one question will suggest the use of a survey or a qualitative approach such as an ethnographic or phenomenological study. Descriptive questions (or the what?) are those where little is known about a topic and the intention is to describe a situation. There is only one variable in a level-one question. The researcher should give a clear concept definition that relates to the way the variable will be defined for the purposes of the study. There should also be an operational definition in a quantitative study that will outline the way it is intended to measure that variable. At this level there is no attempt to establish cause-and-effect relationships between variables (Table 7.1).

A predictive question (or a why question) may also suggest a survey, but the question will be concerned with the pattern or correlation between variables. This level may also involve the collection of physiological measurements through observation or taking samples where at least two different measures from each subject are compared statistically to see if they show a similar pattern or correlation. In a level-two question, more is known about the topic. Here, the purpose of the research is to establish if there is a statistical relationship in the form of a correlation between the variables that have been identified. At this level, although the researcher might have a shrewd idea of what to expect, there is not enough firm evidence from a randomised controlled trial to confidently predict an outcome and so achieve a level-three question.

A causal question (or a how question) will look for a cause-and-effect relationship between two variables, particularly in relation to a clinical outcome. In a level-three question, there will be enough known about the nature of the relationship between the variables in the study to make a confident prediction about

TABLE 7.1			
Type of Question, Approach, Method and Data Production			
Question	Approach	Method	Data
How much, many, often, what do people think, believe, how well are we doing? (Level 1 Question)	Descriptive quantitative survey, audit	Observation, question-naires, interviews, docu-ments	Numeric
What is the lived experience, how do people behave, interpret situations? (Level 1 Question)	Descriptive, qualitative, phenomenological, eth-nographic	In-depth interviews, observation, documen-tary accounts (diaries, etc.)	Words in the form of dialogue, quotes, obser-vation
Which variable is related to another, or series of others? Does this method corre-late with a better outcome than another? (Level 2 Question)	Correlation survey, physi-ological measurement. Quasi-experimental	Physiological tests, mea-surement scales, ques-tionnaires, interviews observation, documents	Numeric
Is this method better than an alternative? Is there a cause-and-effect relationship between an independent and dependent variable? (Level 3 Question)	Randomised controlled trial	Physiological tests, mea-surement scales, ques-tionnaires, interviews observation, documents	Numeric

relationships and outcomes. The purpose is to examine why a relationship exists, or to test a theory. This is achieved by manipulating the independent variable to measure its effect on the dependent variable in an experimental design study such as a randomised controlled trial.

Examining the research questions will also suggest a particular method of data collection that might accurately answer the question. Although in many cases a choice may exist, such as the use of questionnaires or interviews, the nature of some questions will suggest which method might be more appropriate. So, if the question is broad or more abstract, or if it is a delicate or sensitive topic, an exploratory interview will be more appropriate than a questionnaire. Conversely, if the question requires specific and basic information, particularly where the likely responses fall into a small number of choices, a questionnaire will be a more appropriate method of collecting the data on the grounds of speed, cost and ease of analysis. If the question is about behaviour, then, providing it is feasible and acceptable, observation may be more appropriate than depending on memory or the provision of complex details through interviews or questionnaires. A level-three question will usually make it clear that an experimental design will be needed because it involves decisions on what is more effective, appropriate or successful. The question will also suggest the type of data

to be collected. In the main, this will relate to whether quantitative data in the form of numbers will be gathered, or whether qualitative data in the form of words will be necessary.

CONSTRUCTING A RESEARCH QUESTION

How are research questions constructed? Questions can take an *interrogative* or a *declarative* form. The interrogative form is written in exactly the same way as a question. For example, 'What influences women to continue breastfeeding for longer than 4 weeks?' The second, declarative form, is used more often in research reports and is a statement of the purpose of the study. This identifies what particular event, phenomenon or situation the study is to consider and usually starts with such statements as:

- to examine (what?)
- to identify (why?)
- to describe (what?)
- to explore (how?) An example would be: 'to identify some of the factors that influence woman to breastfeed for longer than 4 weeks'

The statement of the aim should allow the reader to picture what will happen to whom in a study. This

	TABLE 7.2		
	Examples of Research Aims		
Study	Aim	Type	Level
Tocque and Kennedy (2021)	This study evaluates whether an established referral Weight Watchers (WW) programme, known to be effective in adults in England, can help mothers-to-be living in North Wales lose weight	Quantitative	Level 2
Nikolopoulos et al. (2017)	This study explored women's experiences with gestational weight gain and their perceptions of discussions about gestational weight gain with HCPs during pregnancy and postpartum	Qualitative	Level 1
Noreik et al. (2021)	This study tested whether referral to one of three online programmes could lead to successful weight loss	Quantitative Randomised controlled trial	Level 3

means there should be an indication of what information or variable is to be gathered or examined, perhaps in relation to another variable, and from whom or what this information will be collected, that is, the sample involved in the study. Table 7.2 illustrates some examples of research aims written in this style.

Precisely worded research questions will provide more direction and clarity for a study. However, although the researcher may start with a clear statement of the research problem, it is important to examine the literature carefully to establish what is known already about the topic. In particular, the researcher should search for known possible relationships between the variables in the study. At this stage, the researcher should examine the way similar studies have framed their questions, and the way in which they have provided concept definitions and operational definitions for variables, as these may be useful in developing a new study.

THE HYPOTHESIS

Some researchers frame their research question around a *hypothesis*. This can be defined as the prediction the researcher makes at the beginning of the study that links an independent variable to a dependent variable; the 'what happened when' questions. As level-one (or what?) questions have only one variable, it can be seen why they do not require a hypothesis. A further definition of the hypothesis is provided by Thomas (2017: 318) as follows:

A hypothesis is a statement that predicts a relationship between an independent (causal) and a dependent (outcome) variable.

The purpose of the hypothesis is to provide a means of demonstrating whether the researcher's prediction or 'hunch' can be accepted or rejected. Researchers do not say that a hypothesis has been *proved* or *disproved*, as it is difficult to be that certain since research always includes a margin of error. From the researcher's point of view, a hypothesis gives the study direction, as the design must take into account how the variables will be measured and the statistical approach to testing the results to see if a relationship between the variables can be demonstrated. Hypotheses force the researcher to think logically and to exercise critical judgement by considering the study within the context of current knowledge and literature. They also believe that stating a hypothesis helps avoid superficiality by challenging the researcher to consider outcomes at the start of a study, and not simply come up with a possible explanation to fit findings where one has not been constructed.

The hypothesis can take one of the following forms:

- directional or 'one-tailed' hypothesis
- non-directional or 'two-tailed' hypothesis
- null-hypothesis

Directional or 'One-Tailed' Hypothesis

Here, a prediction is made about the likely outcome between two variables, e.g. *'women who deliver in a midwifery-led unit will be discharged quicker than those on consultant-led units'*. In this case, the dependent variable is the length of time between the birth and discharge home, and the independent variable is the form of care, i.e. midwifery-led or consultant-led. There is a directional, or *'one-tailed hypothesis'*, because it has predicted the results will be *more than* or *less than* that found in a comparable situation, that is, the researcher has predicted the direction of the result. A study with this kind of hypothesis could be a level-two question where researchers are comparing a group of women under midwifery-led care with a group under consultant-led care and looking for correlation or pattern between the time period between the birth and discharge home and level of intervention, or it could be experimental where researchers randomly allocate women to either a midwifery-led unit or consultant-led unit and the outcome measure would be the time between birth and discharge. In this case, it would be a level-three question, as researchers would be deliberately manipulating the independent variable – the form of care – and looking for a more explicit cause-and-effect relationship with the outcome – the time from birth to discharge.

Non-Directional or 'Two-Tailed' Hypothesis

With a non-directional hypothesis, although a prediction is made, it is not stated in which direction the outcome will be more favourable, e.g. *'there will be a difference in the length of time between birth and discharge home in those women who give birth in a midwifery-led unit in comparison with those who give birth in a consultant-led unit'*. In this example, it could be that those gave birth in the midwifery-led unit will be an in-patient for a longer length of time before going home, or vice versa. All that is predicted is that there will be a difference. This form is called a *two-tailed hypothesis*, as the result could go in either of two directions (or tails). A non-directional hypothesis would be used where the researcher feels there is an association, or pattern, but is uncertain of the exact nature, and so keeps the direction of the findings open.

Null-Hypothesis

A null-hypothesis follows the convention in experiments where the researcher demonstrates an absence of bias by stating that he or she does not expect to find a difference between the two groups in the study, e.g. *'there will be no difference in the length of time between the birth and discharge home between those women who birth in a midwifery-led unit or those who birth in a consultant-led unit'*. The null-hypothesis is known as the hypothesis of no difference and is related to statis-

tical convention where, if a difference is found, then the null-hypothesis (that there is no difference) has to be rejected. In other words, it has been demonstrated that there is a difference between the groups included in the study.

The null-hypothesis is known as the *statistical hypothesis*, as the aim is to establish statistically whether there is sufficient evidence to accept or reject it. If the statistical hypothesis is rejected, then its opposite, the scientific or *research hypothesis*, is accepted. The statistical hypothesis and the research hypothesis are different sides of the same coin, where, in reality, one cannot exist without the existence of the other, its opposite. Which one is 'face-up', or currently accepted, depends on the strength of the statistical evidence to support it. The research hypothesis is another name for the first two examples of the hypothesis examined above, that is, the directional or non-directional hypothesis.

Not all experimental research states a hypothesis; where they are provided, medical research tends to use the null-hypothesis form and midwifery research tends to use the research hypothesis and suggest the direction of the outcome.

Complex Hypotheses

This form of the hypothesis, which is also known as multivariate hypothesis, is very similar to the simple hypothesis except there is more than one dependent variable (Kaur, 2017), e.g. women who give birth in a midwifery-led unit will have a lower level of intervention during the birth and a lower level of analgesia than those who give birth in a consultant-led unit. It is more usual to see hypotheses expressed separately as two simple hypotheses, as this makes them easy to test and understand.

READER ACTIVITY

See if you can identify the dependent variables in the following complex hypothesis:

More postpartum depression and feelings of inadequacy are reported by new mothers who gave birth by caesarean section than by a vaginal birth.

In the example above, the outcome measure, or dependent variables (see Chapter 2), are 'postpartum depression' and 'feelings of inadequacy'. Each of these will form a variable in the study that will need to be clearly defined and operationalised (measured) using some kind of scoring system. The independent variable (see Chapter 2) would be the mode of birth i.e. 'caesarean section' or 'vaginal birth'. It is more usual to see the dependent variables listed separately in a number of hypotheses, as it increases clarity if the results demonstrate that some are rejected and some are accepted.

CONDUCTING RESEARCH

For those undertaking research, the development of the research question is one of the most important steps in the research process (Thomas, 2017). The preliminary stages involve ensuring that a problem area is suitable for research. This concerns the relevance of the topic. It is also important to check that the study is feasible in terms of access to the sample, the resources required to carry out the study, the ethical implications, cooperation from key people involved, and the skills of the researcher, as well as the availability of sufficient time to complete the research.

A thorough review of the literature is crucial, as this will provide valuable background information on the topic, including the possible relationships between variables that might already have been discovered. It is also useful for discovering the way other authors have developed concept and operational definitions for the variables. The literature will help the researcher decide on an appropriate level of question. The methods used in previous studies, including the way the data have been analysed, will also influence the design.

The statement of the research question should be clear. The researcher must be confident that it is possible to answer the research question through data collection. The question should make reference to the sample from whom the data will be gathered, and where there is more than one variable, the nature of any relationships should be made clear.

Once the research question has been constructed, along with the hypothesis if appropriate, it is worth asking, 'Will the information I am collecting allow me to answer the aim?' The final check is to ensure that the research question is not too large to be undertaken in its entirety. Would it be better to take on only one aspect of this problem area and leave the larger questions either to a future project or to someone else?

CRITIQUING RESEARCH

The research question is pivotal to critiquing a research article. This is because so many decisions follow as a consequence of the question wording. The level of the question, for instance, dictates whether the design should be descriptive, correlative or experimental. It is important that the researcher is consistent in the design, which should flow from the aim.

The location of the aim is usually in the abstract under the title in those journals that provide one. It is also commonly found just above the subheading 'method' following the review of the literature in the main body of a research article. Look for the phrase 'the aim of the research was to…'; the words starting with 'to' will form the aim or terms of reference.

If the question is level two or three, there may be a hypothesis, although many researchers omit this. Where a hypothesis is stated, is it directional, non-directional, or a null-hypothesis? Does it indicate a relationship between an independent and dependent variable in a named sample, and is the nature of that relationship stated? Is the researcher looking for an association, or a cause-and-effect relationship between the variables? If it is the latter, then the study should be experimental and the researcher should be responsible for introducing the independent variable.

Whether the researcher is dealing with one or several variables, in quantitative research the researcher should provide concept and operational definitions for each one identified in the aim or hypotheses. Are these clear and unambiguous?

REFLECTION PROMPTS

When you next read a research paper consider:
Has the researcher clearly answered the aim?
Where the researcher stated one or more hypotheses, is there a clear statement as to whether each of these has been accepted or rejected?
Is there a clear conclusion that relates to and echoes the way the aim was worded?
Given the results of the research, do you feel the aim has been adequately answered?

KEY POINTS

- Research studies revolve around collecting information to answer the study aim or research question.
- The way these are constructed will influence the level of the question and the way the study is constructed.
- Research questions must be capable of being answered; they must be feasible and above all relevant to practice or service delivery.
- Predictive (or Relational) and Causal questions may have a stated hypothesis that provides an indication of the prediction the researcher is making between the variables in the study.

REFERENCES

Blaikie, N., Priest, J., 2019. Designing Social Research: The Logic of Anticipation, third ed. Polity Press, Cambridge.

Kaur, S.P., 2017. Writing the hypothesis in research. Int. J. Nurs. Educ. 9 (3), 122–125.

Nikolopoulos, H., Mayan, M., MacIsaac, J., Miller, T., Bell, R.C., 2017. Women's perceptions of discussions about gestational weight gain with health care providers during pregnancy and postpartum: a qualitative study. BMC Pregnancy Childbirth 17 (1), 1–9.

Noreik, M., Madigan, C.D., Astbury, N.M., Edwards, R.M., Galal, U., Mollison, J., et al., 2021. Testing the short-term effectiveness of primary care referral to online weight loss programmes: a randomised controlled trial. Clin. Obes. 11 (6), e12482.

Thomas, G., 2017. How to Do Your Research Project: A Guide for Students, third ed. Sage Publications, London.

Tocque, K., Kennedy, L., 2021. Can Weight Watchers (WW) help address maternal obesity? An audit of weight change in women of childbearing age and mothers-to-be, referred into a commercial slimming programme. Matern. Child Health J, 1–11.

White, P., 2017. Developing Research Questions, second ed. Palgrave MacMillan, London.

8
ETHICS AND RESEARCH

WHAT IS RESEARCH ETHICS?

Research is not simply about the process of data collection; it is also concerned with the conduct of the researcher and the manner in which a study is carried out. Under research governance, this has to conform to set standards in the relationship between the researcher and those participating in the research, as well as the ethical management of the whole project. As with clinical practice, ethics in research must illustrate respect and maintain the trust that people have in health professionals, health organisations and researchers.

Ethical issues are of particular concern where research involves vulnerable groups, such as women in pregnancy and labour, as well as babies who form an even more vulnerable group. Both need their human rights respected and their safety and privacy safeguarded. Midwives work under their code of professional standards and behaviour Nursing and Midwifery Council (NMC, 2018); therefore, they are accountable for the way in which they conduct themselves when carrying out research. In the UK, they must conform to the guidelines laid down in the UK Policy Framework for Health and Social Care Research; Health Research Authority (HRA, 2021a).

This chapter examines the ethical issues raised by research in maternity services. These relate to the protection of fundamental human rights and the obligations and responsibilities of the researcher in carrying out research. The main issues covered include informed consent, confidentiality, justice and an assessment of possible benefits of participation in research balanced against possible disadvantages or 'harm'.

Ethics can be defined as a code of behaviour governed by moral principles. Within a health and social care research context, the (HRA, 2021) provides a strong sense of what is meant by ethical research. The research must be scientifically sound and must be conducted by competent people with integrity and transparency; they must weigh up the benefits and risks of the study with a clear research proposal. It must be compliant with the law and relevant indemnity insurance. It should respect people's privacy and allow people to choose whether to take part in the research. Any interventions should be justified, and the researchers have a duty of care to participants (HRA, 2020).

When planning research in health care, researchers have to anticipate and address the ethical issues that are raised. The increasing complexity and sophistication of research means that ethical issues have become more central to discussions. Ethics are now the part of the research process that the researcher *has* to get right; otherwise, the study will not get approval to take place.

Ethics relate to two groups of people: those carrying out research (who should be aware of their obligations and responsibilities in the way in which they carry out their activities) and the 'researched upon', (who have human rights that should be protected). As with ethics generally, those relating to research provide a basis for deciding whether certain behaviour can be regarded as acceptable, according to agreed principles and values. There are a number of problems implicit in this, as different people may have conflicting views and values on what is acceptable. To overcome this dilemma, research ethics committees (ECs) operate to consider research projects at a planning stage to ensure that they conform to national ethical guidelines and standards.

As medical research has been carried out for far longer and is more frequently conducted than midwifery research, it is not surprising that ethical principles have been developed with medical research very much in mind. This means that ECs often use the experimental approach synonymous with the 'scientific' method as the 'gold standard' against which others are measured. Therefore, in the past, ethical issues have been considered very much in relation to studies with a biomedical approach such as clinical trials, in which the focus is on the potential harm to participants. Moreover, within this biomedical model, the participants can be seen as 'human subjects', rather than active participants in the research. In recent years, there has been increasing awareness that this model of research ethics is inadequate for qualitative research studies. Holloway and Galvin (2016) point out that qualitative research calls for a more holistic approach, which includes a keen awareness of the importance of the participant/researcher relationship and recognition of power imbalances within that relationship. Researchers may be dealing with people who have little sense of agency or real power. This will raise ethical considerations, which must be adequately addressed.

It is important then that all midwives know about research ethics. Firstly, because in making practice research-based, the ethical aspects of a study must also be judged. It is not morally safe to implement research if it does not conform to ethical principles, as it casts doubt on the researcher's honesty and integrity concerning all aspects of the study. Secondly, knowledge of research ethics may also be crucial if the midwife has to act as advocate for an individual mother, baby and family. This may include situations where someone has been invited to take part in research that is not ethical.

DEVELOPMENT OF ETHICAL PRINCIPLES WHICH PROTECT HUMAN RIGHTS

The present guidelines on research ethics have been influenced by a number of internationally accepted codes on the conduct of research. These were developed following the revelation of a number of scientific experiments on humans that were clearly unethical. Following their revelation, it was agreed that society should be protected from anyone who might carry out research that leads to the death or injury of those taking part. Through a series of refinements, the codes outlined in Box 8.1 have influenced present-day research practice in all branches of health care.

The historical background is important because it helps to increase understanding around why ethical principles for research exist and how they apply. In particular, The Belmont Report of 1978 identified the three overarching and ethical principles of research, which protect human rights: respect for the person; beneficence and justice. These three principles remain the foundation of ethical research practice today and underpin current research policy in the UK. Table 8.1 outlines each of the principles, how the researcher demonstrates it has been achieved and, just as importantly, some of the elements that would suggest that basic human rights have been denied.

The following section briefly discusses each of the three principles and in relation to midwifery research.

Respect for Persons

This means that wherever people have capacity, they must be treated as autonomous agents. This is why it is essential to obtain informed consent from participants and ensure that they know they can withdraw at any time if they choose to, without any adverse consequences for the care they receive. The information provided and the approach that the researchers use to gain consent is important because people should have all the information they need to balance benefits and risks; they should come to their own decision and they should never feel coerced. Clearly, it is not a simple matter of someone saying 'yes I will take part in this study'. If consent is truly '*informed*', the following should be evident:

BOX 8.1
MAJOR INTERNATIONAL ETHICAL CODES

THE NUREMBERG CODE

This was developed in 1947 as a result of the human experimentation carried out by the Nazi regime during World War II. The code consists of 10 principles that have been influential in the conduct of research, particularly experimental research, throughout the world. The major principle relates to obtaining informed consent from those involved in research. Although the code relates to physical interventions, account is also taken of psychological and emotional harm. One criticism of the code is that it depends on self-regulation by the experimenter.

THE DECLARATION OF HELSINKI

These guidelines were developed by the World Medical Assembly (WMA) in Finland in 1964 and updated regularly since then, including 2018 (available at https://www.wma.net/policies-post/wma-declaration-of-helsinki-ethical-principles-for-medical-research-involving-human-subjects/). In addition to re-emphasising the principles of the Nuremberg Code, it developed clauses to protect subjects' human rights. An important distinction is made between therapeutic and non-therapeutic research. Therapeutic research relates to situations where the individual may potentially benefit physically from the research, whereas in non-therapeutic research subjects probably will not benefit physically, although others may benefit in the future.

THE BELMONT REPORT

The Belmont Report of 1978 highlighted what has become the three basic ethical principles of research:
1. respect for persons,
2. beneficence,
3. justice.

One of the report's aims was to develop guidelines on the selection of those included in the research. The report emphasises the need for written consent of subjects, and the obligation of the researcher to assess the possible risk and benefits related to participation in research.

- Full disclosure of details about the study.
- A statement that there is no obligation to take part, and that there are no consequences if the decision to participate is 'no'.
- Assurance that the individual can withdraw at any time without any negative consequences.
- Confirmation of confidentiality and anonymity
- Care that all the information concerning involvement is understood.
- Meaningful provision of the opportunity to ask questions.
- Absence of pressure, unfair inducements, or coercion to take part.

However, if a person lacks the capacity to act autonomously, they should be protected. This is definitely something that needs to be considered carefully in midwifery research. For example, newborn babies are people who lack capacity; therefore, consent must be obtained from someone who can legally make a decision on their behalf. This is usually a parent, but sometimes it may be somebody who has been granted parental responsibility or a legal representative. Parents under the age of 18 may also be research participants. In such studies, the law on consent is concerned with the young person's ability to understand and make decisions. Young people aged between 16 and 18 are usually considered competent to give consent by common law. However, for those under 16, the legal concept of 'Gillick competency' will apply. A child/young person's right to give consent is dependent upon their capacity to understand the specific circumstances and details of the research being proposed, which in turn will relate to the complexity of the research itself (HRA, 2021). Nevertheless, it is good practice (if possible) to involve the family in the decision-making process. Although if the young person objects, their wishes should be respected.

READER ACTIVITY

Imagine that someone approaches you and asks if you would take part in their research study.
What information would you want to know before you said yes?
What questions would you ask?

Your answer might be quite a long list, including who the people were, what organisation they represented, what taking part would involve (particularly,

TABLE 8.1		
Issues Involved in Achieving an Ethical Study		
Basic Human Principle Involved	**Achieved Through**	**Denied By**
Respect for individual autonomy	Informed consent	Right to refuse to participate or to withdraw at any point not explained
		Lack of clear written information on the study given to subjects
		Comprehension of information not checked
		Confidentiality and anonymity not assured
		Coerced to participate
		Excessive or unrealistic rewards promised
		Deception regarding study details
		Existing relationship between researchers and subjects exploited
		Covert data collection
Protection of participants (beneficence/non-maleficence)	Risk versus benefit ratio	Risks outweigh benefits
		Unacceptable level of pain, discomfort or distress
		Confidentiality and anonymity not protected
		Access to original data not safeguarded
		No debriefing provided or referral to appropriate agencies offered where appropriate
Justice	Fair selection of sample	Only vulnerable or disadvantaged group included
		Captive group used, or coerced, with no opportunity to refuse or withdraw without application of sanction

if it is anything invasive, painful, risky, or embarrassing), the aim of the project, what will happen to the information gathered and who might have access to that information. Anyone participating in research has the right to expect all of these questions to be answered if autonomy is to be protected. The researcher must ensure that all the details included in Box 8.2 are covered and given to anyone taking part in a study in an information sheet before they can claim that informed consent has been achieved.

Consent

Gaining consent is not simply a matter of giving information; it should be given in words and a language that the individual can understand. A suitably qualified interpreter may need to be used. In some instances, a judgement may have to be made on the person's ability to understand the information and the implications of it, or whether they have the metal capacity to make a judgement as outlined in the Mental Capacity Act 2005 (Department of Constitutional Affairs, 2005).

In midwifery, the timing and circumstances, under which consent is gained, is crucial. It is accepted that

> **BOX 8.2**
> **INFORMATION REQUIRED TO ACHIEVE INFORMED CONSENT**
>
> The identification of the researcher and their organisation
> The purpose of the study
> Potential participants informed they need not volunteer
> Assured they have the right to withdraw at any time
> The nature of the participation (what will happen over what period of time)
> Possible risks or implications of participating, and any anticipated benefits
> Assurance of confidentiality
> Offered the opportunity to ask questions and time to consider the invitation

women should not be recruited into studies when they are in labour, as they are very vulnerable (Vernon et al., 2006). The principle is that women should be provided with all the information and asked if they wish to participate in research in the antenatal period (Royal College of Obstetricians and Gynaecologists (RCOG, 2016)). However, as participants can withdraw their consent at any time, this does need to be confirmed when in labour (Birthrights 2022).

Consideration also has to be given when gaining written consent. Written consent should be obtained following receipt of a clearly written information sheet, explaining the nature of the study. People should then be given a reasonable period of time to consider whether to participate or not. It is this last issue that is problematic if women are asked to participate once in labour, as it allows no time for consideration or reflection.

Confidentiality and Anonymity

A vital component of informed consent is the assurance of confidentiality and anonymity. Confidentiality is a basic ethical principle used in many professional settings (the law and the church) and relates to the researcher, ensuring that unauthorised people do not have access to personal details and data. Anonymity means that steps are taken to protect the identity of an individual by neither giving their name when presenting research results, nor including identifying details that might reveal their identity. This might include such things as personal characteristics or the name of work areas, making it possible to deduce, with reasonable accuracy, the identity of the individual.

Confidentiality does not mean that the information will not be shared with others, as research findings frequently include verbatim comments from respondents; the key is that the person cannot be identified, and so remains anonymous (Wood and Ross-Kerr (2011)). The main issue is that of data security to ensure that others do not have access to the raw data. This involves the researcher storing the data in such a way that no unauthorised person can gain access to it. This applies not only to paper copies of information but also raw data kept on a computer that contains names or identifying details. Here, the researcher must follow the principles of the Data Protection Act (2018). This involves the right of individuals to see the information that is kept on them and their right not to have that information passed on to another party.

Beneficence

This means that there is an obligation to do good and favour the person's wellbeing. It might also be framed as non-maleficence, which means to prevent or minimise harm. This is why it is essential that the benefits and risks of research are carefully considered. Researchers must look at every aspect of the study and try to quantify the risks involved. Again, it is clear to see how this relates to obtaining informed consent. The risks may be clearer in a study, which seeks to conduct a trial of a drug or other intervention, but it may be more easy to overlook risks in a qualitative study (e.g. a study in which participants are interviewed to collect data on their experiences). These may entail an element of intrusion and embarrassment, or in some cases, such as describing a negative birth experience or the loss of a baby, a high degree of emotional distress and pain, as well as anxiety or guilt. Under these circumstances, the researcher must weigh up the costs to the individual very carefully.

Although midwifery researchers are not likely to set out to inflict harm, to some extent, all research involves some risks. Physical, psychological, emotional, social, cultural and financial safety must be considered. The researcher must carry out a risk assessment of the type, severity and likelihood of harm in a study. The extent of any risk should be discussed with those taking part before they enter into a study.

Just because there are some risks, this does not mean that such studies should not be undertaken, as they may benefit others through a greater understanding of the experiences described. For example, if there is an identified risk of emotional distress during data collection, there is a need for the researcher to be sensitive to this element of harm. Whatever the research methods, where an individual is distressed, it will involve identifying whether, in the person's own interests, the researcher should call a halt to the data collection. It also means that individuals should be told beforehand that there might be a possibility of painful memories arising during the course of the study. If there is a likelihood of emotional distress, then the researcher must be in a position to support the individual, or arrange with counselling agencies to accept referrals should the need arise. It is these kinds of details that ECs would expect to see in the outline of intended research projects.

Avoidance of harm also applies to the researchers and the ethics process should also consider the potential risks to those involved in the research, either because they are involved in administering an intervention or collecting data. For example, conducting in-depth interviews with parents who have experienced a still-birth or with women who have been victims of abuse will have consequences for the researcher. It is not just the interview process itself, although that certainly has potential to be extremely upsetting; it is also the fact that the researcher may be immersed in the data for many months. This may involve listening to the recordings of the participants' accounts over and over again. It is difficult not to be affected by this level of involvement with suffering, and the researcher should consider suitable sources of support at the planning stages.

Justice

This relates to treating people fairly. It includes the way people are selected for research studies, as well as justice regarding who benefits from research findings. This is why researchers need to be transparent and provide a rationale for their selection criteria. In selecting the study population, the researcher should ensure that the sampling is inclusive, and those chosen represent the diversity of society in order to promote fairness and equity for those who may benefit from the research. Historically, members of vulnerable groups were overrepresented in potentially risky research and underrepresented in potentially beneficial research. A systematic review by Bonevski et al. (2014) found that there were major barriers to conducting research with socially and culturally disadvantaged groups, including people who are from particular ethnic/racial groups; homeless; on low incomes; from disadvantaged areas; lesbian, gay, bisexual, and transgender (LGBT) community, disabled and those with mental illness. The term 'hard-to-reach' is used in research to describe this issue (Sydor 2013). Barriers to inclusivity include a deep distrust in research and researchers, cultural beliefs and low literacy, which limits the ability to provide informed consent. However, Bonevski et al.'s review (2014) also highlighted that researcher's assumptions and paternalistic beliefs were significant barriers to recruiting from hard-to-reach groups. It is important that the inclusion (or eligibility) criteria for participant recruitment are fair and defendable and not just based on such assumptions and beliefs.

In many countries, there are identifiable groups that are known to be the most at risk during pregnancy, birth and the postnatal period and yet researchers continue to face difficulties conducting research which could benefit people in these groups. In the UK, Black women are four times more likely than white women to die in pregnancy or childbirth, according to Mothers and Babies: Reducing Risk through Audits and Confidential Enquiries (MBRRACE-UK, 2021). Women from Asian ethnic backgrounds face a twofold risk, and women living in the most deprived areas are almost three times more likely to die than those in the most affluent areas. In the past there has not been sufficient research with women in these groups. This is changing, but change is slow. One way to assist in this process is through methods that co-create or co-design research studies with participants. This involves researchers working in partnership with people from hard-to-reach groups, within their community, to understand what their priorities for research are and what questions they want answering. It empowers people to be actively involved in the research process. It also helps to align research findings with service development and change (Greenhalgh et al., 2016; Islam et al., 2021). Not all research would be appropriate for a co-creation/co-design approach, but there are other strategies. Recruitment strategies that have potential to target particular populations like snowball sampling also have an important part to play (see Chapter 14). These are just two examples of how research designs and approaches relate to justice but there are many more.

Researchers are in a powerful position to influence inequities in health outcomes. However, they have to overcome barriers if they are to generate research findings that are representative of all social groups and can be used to deliver guidance and policy that reduce health inequities. Justice then relates to fairness around who is involved in studies and the way in which potential benefits are distributed amongst those taking part. Bias can be built in at any stage of the process. From the planning stages, researchers should have a clear understanding of who may benefit from the research. Justice, as an ethical principle, should provide checks and balances for researchers to examine their own motives for undertaking the research. The most fundamental questions relating to justice should be asked: whether a proposed study is appropriate, necessary and should even take place. There should be transparency around funding and openness regarding potential conflicts of interest. Researchers need to consider whether there is any bias in the way that participants are selected and how their data is collected. They need to examine power relationships between researcher and participant and consider the impact of this on their research. Researchers have an ethical duty to outline the limitations of studies and account for potential sources of bias (Smith and Noble 2014). Bias cannot be completely eliminated in a study; however, researchers, policy-makers and practitioners must consider whether the bias is potentially unethical when they are considering its contribution to knowledge and application to practice.

RESEARCH GUIDELINES, STANDARDS AND POLICY

The three ethical principles outlined above are important, but they are broad and require interpretation in different circumstances. In themselves, they do not provide the detailed guidance on every aspect of the research process. Alongside ethical principles, research must also comply with the law and current best practice. This is why guidelines, standards and policies for research have been developed. Ethical guidelines for nursing and midwifery research were developed much later than those in medicine. In Britain, guidelines were first produced by the Royal College of Nursing (RCN) in 1977, and these reinforced the major ethical issues regarding health-care research and provided guidance on research governance. The guidelines included helpful links to all the sources of information needed to apply for ethical approval at the time. No separate guidelines were produced for midwifery. Moreover, the RCN guidance has not been updated since 2009 and is now out of date. The HRA Policies and Standards (HRA 2021a) now provide the key guidance for all health and social care research in the UK, and it relates to all professions. However, there is a point of view that additional professional guidance on research ethics is valuable. At present, such guidance does not exist in midwifery or nursing. Gelling et al. (2021) holds up the British Psychological Society's Code of Human Research Ethics (2021) as a good example of a profession-specific ethical code and asks if it is time to do something similar in nursing and midwifery.

The UK Policy Framework for Health and Social Care Research (HRA, 2021a) is the current guidance for all health and social-care research in the UK; this benchmarks good practice in research, using the following principles. The framework reflects the relevant UK legislation and takes account the relevant application of this within the four countries that make up the UK. It reflects recognised ethical standards and models of good practice, as they apply to particular types of research. The framework is guided by a clear set of principles, and these are shown in Table 8.2.

Applying for Ethics Approval

In the UK, researchers wishing to conduct research within the National Health Service (NHS) used to make individual research ethics applications to local or regional ethics committees (EC). In 2007, this process was updated and replaced with a UK-wide integrated system, called the NHS National Research Ethics Service (NRES, but now known as RES). It involves an online application process called the Integrated Research Application Process (IRAS). A midwife who wishes to conduct a study involving data collection from NHS service-users or staff, for example, would need to apply in this way. The application process requires that the researcher assess the proposed study's risk level. Low-risk studies, for example, a small qualitative study on barriers to attending antenatal education classes, might be reviewed in a *proportionate* manner by a sub-committee who would make a decision from the information on the application. Studies deemed to be higher risk, for example, a study to trial a new intervention during neonatal resuscitation, would require *full* review and this would be a much more comprehensive review in which the researcher would need to attend an EC meeting and be questioned on their application.

ECs have a very important role to play. They exist to safeguard the rights, safety, dignity and well-being of research participants. The IRAS single integrated application process has helped to make the process more streamlined and consistent for researchers (who also have an important job to do), but this does not detract from the key role of the EC. Their job is to review all the details of a research proposal and give an opinion about whether the research is ethical. They consist of 15 people who all receive training for the role. Some are healthcare professionals and experts, but one third of the committee are lay members. They are independent of research sponsors, funders and the researchers themselves. This ensures that there are no conflicts of interest and enables them to put

TABLE 8.2

Principles That Apply to All Health and Social Care Research

The following statement of principles serves as a benchmark for good practice that the management and conduct of all health and social care research in the UK are expected to meet.

Principle 1: Safety

The safety and well-being of the individual prevail over the interests of science and society.

Principle 2: Competence

All the people involved in managing and conducting a research project are qualified by education, training and experience, or otherwise competent under the supervision of a suitably qualified person, to perform their tasks.

Principle 3: Scientific and Ethical Conduct

Research projects are scientifically sound and guided by ethical principles in all their aspects.

Principle 4: Patient, Service User and Public Involvement

Patients, service users and the public are involved in the design, management, conduct and dissemination of research, unless otherwise justified.

Principle 5: Integrity, Quality and Transparency

Research is designed, reviewed, managed and undertaken in a way that ensures integrity, quality and transparency.

Principle 6: Protocol

The design and procedure of the research are clearly described and justified in a research proposal or protocol, where applicable conforming to a standard template and/or specified contents

Principle 7: Legality

The researchers and sponsor familiarise themselves with relevant legislation and guidance in respect of managing and conducting the research.

Principle 8: Benefits and Risks

Before the research project is started, any anticipated benefit for the individual participant and other present and future recipients of the health or social care in question is weighed against the foreseeable risks and inconveniences once they have been mitigated. (A formal, structured risk assessment is only expected where identified as essential. The risk:benefit ratio will normally be sufficiently described and considered as part of review processes such as research ethics committee review.)

Principle 9: Approval

A research project is started only if a research ethics committee and any other relevant approval body (i.e. the HRA, the Administration of Radioactive Substances Advisory Committee (ARSAC), the Human Fertilisation and Embryology Authority (HFEA) or the Medicines and Healthcare products Regulatory Agency (MHRA)) have favourably reviewed the research proposal or protocol and related information, where their review is expected or required.

Principle 10: Information about the Research

In order to avoid waste, information about research projects (other than those for educational purposes) is made publicly available before they start (unless a deferral is agreed by or on behalf of the research ethics committee).

Principle 11: Accessible Findings

Other than research for educational purposes and early phase trials, the findings, whether positive or negative, are made accessible, with adequate consent and privacy safeguards, in a timely manner after they have finished, in compliance with any applicable regulatory standards, that is, legal requirements or expectations of regulators. In addition, where appropriate, information about the findings of the research is available, in a suitable format and timely manner, to those who took part in it, unless otherwise justified.

Principle 12: Choice

Research participants (either directly or indirectly through the involvement of data or tissue that could identify them) are afforded respect and autonomy, taking account of their capacity to understand. Where there is a difference between the research and the standard practice that they might otherwise experience, research participants are given information to understand the distinction and make a choice, unless a research ethics committee agrees otherwise. Where participants' explicit consent is sought, it is voluntary and informed. Where consent is refused or withdrawn, this is done without reprisal.

Principle 13: Insurance and Indemnity

Adequate (special provision is not expected unless existing arrangements (e.g. professional insurance, membership of NHS Litigation Authority schemes) provide inadequate cover) provision is made for insurance or indemnity to cover liabilities which may arise in relation to the design, management and conduct of the research project.

TABLE 8.2
Principles That Apply to All Health and Social Care Research—Cont'd

Principle 14: Respect for Privacy

All information collected for or as part of the research project is recorded, handled and stored appropriately and in such a way and for such time that it can be accurately reported, interpreted and verified, while the confidentiality of individual research participants remains appropriately protected. Data and tissue collections are managed in a transparent way that demonstrates commitment to their appropriate use for research and appropriate protection of privacy.

Principle 15: Compliance

Sanctions for non-compliance with these principles may include appropriate and proportionate administrative, contractual or legal measures by funders, employers, relevant professional and statutory regulators, and other bodies.

Principles that apply to interventional health and social care research

In addition to the above principles, the following principles apply to interventional research only (i.e. where a change in treatment, care or other services is made for the purpose of research).

Principle 16: Justified Intervention

The intended deviation from normal treatment, care or other services is adequately supported by the available information (including evidence from previous research).

Principle 17: Ongoing Provision of Treatment

The research proposal or protocol and the participant information sheet explain the special arrangements, if any, after the research intervention period has ended (e.g. continuing or changing the treatment, care or other services that were introduced for the purposes of the research).

Principle 18: Integrity of the Care Record

All information about treatment, care or other services provided as part of the research project and their outcomes is recorded, handled and stored appropriately and in such a way and for such time that it can be understood, where relevant, by others involved in the participant's care and accurately reported, interpreted and verified, while the confidentiality of records of the participants remains protected.

Principle 19: Duty of Care

The duty of care owed by health and social care providers continues to apply when their patients and service users take part in research. A relevant health or social care professional (who may or (particularly where the research team is not local to the research site) may not be a member of the research team) retains responsibility for the treatment, care or other services given to patients and service users as research participants and for decisions about their treatment, care or other services. If an unmanageable conflict arises between research and patient interests, the duty to the participant as a patient prevails. The above is taken from the UK Policy Framework for Health and Social Care Research (NHS Research Authority 2021) and may be subject to updates. Check their website for the most up-to-date information.

https://www.hra.nhs.uk/planning-and-improving-research/policies-standards-legislation/uk-policy-framework-health-social-care-research/uk-policy-framework-health-and-social-care-research/

participants at the centre of their decision making. At the time of writing, there were over 80 NHS Research ECs in the UK, reviewing around 6,000 applications a year (HRA, 2020).

Universities also have systems in place for students and staff who wish to conduct research. They will have their own EC who reviews applications and makes decisions on them. Therefore researchers who are attached to academic institutions and wish to collect data in healthcare settings, for example a midwife who wishes to conduct a study as part of a masters or PhD programme, will usually be required to make two applications for ethical approval (the university application and an NRES application).

PROBLEMS IN RESEARCH

The application of principles to practice is never easy, and ethical dilemmas are common in research. One example is that of informed consent. Part of respecting the individual is to ensure that the purpose of the research is made clear so that the individual is in a position to truly give informed consent. However, there are occasions where it is difficult to give comprehensive details of the study without compromising the validity of the results. There are situations where revealing the purpose of the study will influence the expectations or behaviour of the participants. For example, a study of student midwives' hand-washing techniques may not be accurate if the students are told that the thoroughness of their hand-washing technique is being observed. To gain more valid results, the researcher may have to say that they are observing routine procedures, and not draw attention to the importance of hand washing. The argument for this kind of incomplete disclosure would have to be made in the ethics application.

Another problem area for the researcher is that of confidentiality. We tend to think of confidentiality as not sharing information. Clearly, the purpose of research is to communicate and publish the results, without identifying or harming the individual participant. However, at the point of data collection, there are instances where it is not possible to keep confidences, even where this may be expected. One example is where there is a greater obligation on the midwife researcher to inform others of information that has been given in confidence. Clearly, where a respondent in an interview provides evidence of physical abuse by a partner to them or their children, the midwife researcher would have to state that the information could not be kept confidential. The first course of action would be to encourage the respondent to report the matter or to give permission for the researcher to report it. If this option was declined, the midwife researcher would have to report the information. The same would apply to interviews or observation of staff, involving unsafe or unethical practices. The researcher would have to intervene in the activity and report the matter. To overcome any problems in relation to confidentiality, a researcher must be clear in explaining the exact limits of confidentiality during the study. Similarly, if in interviews the respondent uses phrases such as 'between ourselves', or 'I shouldn't be telling you this but', the researcher should caution the individual that certain information would have to be reported.

CONDUCTING RESEARCH AND WRITING THE RESEARCH PROPOSAL

This chapter has identified the main ethical areas to consider when planning research. All NHS research in the UK must conform to agreed standards as set out in the UK Policy Framework for Health and Social Care Research (HRA, 2021a). Other countries may have their own policies and research governance.

The most important principles to address are those of:

- Informed consent.
- Assessment of risks/benefits.
- Confidentiality of material and anonymity of participants.
- Fair selection and treatment of subjects.

At the planning stage, it is important to determine the whole processes involved in carrying out research according to current research policy and how research approval is conducted in your clinical area or organisation. This can be quite a long chain of events, part of which will be ethical approval. The IRAS is accessed online through the HRA website.

The role of the research proposal is key to the application. Most researchers will be required to submit a proposal to their funders and gatekeepers. A research proposal is a structured document, which details the research plan in its entirety. It ensures that the researcher has thought the whole process through step-by-step, stating the question or aim, describing the methods to be used, outlining the practicalities, assessing the resources and costs involved and anticipating any problems. One way to think of it is as a masterplan for the study, and it plays a vital part in informing the ethics application.

In a research proposal, it must be clear that written informed consent will be gained, and that details of the study will be given in writing to those taking part. This will include a clear statement that there is no requirement to participate in the study, and that an agreement to take part is made on a voluntary basis. It should also be clear that the individual can withdraw at any point, without this affecting care. Both the consent form and study information sheet should use clear, unambiguous, plain language and be included in the proposal and the ethics application.

The submission to the EC should demonstrate the major benefit of conducting the study and illustrate how the findings would make a contribution to practice. Careful use of the available literature and details of the local situation should be used to support these claims.

Where the applicant is new to research, it is expected that a supervisor with research experience will be named. This might be someone within midwifery education, or someone with previous research experience. Similarly, where the study will entail statistical analysis, the names of those providing statistical advice and support will be required to provide assurance on the accuracy of the results. Details on how confidentiality and anonymity will be maintained should be included. Information on the arrangements for secure data storage should be outlined. Finally, it is important to ensure that the researcher will not raise expectations that the study will result in the provision of additional services or facilities for those who take part.

Before submitting a proposal it is worth discussing it, particularly the ethics sections, with someone who can give advice on the subject. This may include someone who has had experience of submitting a proposal via the integrated system. The first decision to make is whether ethics approval is required. In the vast majority of cases, it will be. However, if it is considered to be an audit or service evaluation, rather than research, it probably will not need ethics because nothing different is going to happen to the participants. See Chapter 2 for a comparison between audit, service evaluation and research. However, it is not always as clear-cut as it seems. A useful decision tool has been created to help researchers assess whether a study is research or whether it is audit or evaluation (HRA, 2021b).

In addition to ethical application, the research proposal may need to be seen by a local R&D unit who will assess and give advice on the technical or methodological aspects. Support should also be gained from managers, relevant clinicians and any other gatekeepers involved in accessing individuals or data within the research site (s). Written confirmation of their support is to be recommended to ensure that there is clarity on what has been agreed, even if key people 'move on' prior to or during the study.

Permission to start a study is one of the most important steps in the research process. There can be considerable delays and disappointment if this does not go smoothly. Researchers need to ensure that the ethical and methodological sections of their research proposal reach a high standard, and that these are based on sound knowledge and the principles laid down in the most recent standards and polices on research.

CRITIQUING RESEARCH

To some extent, when it comes to critiquing this aspect of the research process, midwives already have some knowledge and experience to draw on. Indeed, Oelhafen et al. (2017) explain that midwives are confronted with ethical issues frequently and acting ethically is a core midwifery competence. Furthermore, the complexity of ethical problems is increasing. Midwives must apply this ethical awareness and knowledge to the evaluation of the ethical issues raised by studies and to the way in which they were resolved by the researcher.

When critiquing research articles, the reader should consider the ethics of the study and specifically look to see if this has been addressed within the article. Although an author may mention some ethical issues in a report, there is not always space to cover all the aspects covered in this chapter. This means that only brief mention may be made of the ethical approval by an EC, the gaining of informed consent, and the assurances of confidentiality or anonymity. Often, the reader is left to assume that things have been carefully thought out and ethical safeguards applied. It is reasonable for the reader to ask the following questions as a minimum:

- Was ethical approval sought and approved prior to the study? Where was it obtained from?
- Is there evidence of freedom from bias in the way the researcher conducted the study? In particular, did anybody or organisation that might have had a vested interest in a positive outcome sponsor the author(s), or could there have been conflicts of interest?
- Was informed consent gained?
- Were there any risks of discomfort or distress involved in taking part in the study not anticipated by the researcher, or not justified by the likely benefits to the individual/others in a similar situation?
- Did the researcher conduct the research in a sensitive manner in regard to the wording of questions and privacy afforded individuals?
- Were any foreseeable discomforts, side effects or potential risks outlined to subjects before they gave informed consent?
- Was a pilot study undertaken that may have identified any risks to the individual?

REFLECTION PROMPTS

Do you think you could explain to someone why researchers need to obtain ethical approval before commencing a research study?

Why might the funding for a research project be an ethical concern?

KEY POINTS

- Research is not simply a process of gathering data; it also involves ethical issues in conducting the study.
- Ethics relate to the protection of the human rights of those involved in research, and the obligations and responsibilities of the researcher. The main human rights the researcher must illustrate are respect for the individual, the protection against harm and justice (fair treatment).
- Informed consent relates to the extent to which an individual agrees to take part in a study, on the basis of a clear understanding of the purpose of the research and the implications of agreeing to take part.
- The 'harm versus benefits' ratio is an attempt to weigh up the possible disadvantages for an individual taking part in a study against the possible positive effects, either for them or others in the future.
- Justice relates to the fair treatment of all those who are potentially or actually involved in the research process.
- All health research requires ethical approval through an approved ethics committee whose role is to protect the public and health staff against harm and exploitation. Indemnity insurance needs to be in place and there may also be a local research and development (R&D) unit that will examine the technical and practical aspects of a study.
- Projects that can be classified as audit or service evaluation are not required to be assessed by an ethics committee, but those responsible should still be mindful of the way the information is collected and the use to which it is put.

REFERENCES

Birthrights, 2022. Can I Change My Mind and Withdraw Consent? [Online]. https://www.birthrights.org.uk/factsheets/consenting-to-treatment/#withdrawconsent (accessed 17 January 2022).

Bonevski, B., Randell, M., Paul, C., Chapman, K., Twyman, L., Bryant, J., et al., 2014. Reaching the hard-to-reach: a systematic review of strategies for improving health and medical research with socially disadvantaged groups. BMC Med. Res. Methodol. 14 (1), 1–29. https://doi.org/10.1186/1471-2288-14-42

British Psychological Society Code of Human Research Ethics, 2021. [Online]. https://www.bps.org.uk/sites/www.bps.org.uk/files/Policy/Policy%20-%20Files/BPS%20Code%20of%20Human%20Research%20Ethics.pdf (accessed 21 December 2021).

Data Protection Act, 2018. https://www.legislation.gov.uk/ukpga/2018/12/contents (accessed 21 December 2021).

Department of Constitutional Affairs Mental Capacity Act, 2005. https://www.legislation.gov.uk/ukpga/2005/9/pdfs/ukpga-cop_20050009_en.pdf (accessed 24 November 2021).

Gelling, L., Ersser, S., Heaslip, V., Tait, D., Trenoweth, S., 2021. Ethical conduct of nursing research. J. Clin. Nurs. 30 (23–24), e69–e71. https://onlinelibrary.wiley.com/doi/10.1111/jocn.16038

Greenhalgh, T., Jackson, C., Shaw, S., Janamian, T., 2016. Achieving Research Impact Through Co-creation in Community-Based Health Services: Literature Review and Case Study. The Milbank Quarterly, 94 (2), 392–429. https://doi.org/10.1111/1468-0009.121

Health Research Authority, 2020. Research Ethics Committee Overview [Online]. https://www.hra.nhs.uk/about-us/committees-and-services/res-and-recs/research-ethics-committees-overview/ (accessed 12th April 2020).

Health Research Authority, 2021a. Research Policy. Standards and Legislation [Online]. https://www.hra.nhs.uk/planning-and-improving-research/policies-standards-legislation/ (accessed 12 April 2022).

Health Research Authority 2021b. Research Student Toolkit [Online]. https://www.hra.nhs.uk/planning-and-improving-research/research-planning/student-research/student-research-toolkit/.

Holloway, I., Galvin, K.T., 2016. Qualitative Research in Nursing and Healthcare, fourth ed. Wiley Blackwell, Chichester. https://www.hra.nhs.uk/planning-and-improving-research/policies-standards-legislation/research-involving-children/

Islam, S., Joseph, O., Chaudry, A., Keane, A., Wilson, C., Begum, N., et al., 2021. 'We are not hard to reach, but we may find it hard to trust' …. Involving and engaging 'seldom listened to' community voices in clinical translational health research: a social innovation approach. Res. Involv. Engagem 7 (1), 46. https://doi.org/10.1186/s40900-021-00292-z

MBRRACE-UK (Mothers and Babies: Reducing Risk through Audits and Confidential Enquiries). 2021. Saving Lives, Improving Mother's Care Report. [Online].https://www.npeu.ox.ac.uk/mbrrace-uk (accessed: 10 January 2022).

NMC, 2018. The Code: Standards of Conduct, Performance and Ethics for Nurses and Midwives. NMC, London.

Oelhafen, S., Hölzli, U., Häsänen, M., Kärema, A., Kasemets, M.T., Bartels, I., et al., 2017. Increasing midwives' ethical competence: a European educational and practice development project. Int J. Ethics Edu 2, 147–160. https://doi.org/10.1007/s40889-017-0033-3

Royal College of Obstetricians and Gynaecologists. 2016. Obtaining Valid Consent to Participate in Perinatal Research Where Consent is Time Critical (Clinical Governance Advice No. 6a). [Online]. https://www.rcog.org.uk/en/guidelines-research-services/guidelines/clinical-governance-advice-6a/ (accessed 10 January 2022).

Smith, J., Noble, H., 2014. Bias in research. Evid. Based Nurs. 17 (4), 100–101.

Sydor, A., 2013. Conducting research into hidden or hard-to-reach populations. Nurse Res 20 (3), 33–37.

Vernon, G., Alfirevic, Z., Weeks, A., 2006. Issues of informed consent for intrapartum trials: a suggested consent pathway from the experience of the Release trial [ISRCTN13204258]. Trials 7, 13. http://www.trialsjournal.com/content/pdf/1745-6215-7-13.pdf (accessed 23 April 2010).

Wood, M., Ross-Ker, J., 2011. Basic Steps in Planning Nursing Research: From Question to Proposal, sixth ed. Jones and Bartlett, Sudbury.

9

SURVEYS AND QUESTIONNAIRES

Gathering data for research is exciting. However, its success depends largely on the method used. This must be appropriate to the research question and should be a reasonable choice for the sample group. In this chapter, the use of the survey, which has traditionally been a popular method of collecting research information, is examined.

The term, survey and questionnaire are often used interchangeably. However, there is a difference. The survey is a research approach which consists of collecting information from a population sample in order to analyse it. A questionnaire is one of the data collection methods used in the survey approach, where participants are asked to respond to a predefined set of questions (Lau, 2017).

This chapter will examine some of the principles involved in the use of surveys and examine the advantages and disadvantages of one method: the use of questionnaires. The principles of questionnaire design will be illustrated at the end of the chapter. The following chapter will examine the use of interviews.

READER ACTIVITY

Access the following published study that uses a survey approach:

Coates, D., Donnolley, N., Henry, A., 2021. The attitudes and beliefs of Australian midwives and obstetricians about birth options and labor interventions. J. Midwifery Women's Health 66 (2), 161–173. https://doi.org/10.1111/jmwh.13168.

Now consider:

- *Why do you think a survey approach was used?*
- *What sort of questions were used?*
- *How did the participants receive the questionnaire?*

THE SURVEY

The survey is a quantitative research design that collects written or verbal information from large numbers of individuals, through either the use of questionnaires or interviews, in an attempt to describe a situation in the form of numbers. It also provides a way of identifying correlation or patterns amongst some of the variables included in the survey. This allows the health researcher to have a better understanding of patterns of behaviour or reactions to the provision of health services that will help in the evidence-based planning and delivery of care. Green and Thorogood (2018) suggest that the survey has become one of the most common approaches of data collection in health-care research, and midwifery researchers have also found this method of collecting data ideally suits many of the questions they wish to answer.

Why are surveys so popular? One reason is that they are very user friendly. They are less intimidating for both the researcher and those participating in comparison to some of the other forms of data collection. They are also a very effective way of collecting a large amount of data, illustrating the very practical reasons for their popularity. They are also an incredibly useful way of filling in gaps in knowledge, such as securing information from a large number of participants, focusing on specific and uncomplicated issues (Denscombe, 2011).

In summary, surveys are widely accepted as a legitimate foundation for decision-making in society. Their use has always been a feature of assessing maternity services, by both health professionals and consumer groups. This pattern is likely to increase in all areas of health care with the importance placed on user involvement under clinical governance.

The basic principle on which surveys are based is that if a researcher wants to know what is going on, then the best way to find out is to ask the relevant individuals. Results are usually quantitative data in the form of numbers. Even thoughts and opinions can be collected as numerical data by using scoring systems and scales (see section on the Likert scale below). However, they can include qualitative data in the form of words and some surveys blend the two to give ideas about the frequency, which is backed up with comments on interpretations, experiences or opinions.

The questions used in surveys can vary in a number of ways, one of the most important being the degree of structure they contain. Very structured questions are useful if the researcher wants to gain some idea of the kind of pattern involved with a certain type of activity, such as the number of women who intend to breastfeed, or the information needs of first-time pregnant mothers. This type of

question has the great advantage that the results are reasonably easy to analyse, as it usually involves counting the number who said 'yes' or 'no' or the numbers choosing each of the options in a list. This method is also a common method within audit, where a snapshot of a particular activity in one clinical arena is produced.

However, the disadvantage of this method, as Green and Thorogood (2018) observe, is that it can be superficial and still leave the researcher asking 'why' in relation to a particular pattern of behaviour or opinion. More in-depth information can be gathered using a less structured data collection tool. However, with a less structured approach, the researcher can be faced with information overload, and the answers may be very different from each other, making comparisons and summaries difficult.

A further variation is the time period examined by the survey. It can cover a 'one-off' collection of data, sometimes referred to as a *cross-sectional survey*, which considers the characteristics, experiences or views of those in a variety of clear subgroups in a population. The same survey can be repeated after a period of time with different groups to identify possible changes. For example, the number of women wanting a home birth could be gathered at one point, and then repeated one or more years later to see if there has been a change. This is known as a *trend survey* and works in the same way as audit where the same measurement is used at different times on different people to gain an indication of changes.

A different form of the survey is the *longitudinal study*, which can follow the same group of people over time and keep going back to them to note any changes. This is sometimes called a *panel study* where the researcher returns to the same group of people over time to identify trends or changes (Cosco et al. 2017). One form of the longitudinal study is the *cohort study*, which follows one specific group of respondents over time (Thomas, 2017). This usually tracks the members of the group to establish possible influences of specific conditions. An example would be the study of a group of babies born to first-time mothers in one maternity unit in one month, who are followed-up over a 10-year period to plot any differences in childhood illnesses that might be influenced by type of infant feeding. The purpose of such studies is usually to identify risk factors for certain conditions. A major problem with all types of studies that include repeated collections of survey data from the same group is people dropping out of the study (called '*study mortality*' or '*attrition*'). Where this results in large numbers of people being lost to the study, it is likely to be difficult to develop any clear conclusions because of the amount of missing data.

There are two further problems concerning the use of surveys: the first relates to the representativeness of the sample, and the second relates to validity, or what is actually being measured. The issue relating to the sample is important, as the researcher frequently wishes to generalise the findings to similar people in the wider population. For this reason, researchers must try to avoid bias in the way the sample is chosen (other methods of sampling will be covered in Chapter 14). Naturally, to get a reasonable picture of what is going on through the survey, the numbers returning questionnaires must be large and should as far as possible be representative of the total group. However, a major weakness of surveys, particularly online or postal surveys, is that response rates can be very low. There is evidence that they have been declining further in recent years due to 'survey fatigue' and privacy concerns (Harrison et al. 2019). This weakens the use of surveys in evidence-based practice, as it is often difficult to know if the results provide a true or accurate picture.

In designing the survey, it is usual to collect some basic 'demographic' details such as age, grade of staff, sex or number of children, so that some comparison can be made with those in the wider population to establish if they are a close comparison. This then gives some indication of how far the sample is representative.

The second question relating to validity is a difficult issue to address. One of the problems in surveys is that the researcher has to accept that the answer given by a respondent is true, despite being unable to test it. There are likely to be some respondents who give socially acceptable answers in surveys, that is, answers that suggest the 'perfect citizen', so the accuracy can never be 100% certain. The only action the researcher can take is to try to reduce the amount of distortion produced by the data collection tool. The pilot study is one method by which this can be attempted.

THE USE OF QUESTIONNAIRES

Questionnaires are a tool of data collection consisting of a series of questions that are usually completed by the participants themselves (self-completing) and can take the form of paper, electronic text sent by email, or online versions. They collect information on such things as personal attributes, attitudes, beliefs experiences, behaviour and activities (Hurst and Bird, 2019), and are probably the most familiar data collection tool in nursing and midwifery research. Most of the population are likely to have completed many questionnaires in their working lives, and perhaps deleted or thrown many more away. This section will examine some of the advantages and disadvantages of this method and outline some of the important principles of questionnaire design.

A large number of research questions in midwifery have been answered by questionnaire. Why are they such a popular method of collecting research data? (see Table 9.1 below for some of the answers).

Although this list suggests that questionnaires are an ideal data collection method, several factors may discourage a response, as Table 9.2 suggests. There are, then, a balancing number of disadvantages to the use of questionnaires. However, people have now received so many questionnaires that their motivation to complete and return yet another may be low, resulting in a poor *response rate*, that is, the number of those returning a questionnaire expressed as proportion of those receiving one (Harrison et al. 2019). Denscombe (2011) suggests that an acceptable response rate varies and is dependent on the method used to conduct the questionnaire (i.e. postal and online questionnaires can have a very low response rate of 10%) whereas questionnaires administered face-to-face can have almost 100% completion rates. However, the lower the response rate, the representativeness of the sample

TABLE 9.1
Advantages of Questionnaires
■ It is cheap to produce
■ It is usually quick and easy to complete
■ It can reach a large geographically spread sample
■ It is easily sent out and returned online
■ It can produce quite detailed data
■ There is a low level of embarrassment or threat to both researcher and respondent
■ Anonymity is protected
■ The fixed-choice questions are easy to answer and to analyse
■ It is a familiar method to respondents

TABLE 9.2
Disadvantages of Questionnaires

- Questionnaires have now saturated the population
- Response rate may be low dependent on feelings on the topic
- Questionnaires are dependent on reading levels, literacy skills and physical ability
- Responses will be influenced by the quality of the design and the motivation used to produce a response
- Online surveys are dependent on internet access and digital literacy
- There is no opportunity for clarification of questions or answers
- There is no support if the recipient becomes distressed while completing the questionnaire
- Fixed-choice questions may not have an appropriate option for everyone
- Creating a good quality questionnaire is a skill to be developed but is important to the response rate and the data it provides

returned can be seriously in question, as there is no certainty that the responses represent the views of all those who were sent a questionnaire. In other words, it may end up with a biased response. Generalisations from this group would then be impossible. Reminders can be sent to increase the final response rate, although the return from this may also be disappointingly low.

Similarly, a further limitation to their use is the often-overlooked assumption that questionnaire recipients can read and write in English. English not being the first language is a significant problem in maternity service users. The global population has been much more mobile over the last decade. In the UK, in areas of high density like London and Birmingham, 9% of the population could not speak English at the time of the 2011 census. This is thought to have been rising since then (Rayment-Jones et al. 2021). While eyesight and physical problems can be an issue this is not likely to be a bigger issue than language for maternity service-users (Rayment-Jones et al. 2021). For this reason, surveys involving the public can omit important opinions because certain groups are excluded through the choice of research method.

In deciding whether the response rate is adequate, the researcher needs to consider:

- Whether the level of response achieved is enough and similar to other comparable surveys?

- Do the non-responders differ significantly from those who did complete and return the questionnaire?

The disadvantages of questionnaires relate to both the researcher and the respondent. A recurring frustration for the researcher is receiving returned questionnaires containing a number of unanswered questions, or incomplete answers. Once returned, it is not possible to clarify answers or probe further. From the respondent's point of view, one irritating feature of questionnaires is to be asked to choose from a range of options where none apply to their own situation. This raises questions of validity where a respondent is not truly describing his or her own views or experiences but merely choosing something the researcher has preselected. A final problem is where the researcher uses value-leaden words such as 'unnecessary', 'painful', 'appropriate', 'satisfied' or 'too long', instead of phrasing questions in a neutral way.

The conclusion is that as a method the questionnaire has a number of advantages and disadvantages. They are surprisingly not an easy option to use in research and have a number of restrictions and limitations. Their success depends on the design, as this will influence whether an individual will complete them or not. For this reason, the next section will consider some of the principles involved in questionnaire design.

QUESTIONNAIRE DESIGN

The first stage in designing a questionnaire is to ensure that it is an appropriate method for collecting the data. Careful consideration should be given to the advantages and disadvantages outlined above. The study aim should also provide some clue as to whether it is appropriate. If the aim depends on finding out what people say or do, or relates to areas where individuals are in the best position to accurately supply the information, then questionnaires would seem a good option. The review of the literature should help to establish whether previous studies have used a questionnaire, and with what success. Once a final decision has been made to use a questionnaire, then the researcher moves into the design stage. A good questionnaire is structured into three main parts:

1. An invitation and motivation to take part
2. Instructions about the aim of the survey
3. The body of the questionnaire

TABLE 9.3
What Should a Researcher Include in an Invitation?

- Who they are and the capacity in which they are writing (e.g. student, member of a clinical team, or manager)
- The aim of the study, in broad terms
- The reason the respondent has been included in the study
- Motivation to return the questionnaire (how they, or others, will benefit from completing it)
- Assurance on confidentiality and anonymity
- Estimate of the time it should take to complete
- Contact address, telephone number and email address, should the respondent want further details or assurances
- If this is a PhD or master's study, include the contact details (e.g. email address of a contact supervisor)
- Confirmation that the study has been given ethical approval

Invitation and Motivation to Take Part

This section has traditionally been referred to as the 'covering letter' but with the variety of ways in which questionnaires are distributed, including web-based and emailed questionnaires, it is better to talk about the invitations and motivation to take part (Table 9.3). This is the first contact potential respondents will have with the study, so it is important that it strikes the right balance that will prompt a reply. It should explain the purpose of the study and why they have been asked to take part. There should also be something that motivates the individual to give up time to participate. This might be by simply suggesting that it will help improve the service for others.

Instructions

The questionnaire should start with a clear title that summarises the purpose. The first section should be clearly marked 'Instructions'. This should simply and unambiguously outline the various ways questions can be answered, such as tick a box, click on an option or add a comment of their own. The pilot study should test the clarity of the instructions as, unless these are successful, valuable data may be lost.

The Main Body of the Questionnaire

The 'business' part of the questionnaire is the body of questions. This section should look attractive and inviting, with good layout and space, as well as clean formatting of the questions and answers on the page. Cluttered and boring-looking questionnaires will not tempt people to answer them. Here, the researcher must ensure a minimum margin for misunderstandings of the questions. The respondent should find it interesting and easy to complete, and the researcher should find that

the replies provide an answer to the study aim. If this is to be achieved, then thought has to be given to:

- choice of questions
- wording and structure of the questions
- method of answering
- analysis of the responses

The Choice of Questions

The choice of the questions will be influenced by the research aim and the thinking that lies behind it. Where the researcher believes that a number of variables such as parity, previous experience and attitudes towards childbirth influence a situation, these should be included in the questions. The review of the literature will also provide some pointers to relevant questions.

At the design stage there is frequently a temptation to include too many questions. The longer the questionnaire, the less likely it is to be returned. Every question should be relevant to the aim of the research. It is worth the researcher asking 'why am I including this question?' If a clear answer cannot be given, the question should be deleted. It is also an advantage to ask colleagues, and particularly 'experts' in the field, for their view on the choice of topic areas and questions.

The Wording and Structure of the Questions

The wording and structure of the questions need special attention. Table 9.4 outlines some of the basic principles of questionnaire design and, although these seem straightforward, they are frequently ignored. One piece of advice is for the researcher to put themselves in the place of the person completing it; will it make sense to them? Are there certain assumptions being made about

TABLE 9.4
Basic Principles in Questionnaire Design

- Give clear instructions on how to answer the questions
- Provide assurances on confidentiality and only ask for name and identifying characteristics (e.g. clinical area if staff) if necessary
- Questions should relate to the study aim
- Avoid long questionnaires
- Avoid long questions; respondents might lose track of its purpose
- Avoid a single question asking more than one thing at the same time; split these into separate questions
- Use simple language and avoid unnecessary or unexplained jargon and abbreviations
- Use a clear layout to make it attractive on the page, and allow realistic space for written comments
- Group questions on the same topic together to form a logical sequence
- Avoid ambiguous questions and vague words such as 'regularly'
- Avoid leading questions and value-loaded words
- Avoid presuming that people do things; ask filter questions first
- Avoid questions with 'no', 'not' or 'never' in the question where the alternative answers are 'yes' or 'no' as it can lead to confusion
- Ensure with fixed-choice questions that there is an alternative for everyone, such as 'not applicable', 'don't know' or 'other'
- If people are unlikely to say 'yes' or 'no' to a question because of social desirability (looking good) then the question is not worth including
- Use Likert scales ('strongly agree', 'often', 'sometimes', 'rarely', 'never', etc.) where the answer may not be simply 'yes' or 'no'
- Include a balance between open and closed questions to avoid repetitiveness
- Leave sensitive, potentially embarrassing or intrusive questions until later in the questionnaire
- At the design stage, think how you will analyse each question, even down to what a table of results will look like
- Get comments on your draft questionnaire from colleagues and pilot it before using it to ensure it works (this should include analysis)

the person's knowledge that may not be justified? In following this advice it may be possible to avoid mistakes such as asking questions that are not answerable. An example would be: *'Do you think the birth of your baby would have been better in a different hospital?'* Not only does this give no indication as to what might count as 'better', it is clearly difficult for someone to evaluate whether there would have been differences if the birth had taken place in a different setting.

Vague words are a further problem in the wording of questions. There is a need for clarity of thought that should lead to precision in the wording of questions. Words such as 'regularly' should be avoided as in *'since the birth of your baby are you able to go out regularly?'*. This does not explain the context in which 'going out' is placed. Does it mean shopping, visiting people or social activities? Nor would it be meaningful as a 'yes' or 'no' response, as 'regularly' could mean vastly different things to different people.

As can be seen from the list of principles in Table 9.4, simplicity is one of the keys to questionnaire design. It is important to use simple words and to avoid jargon or technical terms such as 'primiparous' and 'multiparous' to non-medical people. Here, the reading level of the questionnaire needs careful assessment to ensure that people can understand each question (Denscombe, 2011). The structure of each question should be simple and short and avoid asking more than one thing in a single sentence, such as:

Have you more than one child and were any of these born at home? ❑ *YES* ❑ *NO*

This should be divided into two; first it should ask 'have you more than one child' and then as a further sub-question: 'If 'yes', were any of these born at home?' This would then appear as follows:

5 a) *Have you more than one child?*
   ❑ YES ❑ NO

   b) *If yes, were any of these born at home?*
   ❑ YES ❑ NO

It is also important to avoid biasing the individual's response with leading questions or emotive words that suggest the appropriate answer, for example:

Would you agree that the midwife kept you fully informed during the labour? Would it be more convenient for you to attend antenatal classes in a health centre near your home rather than in hospital?

This last question would be better asked in a more neutral way such as:

If you had a choice of where you could take part in antenatal education, which would you choose?
a) ❑ *Those at my local hospital*
b) ❑ *Those at my local health centre*
c) ❑ *Either one would be acceptable*
d) ❑ *Neither one would be acceptable*

The Method of Answering Questions

The method of answering questions can take a number of forms. The final example above is called a multiple-choice question where the respondent chooses one of the alternatives offered. This falls into the category of *closed questions* as opposed to *open questions*. In open questions, the respondent is not offered options to choose from but is left to express the answer in his or her own words. An example of an open question would be the following:

What did you hope to gain from a home birth?

Open questions work well where respondents are used to expressing themselves in writing. They will not work well or be productive with everyone. Open and closed questions have their advantages and disadvantages. For instance, although closed questions have the advantage of simplicity, they may influence the respondents by suggesting answers that they may not have thought of without the prompt of the fixed-choice options. The open question has the advantage of the respondent using terms and options that they feel describe their own experiences or views, rather than using those offered by the researcher. The disadvantage of open questions is the large amount of data that has to be analysed and coded before any kind of summary or identification of issues takes place. The ideal compromise is to have a mix of open and closed questions, which maximises the advantages of both forms of question (Denscombe, 2011).

One method of increasing the sensitivity of closed questions is the use of a range of scaling techniques. Although closed questions are considered to have a yes or no answer, where attitude or opinion is concerned how people feel about an issue or statement may lie anywhere along a continuum. This can be dealt with using a *Likert scale*, which is named after the American,

Rensis Likert, who first introduced them in the 1930s. These can take three forms and relate to:

- agreement
- evaluation
- frequency

In the case of agreement scales, statements in a broad mix of positive or negative forms are given and the respondent is asked to make a choice between five choices ranging from 'strongly agree' to 'strongly disagree'. Fictional examples are shown below:

1. Agreement
   I feel that pain relief in labour should be taken as a last resort
   ❑ Strongly agree   ❑ Agree   ❑ Undecided
   ❑ Disagree   ❑ Strongly disagree
2. Evaluation
   The information I received from the midwife about the alternative forms of pain relief was
   ❑ Excellent   ❑ Very good
   ❑ Undecided   ❑ Poor   ❑ Very poor
3. Frequency
   I get feelings of panic when I think about looking after a baby
   ❑ Always   ❑ Sometimes
   ❑ Rarely   ❑ Never

In the last example, four choices have been used, as these seem to cover the main possibilities. The inclusion of 'never' removes the necessity to include a neutral mid-category. Some people argue that with examples (1) and (2) above, the mid-category of 'undecided' should be removed to prevent people choosing a neutral option and sitting on the fence, although this is not always appropriate (Taherdoost, 2019). It should also be remembered that there must be an option that applies to everyone; there are occasions when a mid-category could be a legitimate choice and should be respected.

The statements or 'items' in the Likert scale should be a mix of those expressed positively and those expressed negatively to prevent respondents simply putting a tick in the same column each time without really thinking about the question. So, for instance, the following two examples may be used in a satisfaction questionnaire.

The midwife was too busy to answer my questions (negative item)

I felt confident with the midwife who conducted the birth (positive item)

The order of these statements should not follow a set pattern, for instance, alternately positive and negative; providing there is an equal number of each kind of statement, they should be presented in a random order.

An alternative technique to the Likert scale is to use a visual analogue scale (VAS) which is a line drawn across the page, usually 10 cm in length, with opposite words at each end. Respondents are asked to place a cross on the line to correspond with how they feel.

'On a scale of 0 to 10, with 0 being no pain and 10 being the worst pain you've ever felt, please rate your pain today'

0....1....2....3....4....5....6....7....8....9....10

(No Pain Mild Discomfort/Pain Moderate Pain Significant Pain Severe Pain)

This can either be calibrated with lines at centimetre points or can be assessed during the analysis by overlaying a calibrated piece of clear plastic on the line. This approach is often used in relation to pain assessment in health care (as above).

The Analysis of the Responses

The analysis of both the Likert scale and the VAS is treated in a similar way, by allocating a numeric value for the chosen response. In the case of the Likert scale a score of 5 is allocated for 'strongly agree' answers, 4 for 'agree', 3 for 'neither agree/disagree', 2 for 'disagree' and 1 for 'strongly disagree' when the statement is in the positive. When the statement is expressed in the negative, the reverse order of numbering would be applied (i.e. strongly disagree to the statement '*the midwife did not have time to answer my questions*' would be scored 5 to show there was a positive response to the midwife). An overall score for all the Likert questions can then be calculated for each person. It is also possible to give an average score for everyone in the sample. So, for instance, an average of 4.2 for the statement '*I felt confident with the midwife who helped me give birth*' would suggest that there was a high degree of satisfaction as the average was between the 'agree' and 'strongly agree' point on the scale. In the same way, the

points on the VAS could be divided into 10 sections with each section given a score from 1 to 10, where 10 could be allocated to the positive end of the scale and 1 to the negative.

In questions requiring a 'yes' or 'no' answer, the responses can be expressed as a proportion of the total in terms of the percentage giving each response. The method of analysis should be carefully thought out at the design stage and tested in the pilot and not left until the questionnaires start arriving back.

DETAILS OF HOW TO RETURN QUESTIONNAIRES

Although this section has covered the three main parts of a questionnaire, researchers should also give thought to instructions on how to return the questionnaire to the researcher. If it has not been included in the instructions, the questionnaire should end with a 'thank you'. Online questionnaires should indicate the end of the questionnaire has been reached and allow the respondent to 'submit', again with a 'thank you' post-submission. Paper questionnaires should clearly say how the questionnaire should be returned. This should be as simple as possible and should not involve the respondent in a complex or costly activity; there could be a prepaid return envelope included with the questionnaire package, for example. It is this aspect that will influence the response rate and so should also be part of the pilot study to ensure it works smoothly.

ONLINE SURVEYS

Finally, what is the future of surveys and the use of online questionnaires, which have become very popular. The trend was already moving towards online before the pandemic, but the Covid pandemic seems to have been responsible for making a further leap to online surveys (Hlatshwako et al. 2021). Although this approach to data collection can be rich and valuable, as with all methodological issues, this approach has both advantages and disadvantages. Firstly, advantages would include the ease and speed of reply, both for the respondent and the researcher (Evans and Mathur, 2018). The number of people reached through such methods can be considerable and even world-wide.

The method of analysis is also easier as data does not have to be retyped but can be imported directly into a database for analysis and can give very fast results.

Clearly, there will be a number of disadvantages to the system, as it is still a relatively new medium and lessons are still being learnt. However, researchers are already sharing their experiences and offering useful advice (Hlatshwako et al. 2021; Lagan, 2010). As with postal questionnaires, there are concerns that the medium has in-built biases, such as the cross-section of potential respondents all need easy access to a computer, and essential computer skills. Respondents will still require reading, literacy and hand dexterity skills and this may form a barrier for some. Although postage costs are reduced compared to mailed questionnaires, there can be a design cost to such tools and technical knowledge skills related to Internet mediated research (IMR). Some reviews have suggested that online surveys tend to have a lower response rate (Daikeler et al. 2019). However, this will continue to develop as a productive and growing area of midwifery research.

REFLECTION PROMPTS

Reflect on any surveys you have been approached to take part in recently.

- What was its purpose?
- Did you complete the questionnaire?
- If so, why?
- If not, why not?

CONDUCTING RESEARCH

Although a survey provides quick and easy access to a large amount of data, the researcher should be cautious in the use of the questionnaire. This is because it is not always appropriate for those for whom writing is either not easy or not a welcome mental activity, or for those who have physical conditions, such as visual or handwriting problems. Even for those used to expressing themselves in writing, questionnaires have almost reached saturation point, and the motivation to complete and return a detailed questionnaire may be low (Stedman et al. 2019).

Consideration must be given to the research aim, the sample, and the possible advantages of using another method, such as interviews. Ethical issues exist, and thought needs to be given to the possible harm through upset, anxiety or guilt caused by certain kinds of topic areas. These may include the loss of a baby, or the birth of a baby with a medical problem that may be thought to relate to maternal behaviour, such as smoking or dietary intake. Care should be taken, then, where the respondent may confront emotionally sensitive issues when they may be in a vulnerable mental state and may have no one to help them through the distress caused by the questionnaire.

Where the decision to use the questionnaire is appropriate, it is important to avoid believing that designing appropriate questions is easy. The three elements, invitation to participate, instructions and main body of the questionnaire, need careful planning and design. The review of the literature will help identify appropriate topic areas and may even give some pointers as to the kind of questions that have worked well in other studies. In selecting the wording of the questions, the researcher must keep validity and reliability in mind. The two important questions that need to be constantly addressed are:

- What am I trying to measure (validity)?
- How accurately will this question measure it (reliability)?

The basic principles of questionnaire design (see Table 9.4) should then be rigorously followed. Decisions on how the data resulting from each question are to be presented in a report/article should be considered at the question design stage. If the researcher needs statistical advice, it is at this stage it should be sought (see Chapter 13).

Questions should be as clear and as straightforward as possible. This means using simple language and simple sentences. Midwifery or medical jargon and abbreviations should be avoided as much as possible. It is not always easy for the researcher to identify any vague terms and ambiguity, as they have designed the questions and are not confused by their meaning, so it is important to ask others to comment at the design stage.

Respondents should find a questionnaire interesting and enjoyable to complete. There should be variety in the way the questions are asked or required to be answered. The most frustrating experience for a respondent is to find that the choice of words clearly betrays the researcher's preconceived assumptions or personal agenda. This can be revealed through the use of emotive words such as 'better' 'disappointed', 'acceptable', and so on.

Using a questionnaire from a previous study is a big advantage; however, especially where a questionnaire has to be designed, a pilot study should be undertaken. In the pilot, it is important to have a good cross-section of the kinds of people who will be included in the main study. This is perhaps just as important as the size of the sample. The main questionnaire should be accompanied with a short questionnaire asking pilot respondents to identify any particular strengths or weaknesses in the main questionnaire. Relevant questions include:

- How long did it take you to complete the questionnaire?
- Were there any questions you had particular problems with?
- Was there any particular wording you had difficulty with?
- Are there any questions you feel were missing from the questionnaire?
- To sum up, what did you feel were the strengths of the questionnaire?
- What areas do you feel could be presented differently?

A 'practice' report based on the analysis of the data from the pilot should be produced to provide experience of moving from raw data to data presentation and analysis. At this point, serious shortcomings in the design of some questions, especially the method of answering, can be revealed.

CRITIQUING RESEARCH

Surveys using questionnaires are a popular method of data collection in midwifery; they have become so familiar that they are rarely challenged as to their use. The researcher must give a clear rationale for selecting a questionnaire rather than the usually more effective method of interviewing. Where the sample is geographically spread, or where an existing relationship between the researcher and participants may compro-

mise the use of interviews, then questionnaires are an appropriate choice. It is worth considering any ethical issues raised by the use of the questionnaires with the topic, and whether the researcher has addressed these. For instance, a reader would be unhappy to review a paper where a questionnaire was used to explore feelings about the loss of a baby, or similar subjects that may result in upset, anxiety or needlessly raising feelings of guilt, confusion or regret.

The space provided in some journals does not permit the inclusion of an entire questionnaire, so it can be a challenge to judge each question. Sometimes, tables provide a clue as to the content and wording of the questionnaire. Where possible, the reader should consider the perspective of the respondents and ask was there any possibility of ambiguity or misunderstanding? Are the questions in any way leading, for instance, the use of emotive words that suggests how the researcher felt about the topic?

What evidence is there that the researcher addressed the issue of reliability of the questions, especially if they were designed for the study and had not been used in previous studies? Was the accuracy of the questions tested through a pilot study? In regard to validity, how does the reader know whether the questions were measuring what they were supposed to measure? Did the researcher develop some of the questions from previous research, or were experts in the field approached to comment on the appropriateness of the topics for the study?

Finally, readers should consider the researcher's interpretation of the results. Are the results strong enough to support the statements made by the researcher? It is also important to be aware that what people say they do may not be what they do in practice. In other words, the reader should always be somewhat cautious in treating self-reported data as if it were 'the truth'.

KEY POINTS

- A survey is the term given to describe a process of using questionnaires and other data collection methods to find out more about a specific group. A questionnaire is not a survey in itself, but it is part of a survey. Think of the questionnaire as the *physical sheet of questions*. A survey always contains a questionnaire, but a questionnaire doesn't have to be part of a survey.

- Survey response rate is variable: where it falls under 50%, it is difficult to be certain that the responses received are representative of the sample as a whole.
- Increasingly, surveys are conducted using online platforms; however not everyone has access to a computer or has reliable Wi-Fi, which may negatively impact on response rates.
- Questionnaires can be used to collect data in many different types of research studies. They enable a large amount of data to be collected quickly and cheaply. They have the advantage of being familiar to a majority of the population, and compared to other forms of data collection, are a non-threatening medium for both the researcher and respondent.
- Questionnaires have been used so often in the past that people are now less likely to return them. So researchers should consider whether this is the most appropriate method. In particular, the ethical issue of harm should be considered where the questions could produce emotional upset, regret, anxiety or confusion.
- Designing a questionnaire involves three elements: the invitation, the instructions and the body of the questionnaire. There are clear guidelines that should be followed in the construction of questions. The importance of avoiding bias and ensuring reliability and validity must be stressed.
- The basic premise of questionnaire design is that the respondent can read and write, and is fluent in the English language. For several reasons, there is a proportion of the population who will always be excluded in studies using questionnaires.
- A pilot study, or the use of a previously used questionnaire, is a good indicator of rigour in the use of questionnaires.

REFERENCES

Cosco, T., Kaushal, A., Hardy, R., Richards, M., Kuh, D., Stafford, M., 2017. Operationalising resilience in longitudinal studies: a systematic review of methodological approaches. J. Epidemiol. Community Health 71 (1), 98–104.

Daikeler, J., Bošnjak, M., Manfreda, K.L., 2019. Web versus other survey modes: an updated and extended meta-analysis comparing response rates. J. Surv. Stat. Methodol. 8 (3), 513–539. https://doi.org/10.1093/jssam/smz008

Denscombe, M., 2011. The Good research Guide for Small-Scale Social Research Projects, fourth ed. Open University Press, England.

Evans, J., Mathur, A., 2018. The value of on-line surveys: a look back and a look ahead. Internet Res. 28 (4). https://www.emerald.com/insight/content/doi/10.1108/IntR-03-2018-0089/full/html?fullSc=1&mbSc=1&fullSc=1

Green, J., Thorogood, N., 2018. Qualitative Methods for Health Research, fourth ed. Sage Publications Ltd, London.

Harrison, S., Henderso, J., Alderdice, F., Quigley, M., 2019. Methods to increase response rates to a population-based maternity survey: a comparison of two pilot studies. BMC Med. Res. Methodol. 19 (1), 65. https://doi.org/10.1186/s12874-019-0702-3

Hlatshwako, T.G., Shah, S.J., Kosana, P., Adebayo, E., Hendriks, J., Larsson, E.C., et al., 2021. Online health survey research during COVID-19. Lancet Digit. Health 3 (2), e76–e77. https://doi.org/10.1016/S2589-7500(21)00002-9

Hurst, P., Bird, S., 2019. Questionnaires. In: Bird, S. (Ed), Research Methods in Physical Activity and Health. Routledge Press, London.

Lagan, B.M., 2010. Internet-mediated research: a reflection on challenges encountered and lessons learnt. Evid. Based Midwifery 8 (1). https://link.gale.com/apps/doc/A221919492/AONE?u=anon~ed6d11af&sid=googleScholar&xid=4a517ad7

Lau, F., 27 February 2017. Chapter 13: Methods for Survey Studies. In: Lau, F., Kuziemsky, C. (Eds.), Handbook of eHealth Evaluation: An Evidence-based Approach [Internet]. University of Victoria, Victoria, BC. https://www.ncbi.nlm.nih.gov/books/NBK481602/

Rayment-Jones, H., Harris, J., Harden, A., Silverio, S.A., Turienzo, C.F., Sandall, J., 2021. Project 20: interpreter services for pregnant women with social risk factors in England: what works, for whom, in what circumstances, and how? Int. J. Equity Health 20 (1), 1–233. https://doi.org/10.1186/s12939-021-01570-8

Stedman, R.C., Nancy, A., Connelly, N.A., Heberlein, T.A., Decker, D.J., Allred, S.B., 2019. The end of the (research) world as we know it? understanding and coping with declining response rates to mail surveys. Soc. Nat. Resour. 32 (10), 1139–1154. https://doi.org/10.1080/08941920.2019.1587127

Taherdoost, H., 2019. What is the best response scale for survey and questionnaire design; review of different lengths of rating scale/attitude scale/likert Scale. Int. J. Acad. Res. Managem. 8 (1), 1–10. https://ssrn.com/abstract=3588604

Thomas G., 2017. How to Do Your Research Project. A Guide for Students, third ed. Sage Publications Ltd., London.

10 INTERVIEWS

Interviews have a great deal to offer midwifery research as the type of data produced tends to be richer and has more depth than is generally possible with questionnaires. Interviews also make use of the midwife's professional skill of sensitively, collecting information through a conversational medium. It can also increase the variation in the range of people included in a study.

In this chapter, we examine some of the features of interviews, especially their advantages and disadvantages, and consider some of the skills involved in interviewing.

DEFINITION

Interviews consist of data gathering through direct interaction between a researcher and respondent where answers to questions are gathered verbally. They can be conducted face-to-face, online or by telephone. Although usually conducted on a one-to-one basis, they can be carried out with a group of individuals in the form of a *focus group*. These are small groups of individuals who are facilitated, by the researcher, to discuss certain topics and experiences.

There are occasions when interviews are used for quantitative research. This is when highly structured questions, for example multiple choice questions, are used as part of a survey which is administered by a researcher or research assistant. Much more often interviews are used as part of a qualitative approach and this chapter is written with quantitative approaches in mind.

The research question and approach will influence the type of data collected and method of data analysis. Interviews have the ability to describe, explain and explore issues from the individual's perspective. The strengths of interviews for data collection are that they provide a way of gaining insight into the participants' perspectives on important issues or personal experiences. However, from the researcher's perspective, they present some of the greatest challenges and the need for a high level of skill in their use. To a large extent, the researcher *becomes* the tool of data collection in studies using this method. This is because although interviews may be recorded in writing on a printed form or in a notebook, or verbally on audio equipment and later transcribed, it is the researcher's skills and personality that will encourage or discourage the interviewee to open up and select the information they feel willing to disclose. During interviews, it is also the researcher's ability to know when to seek clarification or illustration that can make all the difference to the quality of the data collected.

INTERVIEW STRUCTURE

Interviews can be categorised by the degree of structure they contain. This can range from a highly structured format of questioning, where they virtually take the form of reading out questions from a questionnaire and recording the answers, to in-depth, unstructured interviews. The former approach is used in survey designs that concentrate on the production of quantitative data. The advantage of this format is that the questions are standardised in the way questions are asked and recorded. This increases the accuracy of the results and also makes analysis easier and more compatible with statistical computer analysis programs. The disadvantage of a highly structured approach is that there is little scope for spontaneity and depth of information. This can result in them being somewhat superficial, leaving us with little understanding of a situation. We must also remember that, as a self-report method, we have to assume that what someone states in an interview is accurate.

At the other end of the interview structure continuum is the unstructured or minimally structured interview where questions develop as appropriate, allowing the participant to talk about what they see as important in their own words, providing an insider's description of events and issues. Such interviews provide thick data with rich description (Bearman, 2019). The purpose of these in-depth interviews is not to test a hypothesis or evaluate something, it is to understand people's lived experience and the meaning they make of that experience (Seidman, 2019). Such interviews have very few prepared questions and instead use an *interview guide*; the rest will be requests for more detail or illustration. They may just start with a trigger question such as, 'So what happened once you went into labour?'

The disadvantage of the approach is that it requires a great deal of personal skill from the researcher and generates a large amount of data to be analysed and coded, and so can be very time consuming and costly.

Somewhere between these two extremes are *semi-structured interviews*. They contain some fixed questions covering a key issue or issues, which are asked of everyone, yet they are versatile, flexible and reciprocal. This is because the interviewer has some freedom to explore areas that seem appropriate to the interviewee (Kallio et al., 2016). The design of the questions is important and leading questions should be avoided, for example: '*Did you have a lot of pain during your labour?*' This question not only makes assumptions, but it is also a closed question as the answer could just be 'yes' or 'no'. Open questions encourage participants to talk freely about their experience or share their thoughts and feelings. The semi-structured approach ensures that important areas are covered, but still allows other areas to arise spontaneously and still enables the collection of rich, *thick* description. Thick description is description which captures the contextual, cultural and social meaning behind an experience (Hennink et al., 2020: 240).

ADVANTAGES AND DISADVANTAGES OF INTERVIEWS

Why choose interviews as a data collection method? There are a number of very clear advantages to using interviews, as can be seen from Box 10.1. They are suitable for a wider variety of individuals than questionnaires, are less likely to lead to misinterpretations of the questions and provide much richer, more detailed data. The presence of the interviewer can also be an asset as they can clarify questions and answers and gently probe where more information may be needed to gain a complete and accurate answer. Interviews have a particular relevance in midwifery as they provide an opportunity to pursue a woman-centred approach to issues and situations. This is particularly the case in semi-structured and unstructured interviews, as their purpose is to hear 'the voice' of the participants, gaining insight into their situation and gaining an understanding of their perspective.

As with all the other methods of data collection presented in this book, we have to be aware of their disadvantages. The main issues are outlined in Box 10.2. One of the main issues is that successful interviews not only depend on the high skill levels of the interviewer, but also depend on the interviewee being able to articulate and reflect on their experiences. A number of other issues relate to the practicalities of the technique. They require a great deal of time per interview in terms of both gathering the data and their analysis, particularly where the interview is semi-structured or unstructured. This naturally increases the cost of such research.

A further problem is the influence of the interviewer on the information produced. The fact that this is a social situation means that the characteristics of each of the individuals concerned can play a part in the reliability and validity of the information produced. There is inevitably a conscious or subconscious influence on the selection and editing of information by the participant. Where the interviewer is a midwife or other health professional, no matter how much they encourage participants to see them as just someone interested in their experiences, there is a hierarchical position of the interviewer over the interviewee that may influence the outcome of some interviews. For example, 'socially desirable' answers (those that put the person in a positive light) may be selected to impress

or avoid possible criticism or rebuke from health staff. One other problem is where the participants 'second guess' the answers on the basis of what they think the interviewer wants to hear. All these elements will have a negative effect on the validity of interview data. The issues around the researcher/participant relationship are explored further in the section on *reflexivity* a little further on in this chapter.

PRINCIPLES IN THE USE OF INTERVIEW

Interviewing is a difficult skill to learn as it is usually done in private. It is therefore outside the gaze of those who need to learn from those who do it well. Although asking questions and receiving answers sounds deceptively easy as a method of data collection, like everything else in research, things are never that simple. However, it is possible to overcome some of the difficulties through knowledge of the pitfalls and by following some essential principles.

A major step is to recognise that research interviews are not like ordinary conversations, as their purpose is to elicit research data. Careful preparation of any questions to be used in the interview schedule is needed and testing them through role-play with colleagues can be very helpful. These could be recorded for playback later to identify appropriate skills and areas that need developing. This should, of course, be followed up later with a pre-test study or pilot with members from the group in whom the researcher is interested.

Interviews can be in person or remote. If in person, a major consideration in carrying out an interview is the location and characteristics of the environment in which the interview takes place. The participant should feel relaxed and comfortable. There should be as few disturbances and distractions as possible whilst the interview takes place. Although many people provide the best information in their own home, the interviewer's control over the setting is drastically reduced. Despite interruptions having an impact on the flow of information, sometimes this has to be accepted and may be inevitable, especially with a young baby around. In Menage et al.'s (2020) research on compassion in midwifery the interviewer found that interviewing women in the postnatal period could take a long time and required patience as the interview would frequently have to be paused for example, when the baby needed to be fed, settled or changed, and then started again when the woman was ready.

Interviews in a participant's home also raise issues of personal safety. Researchers are encouraged to do a risk assessment for their data collection activities. Depending on where they are conducting interviews and who they are interviewing, the level of risk may vary. It is wise for researchers to ensure that somebody else knows where they are and the timetable they are following. All reasonable precautions should be taken to stay safe. They should ensure they have a mobile phone and might consider an alarm to enhance personal safety.

Wherever the interview takes place, simple things such as ensuring that the sun is not shining in the participant's eyes and that they are comfortable are important, as this will affect the quality of the information produced. The interviewer's appearance also needs careful thought so as to reduce producing socially desirable answers. The way the interviewer is dressed or the accessories worn could act as distractions, or indications of possible personal beliefs and values. Where possible, the interviewer's appearance should be relatively nondescript. In terms of etiquette, it is also important that the interviewer states the approximate length of time the interview may take and ensures that respondents are not worried about other responsibilities or obligations that may distract them as the interview lengthens.

The nature of the interview will also be influenced by the method of recording the answers. The options are making written notes as the interview unfolds or using an audio recorder or (less often) video. Interviews carried out using online platforms with video links are popular and these can easily be recorded. In relation to writing or recording data during in-person interviews, both have their advantages and disadvantages. Written notes are not as intimidating as using an audio recorder and the interviewer does not have to worry about background noise affecting the recording. There is also little risk of technology letting the researcher down. The big disadvantage of writing is the inability to maintain eye contact with participants. This can be difficult for both interviewer and participant. It can feel more like making a police statement rather than an interview. There is also an inevitable loss of information as it is rarely possible to listen as carefully when writing and to write down everything that is said when trying to maintain the flow of the interview. The main difficulties for the researcher are multitasking as they try to cope with the practicalities of thinking about the next question, remembering what has just been said, writing (or typing on a laptop or tablet) quickly and legibly and making a mental note of interesting comments that have just been made that will need to be probed or followed up later.

Audio recording has the advantage of leaving the interviewer free to concentrate on the conversation rather than trying to speed-write everything. The ability to maintain eye contact can also be very important in interviews on sensitive topics. Apart from the problem of background noise, audio recorders are successful in capturing almost all of the comments from the participant in their own words. They capture the participant's tone of voice and emphasis and they can be listened to again and again, to check meaning. This can be a crucial advantage in qualitative research. The disadvantages of audio recorders include the fact that participants may find them intimidating. They are an additional worry for the interviewer, in case something goes wrong with them, such as batteries running out or recordings being lost. Almost every researcher has their 'bad experience' story of 'lost' interviews. In addition, transcribing interviews from recordings is very time consuming.

INTERVIEWING REMOTELY

Many studies have successfully used interviews from a distance by using online platforms or telephone. They work well in a quantitative design. For example,

Thompson et al. (2019) used Skype audio calls to interview parents about their decision-making regarding the mode of breech birth at term. Participants (both mothers and their partners) were recruited via social media platforms and thus there was a very wide geographical reach. Therefore audio calls provided a convenient and cost-effective method of qualitative interviewing which was conducted at a tiny fraction of the cost of travelling to interview participants. This method of interviewing can be helpful for health professionals and health care recipients with little time for interviews. In addition, they provide anonymity for participants, and also make good use of project time.

These advantages should be weighed against the potential disadvantages.

READER ACTIVITY

Make a list of the possible disadvantages to conducting interviews by telephone.

Telephone interviews may not be a good medium for pursing very sensitive issues. If may be more difficult to detect if the participant is becoming upset or distressed or to support participants appropriately if they do. The lack of visual cues also means that the researcher can be unaware of misunderstanding or confusion. Those involved may also feel less engaged with the interview process, and that this can have an impact on the quality of data compared to the face-to-face interview.

The conclusion is that, as with other tools of data collection, the choice of online or telephone interview has to be matched with the research question, the sample, the type and extent of data required and comparisons made with the advantages of other forms of data collection.

Interviews that use virtual meeting platforms have become popular and it is highly likely that this will continue. It is not surprising given that interviewing in a virtual space where the interviewer and interviewee can see and hear each other appears to have the advantages of the face-to-face interview (increased rapport and ability to pick up on non-verbal cues) and the telephone interview (convenience, save on travel, time and resources) combined. The popularity has been growing over the last decade but with the Coronavirus pandemic which arrived in the UK in early 2021, bringing severe restrictions on face-to-face meetings, these platforms became much more widely used for work and leisure. For researchers, the ability to continue with important research studies during the pandemic owes a lot to virtual meeting platforms. No longer able to rely on the ability to actually meet with participants to conduct interviews, other ways to connect have been elevated to new heights. Increasingly, studies offer participants a choice. For example, Anderson et al. (2021) carried out research into pregnant women's experiences of social distancing behavioural guidelines during the Covid-19 pandemic 'lockdown' in the UK and participants were given a choice of interview by either telephone or video call.

INTERVIEWING SKILLS

The success of this type of research is greatly influenced by the interviewing skills of the researchers. Midwives have many of the skills that are needed as they are used to 'interviewing' women in other contexts. This section is intended to assist midwives to use the skills they already have and remind them what they should pay particular attention to when conducting a research interview.

What makes a good interview? Good interviews are the result of more than asking the questions clearly, although that does help. One key to successful data collection through interviews is to establish *rapport* with participants (Hennink et al., 2020: 128; McGrath et al., 2019). This is something that midwives are used to doing with the women and families they work with. Rapport is a trusting relationship between people which has an empathic quality (Prior, 2017). This means producing a friendly atmosphere where individuals feel respected and sufficiently comfortable with the researcher to trust them with sensitive information without fear of judgement or criticism. McGrath et al (2019) advocates that researchers develop a spirit of *open curiosity* towards the interviewee to show that they are interested in what they have to say, in order to build and maintain rapport.

The seating position of the interviewer in relation to the participant makes a difference when interviewing; if they are square-on, almost in a head-to-head position, the participant may feel it is more like an interrogation rather than a relaxed conversation. Sitting slightly to the side of the individual, where eye contact can be made, helps to establish the right atmosphere. It is important that this is at a comfortable distance from the individual, so that they do not feel that their personal space is being restricted or invaded.

Body language and other non-verbal skills are important. By making eye contact and leaning slightly forward the researcher indicates that they are listening and this also encourages rapport. Interviewers should avoid crossing their arms or legs, as this might suggest they are nervous, or keeping information secret from the respondent. The key principle is to relax; if the interviewer is relaxed, it will encourage the participant to relax also.

It is also important to consider the process of closing the interview. The researcher should thank the respondents and ask them if there are any things they feel have not been covered or said so far. The researcher should offer the participant the opportunity to ask any questions of the interviewer. This allows any concerns or important questions that may have come to the participant's mind during the course of the interview to be identified. This is a clear demonstration of the kind of reciprocity or balance of 'give and take' that should exist in interviews, where the researcher should share any expertise or knowledge with the participant.

INTERVIEWING IN FOCUS GROUPS

A focus group is a small group of participants (usually 5 to 8) brought together so that the researcher can obtain the participants' perceptions of a specific topic in a non-threatening and open-minded way (Gray, 2019: 79). It is thought that the group dynamics aid the process and help participants to feel more relaxed and not as 'put on the spot' as in a one-to-one interview. The skills of interviewing with focus groups are somewhat different, as the setting and issues that arise are not the same as with individual interviews because of the group context. Some research designs use focus groups alone and others use focus groups in conjunction with other data collection methods such as questionnaires or in-depth interviews. In focus groups, the researcher must find a way of facilitating group discussion which enhances participation and com-

munication and also stays on-topic. This has its challenges. For instance, one problem is that inevitably one dominant or more vocal participant will emerge in the group (Hennink et al., 2020: 160–162). Their view is valued but they should not be allowed to dominate to the extent that they prevent others from contributing. Conversely, some participants may be extremely quiet and reluctant to contribute and yet their contribution is just as important. Therefore, gentle encouragement may be needed. A further problem is how to keep track of who has said what, especially where groups are audio recorded. Hennink (2020: 154) suggests that focus groups are conducted with a moderator who sets the tone and enables the discussion and a separate note taker. A note taker records the key issues discussed in the conversation and other details like body language (Hennink et al., 2020: 154; Krueger and Casey, 2015). A tracking sheet can be used to identify individual responses so that variations in experiences and views can be attributed to those within the group without confusing who said what. However, where there are rapid exchanges of conversation, keeping track of who is speaking and marking this on a sheet can be very difficult. Video recording focus groups gets around this to some extent but it may increase the participants' self-consciousness which may be a barrier to open and authentic participation. Focus groups can also be conducted very successfully using online platforms such as Zoom or Microsoft Teams which makes recording straightforward and also has obvious advantages when recruiting participants from different geographical areas (Richard et al., 2021).

RESPONDENT VALIDATION

Respondent validation (sometimes called member checking) is the process of returning interview transcripts back to participants for checking and agreement. Respondent validation is often favoured in feminist research, as a means of increasing the participant's control over the data. It provides participants with another chance to be clear about what they have said. And they can indicate anything that they wish to remove and anything they wish to amend or add. However, member checking runs the risk of participants self-consciously censoring and changing their transcripts beyond recognition. Another consideration is that when people are being interviewed about distressing experiences the continued reflection on what the participant said may start to feel like a therapeutic process. Koelsch (2013) has described how this continued engagement with the transcript can blur the boundaries between therapy and research as participants reflect on their stories and enter into a prolonged relationship with the researcher. Therefore the decision to use respondent validation should only be made after careful analysis of its risks and benefits.

REFLEXIVITY

All researchers will inevitably have their own preconceived ideas and ways of looking at the world and the topic they are researching. They may have every intention of putting this to one side, something called *bracketing*, as they conduct interviews. However, who the researcher is will make a difference to the study (Dodgson, 2019). They come to the study with their own life-experience and prior knowledge which cannot be simply erased. Instead, one method of dealing with this which is widely advocated in qualitative data collection is something called *reflexivity*. Reflexivity is a continuous process of self-awareness and reflection that the researcher engages in (alongside data collection and analysis) to acknowledge and declare any pre-conceived ideas or views which could impact on the study (Dodgson, 2019). Qualitative interviewers may be encouraged to write or record a reflexivity journal and to share this with another researcher or their supervisor as a means of dealing with subjectivity.

One important consideration when gathering data on a particular experience is whether the researcher's position is an *insider*: someone who has shared this experience in some way, or an outsider: someone with little or no experience regarding the study topic (Burns et al., 2012; Berger, 2015). This is because it is likely to impact on the research process and is important when assessing the similarities and differences between the researcher and the participants. Being an *insider* researcher can potentially be a more emotional and problematic experience for the researcher and can make it difficult to maintain the researcher role. For example, if a midwife is interviewing women as a researcher, it is not always easy or even possible for the

researcher to de-activate their midwifery role. This can lead to role confusion (Burns et al., 2012) and strategies to mitigate this should be considered well in advance. However, insider knowledge can be useful, particularly in developing good rapport and picking up subtleties that might be missed by a researcher unfamiliar with the setting (Ross, 2017).

Reflexivity applies to the entire research process but it is of particular significance when interviewing as this is when the researcher and participant are in a form of relationship with one another and that relationship is integral to data collection. Part of reflexivity is to provide openness and transparency about who the researcher is in relation to the participants and the context. The context refers not only to the environment and situation but also to factors, such as race, socio-economic status, age, cultural background and sexuality (Berger, 2015). To be reflexive, the researcher should continually consider this and engage in internal dialogue and critical self-evaluation of their position in the research (Mitchell et al., 2018).

REFLECTIVE PROMPT

If you were conducting a study which involved interviewing student midwives about their experiences in clinical placements, would your position be an outsider or an insider?

What impact might your own experiences have on the interviews?

CONDUCTING RESEARCH

Interviews should be considered when the research question suggests a self-report method appropriate to a face-to-face setting, either one-to-one or in a focus group. Focus groups are useful for establishing how a specific group talks about and experiences issues in which the researcher is interested. One of the advantages of the focus group, compared with individual interviews, is that in a group process people can sometimes find it easier to identify and clarify their views. Although interviewing a group may seem a more cost-effective method than interviewing the same number individually, they are used for different reasons and will not always achieve the same outcomes. Both one-to-one interviews and focus group interviews are useful where the individual may not have considered the subject in any depth or may not feel their views are important enough to return a questionnaire. Similarly, they should be considered where the topic might need to be explored with the help of the researcher, or one that may produce some depth that could not be captured by a questionnaire. Interviews are a good choice where the aim of the study is to explore a topic through the eyes of the participant and the researcher wants participants to recount their experiences in some depth in their own words. They are also suitable for topics that may be very sensitive and demand a high degree of trust and privacy.

One special situation requiring a lot of thought is interviews conducted with health professionals, particularly where those to be interviewed know or are known by the interviewer. This is a very different situation from interviewing strangers, as past histories can interfere with the quality of data produced and where the social distance needed to explore certain topics with strangers does not exist. See section on Reflexivity above.

Once the interview has been chosen as the appropriate data collection tool, they must consider the degree of structure it will contain, ranging from structured through to semi-structured and unstructured. The more unstructured options are often chosen where little is known about the topic and the researcher does not want to use questions that make assumptions or suggest a particular perspective. Whichever degree of structure, researchers must ensure they are fully trained and experienced in undertaking the role of interviewer and rehearse with colleagues using an audio recorder to listen for strengths and areas for improvement. The interviewer should be relaxed and establish rapport so respondents are put at their ease and feel that they can talk honestly. However, it is a difficult role to get right. Although listening and valuing what the person is saying, the interviewer is not passive. They must simultaneously analyse (in real time) the contribution this is making to the research question. For example, should they consider asking for more detail, or try to change the topic? This is why the interviewer is the tool of data collection and it requires tremendous skill, focus and awareness if the participant's time is going to be fully respected.

The body language of the interviewer is fundamental in helping the participant to relax in a potentially stressful and intimidating situation. There are many skills involved in the interview, for example, active listening and avoiding rephrasing the participant's answer in one's own words, as this can lead to bias. In addition, where it is clear that the participant has decided to describe a particular topic or account rather than an alternative, the interviewer must consider whether to bring them back to that point later and explore the alternative. Where an interruption or deviation in conversation occurs, the interviewer may have to help the respondent to return to the place reached before the interruption or change in direction.

Anything can happen in a free-flowing interview. Sometimes, while telling their 'story', respondents can relive painful memories, and experience heightened emotional responses. If a memory is stressful or painful, the respondent may exhibit anger, fear, sadness or distress. Under these circumstances, a decision has to be made on whether the interview should be abandoned or delayed until the participant recovers. However, some people find these emotional moments therapeutic. Individuals can sometimes feel grateful for the opportunity to have someone at last listen and acknowledge their experiences and feelings.

Where an interview is particularly intense, it is possible for the feelings of closeness with the interviewer to lead to the participant revealing 'secrets'. It should be remembered that where the interviewer is a midwife, the Nursing and Midwifery Council (NMC) professional code of conduct (NMC, 2018) does not allow all information to be kept secret (see Chapter 8 on ethics). Examples would be abuse or neglect, or a report of poor or unacceptable professional conduct. Under these circumstances the midwife cannot continue in the researcher role of keeping the information confidential but has a duty to report it. If the situation arises where a participant indicates that they want to share something that they declare is confidential, the midwife interviewer must stop them and make the researcher's own position clear before the participant says something that might be regretted later.

These points emphasise the demanding nature of interviews, especially those relating to very sensitive areas. It is possible for the researcher to absorb a great deal of other people's emotions that must then be dealt with. For this reason, interviewers should only conduct a small number of interviews per day and have a good research supervisor or mentor who can help deal in a positive way with the emotional after-effects of interviewing. Finally, interviews may involve entering into someone's emotional life and therefore the decision to use this method should not be taken without careful consideration. The researcher can feel a sense of betrayal and exploitation in sharing data or experiences where they have arisen in very poignant and private circumstances. Despite these words of warning, interviews can be exhilarating, richly rewarding and provide real insights into key areas of life that cannot easily be gained using other methods.

CRITIQUING RESEARCH

In critiquing a research article based on interviews, the first question to ask is, 'was it an appropriate choice of data collection tool?' In other words, given the study question or aim, are interviews an appropriate tool for data collection? Weighing up the advantages and disadvantages of interviews, would an alternative method have been more appropriate? We also need some indication of the degree of structure in the interview that may have encouraged or curtailed the views of the respondent, and the language in which they could respond; the more the interview was structured, the less it is possible to express views in the participant's own words.

One problem with many research reports is that it is difficult to get an idea of the conditions under which the interview took place. We frequently have no idea of the possible strength and weakness that may have influenced the reliability of the interview. In most instances, although the person undertaking the interview might be named, we have little idea of their appearance at the time of the interviews, and how they were dressed. Where the interviewer was a midwife, did the participants know them, and were they in uniform? Both these factors might influence the findings.

We should look for some assurance that the researcher followed principles to increase the quality of the data; for instance, did he or she practice the interview with either colleagues or test out the interview design in a pilot? Did they return some interviews back to those involved for validation (see section above on respondent validation)? The method of analysis of the findings should also be described and be credible, for example, naming a type of data analysis or the particular process used, for example thematic analysis or interpretive phenomenological analysis (IPA).

The presentation of results should also be examined. Although selection and editing are inevitable, it is still important that themes and key examples of issues are relevant to the aim of the study and based on a cross-section of those contributing to the study.

Finally, remember, as with questionnaires, that interviews are self-report methods and rely on the accuracy of what people say and the extent to which this truly reflects actions and beliefs. For this reason, generalisations are not usually made from interview data. Interviews provide insight and aid understanding and findings drawn from their analysis may be transferable or applicable to other settings but it would be inappropriate to consider such findings generalisable.

KEY POINTS

- Interviews have many advantages over questionnaires. In midwifery, they also have the advantage of being compatible with a woman-centred approach to care. They are predominantly used to collect qualitative data using a semi-structured or unstructured format. They can sometimes be used for quantitative research if questions are highly structured (such as multiple choice) and it is helpful to call these *survey interviews* to avoid confusion.

- Semi-structured and unstructured interviews have the advantage of collecting rich data through the interactive form of the interview. They provide a unique view of events as seen by those receiving services or those experiencing parenthood. The results are frequently unexpected, illuminating and can differ from the perspective of health professionals.

- There are a number of disadvantages to interviews. They are costly and time consuming. The physical presence of the researcher can also be intimidating to some participants, and the resulting data can be consciously or subconsciously skewed in the direction of socially desirable answers. They also require a high level of skill on the part of the interviewer to avoid some of the pitfalls outlined.

- The time-consuming nature of interviews means that sample size is frequently smaller than that possible with questionnaires. However, this does not automatically limit their usefulness, especially within qualitative research.

REFERENCES

Anderson, E., Brigden, A., Davies, A., Shepherd, E., Ingram, J., 2021. Pregnant women's experiences of social distancing behavioural guidelines during the Covid-19 pandemic 'lockdown' in the UK, a qualitative interview study. BMC Public Health 21 (1), 1202. https://doi.org/10.1186/s12889-021-11202-z

Bearman, M., 2019. Focus on methodology: eliciting rich data: a practical approach to writing semi-structured interview schedules. Focus Health Prof. Educ. Multi-Professional J 20 (3), 1. https://doi.org/10.11157/fohpe.v20i3.387

Berger, R., 2015. Now I see it, now I don't: researcher's position and reflexivity in qualitative research. Qual. Res. 15 (2), 219–234. https://doi.org/10.1177/1468794112468475

Burns, E., Fenwick, J., Schmied, V., Sheehan, A., 2012. Reflexivity in midwifery research: the insider/outsider debate. Midwifery 28 (1), 52–60.

Dodgson, J.E., 2019. Reflexivity in qualitative research. J. Hum. Lact. 35 (2), 220–222. https://doi.org/10.1177/0890334419830990

Gray, J., 2019. Introduction to qualitative research, seventh ed. In: Grove, S.K. Gray, J. (Eds.). In: Understanding Nursing Research: Building an Evidence-Based Practice, Chapter 3 Elsevier, St. Louis.

Hennink, M.M., Hutter, I., Bailey, A., 2020. Qualitative Research Methods, second ed. SAGE Publications, London.

Kallio, H., Pietilä, A.-M., Johnson, M., Kangasniemi, M., 2016. Systematic methodological review: developing a framework for a qualitative semi-structured interview guide. J. Adv. Nurs. 72 (12), 2954–2965. https://doi.org/10.1111/jan.13031

Krueger, R.A., Casey, M.A., 2015. Focus Groups: A Practical Guide for Applied Research, fifth ed. SAGE, California.

Koelsch, L.E., 2013. Reconceptualizing the member check interview. Int. J. Qual. Methods 12 (1), 168–179.

McGrath, C., Palmgren, P.J., Liljedahl, M., 2019. Twelve tips for conducting qualitative research interviews. Med. Teach. 41 (9), 1002–1006. https://doi.org/10.1080/0142159X.2018.1497149

Menage, D., Bailey, E., Lees, S., Coad, J., 2020. Women's lived experience of compassionate midwifery: human and professional. Midwifery 85, 102662.

Mitchell, J., Boettcher-Sheard, N., Duque, C., Lashewicz, B., 2018. Who do we think we are? Disrupting notions of quality in qualitative research. Qual. Health Res. 28 (4), 673–680. https://doi.org/10.1177/1049732317774889

NMC, 2018. The Code: Standards of Conduct, Performance and Ethics for Nurses and Midwives. NMC, London.

Prior, M.T., 2017. Accomplishing 'rapport' in qualitative research interviews: empathic moments in interaction. Appl. Linguistics Rev. 9 (4), 487–511. https://doi.org/10.1515/applirev-2017-0029

Richard, B., Sivo, S.A., Ford, R.C., Murphy, J., Boote, D.N., Witta, E., et al., 2021. A guide to conducting online focus groups via reddit. Int. J. Qual. Methods, 20. https://doi.org/10.1177/16094069211012217

Ross, L.E., 2017. An account from the inside: examining the emotional impact of qualitative research through the lens of 'insider' research. Qual. Psychol. 4 (3), 326–337. https://doi.org/10.1037/qup0000064

Seidman, I., 2019. Interviewing as Qualitative Research: A Guide for Researchers in Education and the Social Sciences. Teachers College Press, New York.

Thompson, E., Brett, J., Burns, E., 2019. What if something goes wrong? A grounded theory study of parents' decision-making processes around mode of breech birth at term gestation. Midwifery 78, 114–122.

11

OBSERVATION

In the last two chapters, questionnaires and interviews have been described as methods that gather data on what people do and think by asking them directly. One of the major difficulties of these two methods is that researchers have to assume that what people say they do is accurate. Observation differs in that it collects information first-hand, based on what people are seen to do by the researcher.

READER ACTIVITY

Can you find an example of a midwifery-focused
   observational study?
Why did the researchers choose this methodology?

The aim of this chapter is to consider the reasons for using observation as a method and to identify some of its advantages and disadvantages. Two approaches to observation will be highlighted. Firstly, the quantitative method of checklist observation will be briefly mentioned. Secondly, qualitative approaches to observation will be outlined in more detail. Although observation is used less frequently than questionnaires and

interviews, there are an increasing number of well-designed observational studies in the midwifery literature, a few of which are included within the narrative of this chapter.

WHAT IS OBSERVATION?

Individuals are observing the world around us all the time, so what is the difference between 'looking' and 'observing' in research terms? The answer, according to Thomas (2017: 226), is that observation in social research, *'means watching carefully'* (i.e. it becomes a research method when it is systematically planned and recorded and when the results are checked for their accuracy). In other words, observing is different from looking when it is carried out systematically for the purpose of answering a research question to develop knowledge. Observation can be defined as the collection of data that are visible to visual sensors, whether that consists of the researcher's eyes or the use of some means of visual recording. Watson et al. (2010: 382) add that as a tool of data collection, *'observation is an active process by which data are collected about people, behaviours, interactions, or events'*.

As with interviews (see Chapter 10), observation varies depending on the amount of structure used to record the data. At one extreme is the highly *structured observation* checklist of set variables that produces quantitative data, and at the other extreme is the *unstructured observation* of situations that are used to produce qualitative data.

In the last chapter, researchers were seen as the tool of data collection in the way they channelled the verbal information in the form of an interview. In this chapter, researchers are again the tool of data collection in the way in which they select and record the data they 'see', to answer the research aim.

WHY USE OBSERVATION?

Researchers have repeatedly noted that although they can ask people about their behaviour, actions or beliefs (i.e. what and why they do or believe something), they may not always get an accurate answer. This is because people are not always aware of what they do, or they are unable to accurately describe or articulate their actions. Some actions are carried out at a subconscious level and are difficult to describe or write down. Explaining how to tie a shoelace to someone, over the phone, is a good example. Data gathering, using observation, can overcome the problem of verbal descriptions because it draws on eye witness accounts and is therefore more direct (Denscombe, 2011). It can be applied to numerous midwifery activities where the best way to find out how someone does something or 'what happens' in certain situations is to watch it unfold.

One example of this is the work by Sosa et al. (2018) who observed 30 births, focusing on midwifery support in labour in three different birth settings (i.e. an alongside midwife-led unit), a freestanding midwife-led unit, and women's homes. They aimed to explore midwifery one-to-one support in labour in a real-world context of midwife-led birth environments. It would have been difficult to only observe the midwives' interactions with women, so semi-structured interviews were also conducted post-birth with the midwives involved. This is also a good example of *triangulation*, that is, the use of more than one data collection tool to increase the validity of the results.

Another example is Newnham et al. (2017) who used interviews and observation in their study. The researchers were interested in several aspects – the personal, social, cultural and institutional influences – on women's decision-making around using epidural analgesia in labour, especially around the gaining of consent for an epidural in labour. They used interviews with the women and observation of practice environment, again to increase the validity of their findings and inform midwifery practice.

STRUCTURED OBSERVATION

The next two sections will look first at the use of structured or systematic observations, followed in the next section by the use of unstructured observation. In structured observation, it is assumed that social activity can be separated into behaviours (set variables) that can be counted, and initially the researcher is required to define what these are. Next, the researcher devises a way to count the variables (e.g. recording during a set time period), frequency count recording (or event sampling) and interval recording (Thomas, 2017). The data is then imputed onto a checklist observation sheet that itemises the kinds of activities to be observed. The researcher will indicate, often with a tick, each time one of the items on the list occurs (e.g. a checklist of the times in an antenatal group setting a midwife asks a direct question as a way of gaining involvement from those present). The results are usually presented numerically, in the form of the number of occasions (*frequency distribution*), a percentage, or displayed in a table or figure such as a bar chart.

The set variables to be recorded need clear and unambiguous *concept definitions*, which are precise descriptions of its meaning or form to ensure accuracy of recording, especially when a number of observers are involved. This helps to reduce the problem of the observer having to make a large number of inferences regarding an item, such as 'gives emotional support'. What exactly does that mean in terms of what would be observed? The greater the degree of inference required, the less reliable the outcome. The ideal type of item for checklist observation includes those capable of being explicitly defined so that there is no question in the mind of the observer as to whether or not they have been identified.

As events and activities unfold so quickly, there is a limit to the number of different aspects the researcher can observe at once. Care has to be taken to avoid the checklist becoming too complex. For example, it may not be possible to accurately record the type, duration and form of touch between a midwife and woman in labour, as well as the duration of eye contact and any additional non-verbal forms of interaction.

Not only should the optimum number of elements be considered in the checklist but also the form of recording must be simplified to enable speed and accuracy. Simple ticks or crosses are the best form of recording items on hard copies or selected from an electronic checklist using a tablet or handheld device. Before using a checklist, the researcher should thoroughly practice with a pilot study. This may suggest ways of reducing the complexity of the list, as well as providing the researcher with an opportunity to develop the skill of observing and recording at the same time.

The limitation of an observational checklist is the depth of information that can be achieved and the limited complexity of interactions that can be accurately observed. This type of approach is also restricted to predicted behaviour and does not cope well with unexpected activities not included on the checklist. This means this form of observation is not appropriate where the researcher knows little about what will be observed.

UNSTRUCTURED OBSERVATION

In contrast to the checklist approach of structured observation are the unstructured methods found in qualitative studies. This means that the researcher records the events and behaviours they 'see', in a more open and flowing way. Anthropologists and sociologists first developed this form of observation to examine the actions and interactions of people in their natural social world (Stellmach et al., 2018). Observational research, when used in midwifery, sees midwife researchers collecting data that is non-interventional and non-experimental to answer research questions around how mothers and midwives respond and behave in specific circumstances.

The different roles vary in the extent to which the researcher becomes directly involved with those observed, that is, whether the role is participant. Participant observation is where the researcher participates in the research either openly or covertly and interacts freely with the participants. Advantages of participant observation include less impact, increased closeness to the situation and non-interference with the situation being observed. It is also thought to provide a better understanding and good quality insights into complex environments. However, it can cause disquiet to the reliability of the findings due to concerns over objectivity and so requires significant reflexivity in the researchers (Denscombe, 2011).

An example of this would be the study by Nilsson et al. (2019), which is an ethnographic study that aimed to enhance the understanding of the midwives' ability to practice as autonomous professionals within an obstetric unit in Sweden. They used participant observation by midwives to collect their data; this was subsequently analysed through interpretation, which was grounded in reflexivity and described within ethnographic accounts.

Non-participant observation is where the researchers may be present, but they do not interact directly with the participants. This is thought to enhance objectivity and neutrality but may increase bias due to the impact of being observed by an unknown researcher and through biased researcher interpretation of what they have observed. An example of this would be the study by Norris and Murphy (2020) who observed the learning and teaching between midwife mentors and student midwives in a midwifery-led environment. They found that there was a model of midwifery practice supported by a knowledge and understanding of physiological birth, which enhanced and underpinned the learning experience of student midwives.

A further variation is the extent to which the observed are aware that they are being watched. The term 'overt' signifies that those in the setting are aware of the observer's role, and 'covert' signifies situations where they do not know that observation is taking place. Most healthcare research now takes the overt approach because considerable ethical issues are raised by the concealment of data collection, whereas in covert research, the individual has not given their informed consent to take part. This is despite the possible advantage of reducing the 'observer effect', which is people changing their behaviour because they know they are being observed (Choi et al., 2019; Demetrious et al., 2019). Interestingly, the Internet is providing new opportunities for overt non-participation observation. Researchers may browse web-pages, create avatars in digital worlds or subscribe to email lists to collect their data.

An example of unstructured observation is the ethnographic study by Baron and Kaura (2021). The aim of the study was to explore and describe the contextual realities within an antenatal clinic (ANC) environment that influenced waiting times. It was a qualitative study, which collected data through unstructured observation and semi-structured interviews with pregnant women and midwives. The researcher would typically follow and observe the participants throughout their ANC visit, using an unstructured observation tool. During the observation, the researcher also wrote field notes of the waiting times, the activities and procedures that the women underwent, and the duration of the consultation and contact times. This kind of study illustrates the richness of data developed through ethnographic work. It contrasts with checklist observational studies because the researcher is interested in more in-depth information that does not necessarily follow a clearly anticipated path. There is also a great emphasis on discovering the form of behaviour found in natural settings, such as maternity care environments.

RECORDING IN OBSERVATIONAL STUDIES

One issue for the observational researcher is how to record the observations. Checklist designs are easiest to imagine, as the observer uses an electronic check list or pre-printed sheets consisting of columns or tables of items in which a tick is placed if an activity or event is observed. Where a study involves a number of observers, inter-observer reliability has to be demonstrated, that is, ensuring that the same event or item is recorded in the same way by each person carrying out the observations. This is where the training of observers plays a vital role in achieving consistency between observers (Watson et al., 2010).

Qualitative observational methods are more complex and raise greater issues for the researcher. Field notes are the major form of recording observations in qualitative studies. These are narrative accounts of events and situations and can be made while activities are in progress, or they can be written up some time later. Each alternative has its advantages. The researcher may draw attention to themselves if they write their observations during events; however, there is a greater dependency on the accuracy of memory where notes are written up later. The method chosen will depend on the many factors that researchers find in a setting, although the tendency is to make at least some rough notes at the time and to develop these later.

ADVANTAGES OF OBSERVATION

Observation is the most appropriate way of collecting research data in many situations, as the researcher is able to see what actually happens and does not depend on reports that may be distorted by memory or perception. In other words, they record what people actually do as opposed to what they say they do. In checklist studies, using structured or systematic observation, the frequency of events can be quantified and relationships and correlation can be established. Using observation is an efficient way of producing large amounts of objective pre-coded data that is reliable with high levels of inter-observer reliability (Denscombe, 2011). However, it may over-simplify behaviour or miss contextual information, as well as observe behaviour but not observe intention (Denscombe, 2011).

It is in the area of qualitative research that observation can be particularly appropriate to midwifery research: they are particularly useful in providing a holistic view of a setting and suggest that health professionals as observers have an advantage as an insider as they can ask the kinds of questions that would not occur to an outsider. However, it is possible to argue the reverse of this, where an outsider may ask questions that the insider would not think to ask, due to familiarity with the setting. The important point is that as observation takes place in a natural setting; it can provide an accurate picture of what actually happens. It can also take into account quite a large canvas of activity in the form of a description (e.g. a birth spread over a long-time period). Qualitative observation also provides flexibility, meaning the focus of attention can change as a result of early observations.

Observational studies are not frequently found in midwifery research, although they clearly have much to offer in gaining answers to questions that are not amenable to other forms of data collection. As with interviews, they can be used in both a quantitative and qualitative approach and appear to be extremely suitable for midwifery research, either as a single method but more often used in conjunction with other forms of data collection (Johnsen et al., 2018).

DISADVANTAGES OF OBSERVATION

Despite the positive aspects of this method, there are a number of pitfalls. Ethical problems are a major concern for the qualitative researcher, especially where covert observation is being used. The issue is one of observing individuals who have not given their permission to be included in a study. This goes against the basic principles of informed consent discussed in Chapter 8.

However, one of the difficulties in observation is the problem of *reactivity*, when people who are told what is being observed may change their normal behaviour and so distort the accuracy of the results. For instance, take the example given in Chapter 8 of observing student midwives' hand-washing techniques and imagine indicating to a student that their technique is about to be observed. The result may be that their technique is surprisingly good but may be far from an accurate picture of normal activity.

The question of ethics is also raised in situations where the observer sees an activity that may put individuals at risk or is an unprofessional act carried out by a member of staff. Although the researcher tries to maintain a confidential relationship with subjects, in certain circumstances it is not possible to honour this. One example would be where the observer has a public duty to disclose information, as in the case of observing unlawful or unprofessional activity or something that may potentially put a child at risk. In such situations, the researcher is obliged to report these observations and must abandon the researcher role for that of the midwife (see Chapter 8 for a discussion of these issues).

From a practical point of view, observation is a very time-consuming and therefore an expensive method. It also requires a great deal of interpersonal skills on the part of the observer, who should have training and experience with this method. Where more than one person is involved with the data gathering, there is also the problem of inter-observer reliability. This concerns the extent to which different observers select, interpret and record events in different ways.

One of the most obvious problems already referred to is that of *reactivity*, where people act differently because they know they are part of a research study. This seems an inevitable feature of observations made in the early stages of a study or in early interactions with individuals. This raises the issue of validity. The observer has to consider the extent to which the observations are a true picture of what is going on. The 'ironic' tone of the authors' description indicates that it is usually clear to the researcher when observations are not a true reflection of activities. This challenge to the reliability of the method and validity of the results is reduced where the observation extends over a longer time period, where people relax more into their usual way of behaving.

A further problem for the midwife researcher is the difficulty of being able to stand back from the familiar taken-for-granted routine of the maternity setting and ask, 'why do things happen like this?' In anthropological terms, this is called establishing '*cultural strangeness*', where the aim is to see things from an outsider's point of view. However, the longer the researcher is in the field setting, the greater the danger of what is referred to as '*habituating*'. This term has its origins in anthropological studies, where over an extended period of observing isolated indigenous communities, researchers would become so at home with the new culture that they would stop seeing activities and customs as 'strange', or noteworthy. In qualitative research, it refers to the researcher becoming overfamiliar with the research setting and no longer noticing the kind of elements that need to be included in the observations. This results in a loss of objectivity and observations become subject to researcher bias (Denscombe, 2011).

A major problem for researchers is one of selectivity. As it is not possible to observe everything that is going on or see things from every angle, decisions have to be made on where observers will place themselves and what they will attempt to observe. This will inevitably lead to some things being observed and others left out. In the same way, it is not possible to record everything, and some details will be omitted. No two observers will observe the same things or observe in the same way, which illustrates that observation is open to some variation and in its 'open', form will, at least to some extent, be influenced by the observer. In some situations there is also the possibility of misinterpreting what is going on. This is particularly true when observing a long-established relationship where subtle patterns of communication styles have been developed and understood between people. These can appear strange or alien to the observer. The difference between cajoling someone to do something and apparently being hostile or unsympathetic can easily be misinterpreted by the researcher, unaware of the usual pattern of conversation between people.

Observer bias is a further concern, where researchers may be inclined to look out for certain activities and ignore others that do not fit in with their views or expectations. Where each period of observation is lengthy, *observer drift* can also be a problem. This is when observers lose concentration after a time, find themselves thinking of other things and lose awareness of what is happening. This will clearly affect the quality and accuracy of the data (Griffiths and Rafferty, 2010). In some situations, time sampling is carried out so that the observation period is broken down into shorter segments, and the researcher attempts to sample across all the time periods. This allows the researcher to remain relatively fresh throughout the period of observation. Where the researcher is concentrating on events, such as a birth, this is not always a viable alternative, and an awareness of the danger of observer drift is the only precaution possible.

CONDUCTING RESEARCH

As with each of the methods of research covered so far, the researcher must ensure that observation is the appropriate choice for the study aim (Fry et al., 2017). In situations where self-reports may be inaccurate or where there is a need to consider a holistic view, then observation may be the best method.

The decision on which type of observation should be used is based on the requirements of the research question. Where the question relates to a quantification of results, such as 'how often', or 'how much', or where the question is related to establishing whether something happens or not and with what frequency, a checklist design will be appropriate. This will take the form of a structured sheet that looks like a spreadsheet or grid to allow ease of completion in the form of ticks, code numbers, or letters. Where the research question does not imply a quantitative approach but is more concerned with developing a broad understanding of how people act in a natural

setting, as in an ethnographic study, then a participant or non-participant observation study should be designed.

The exact role the researcher will play in this kind of research will require thought. The variation in role from participant to non-participant observer should be considered. This does not necessarily mean that the researcher will stay within one role. However, the consequences of the different types of researcher role must be considered in relation to their influence on those observed and the consequence for the data gathered.

At an early point, the ethical implications of the study need to be considered. Where an ethics committee is involved, informed consent and the issue of possible deception should be addressed in a way that will satisfy the committee that consent has been considered, and harm will be avoided.

There are a large number of skills required of the observer. Researchers have to work out what is going on in a situation, without using their own stereotypes and preconceptions. Rather, they should try and see things through the eyes of those observed. In terms of the practical activities concerned, researchers must decide on the issues of what to record and how. It is important in observation to have clear concept definitions for the items that will be recorded. This is true of checklist observation, as well as qualitative observational approaches.

The how of recording will depend on the extent to which contemporary recording may disrupt the flow of activities being observed. The main alternatives will be note taking at the time or sometime later or the use of an audio or video recorder. The exact details of what is recorded will change during the course of observation. Early notes may be very broad and will try to establish some ideas of the kind of pattern of activity taking place. They will then become more focused, depending on earlier observations and the questions arising from the field notes.

The analysis stage of this kind of data is a very sophisticated activity. As with the analysis of quantitative data, advice and help should be sought from those with previous experience. In presenting the qualitative report or article, the structure is very different from that of a quantitative report or article. Some of the sources of work referred to in this chapter should be considered as a guide for writing the report in order to do full justice to the information collected.

CRITIQUING RESEARCH

In critiquing observational research articles, readers have to decide whether this was a suitable method to answer the research question. It is important to determine what the researcher was observing and how. In both checklist and qualitative approaches, does the researcher give a clear concept definition for the items being observed?

Perhaps only second to experimental design, observation raises a number of ethical issues, so an important element it to ensure that an ethics committee approves the study. Was the research overt or covert, that is, were people aware that they were being observed or not? Was permission sought from subjects where it was overt? Where permission was not sought, does the researcher provide a convincing justification for not securing this?

Where the researcher is present in the research setting, as opposed to the use of cameras, they must consider the extent to which the researcher may have had an influence on the people and events observed. What did the researcher do to try to minimise the reactive effect on subjects? In good qualitative studies, researchers are expected to provide a clear description of how they presented themselves in the setting in terms of dress and behaviour. Do the researchers appear to display any bias, emotions and prejudices in their dealings with those observed, which may have influenced the quality of the data collected? Do the researchers appear to gravitate towards certain people in the study, and avoid others? In other words, has there been a bias in who was observed that might have produced untypical results?

Where more than one observer was responsible for the data collection, how was inter-observer reliability achieved? Even where there is only one observer, it is important to establish if any training was received or a pilot study undertaken.

Has the researcher included other methods of data collections, such as structured or unstructured interviews or the use of diaries or other form of documentary methods? Is the interplay between the different methods explained? In unstructured observation, the researcher using a qualitative approach should have produced 'thick', or 'rich', data. Does this enhance credibility so it almost feels as if you are there?

When it comes to analysis, do the researchers leave a decision trail so that the reader can audit the way they have moved through the data collection to the establishment of the categories used to present the findings? Overall, do the researchers convince the reader that they have tried to be as rigorous as possible throughout the study?

REFLECTION PROMPTS

What would be your thoughts and feelings if you were involved in an observational study where you were being observed providing midwifery care?

KEY POINTS

- Observation can be used to produce quantitative or qualitative data.
- Although it is not used as often as some of the other methods, observation can play an important part in answering important questions in a holistic and woman-centred way.
- In observation, the main issues concern the degree of structure in the data collection and the influence of the observer's presence on what is observed.
- There are a large number of decisions to make prior to the study by researchers. These include the nature of the role they will play, the amount of interaction they will have with those observed, the method of recording, the extent of recording and the method of analysis.
- The time period needed for some studies makes this a costly method of collecting data, and one that requires a large amount of personal skills, as well as research expertise. However, the benefits of such an approach are considerable.

REFERENCES

Baron, J.C., Kaura, D., 2021. Perspectives on waiting times in an antenatal clinic: a case study in the Western Cape. Health SA (Online) 26, 1–9.

Choi, W.J., Jung, J.J., Grantcharov, T.D., 2019. Impact of hawthorne effect on health care professionals: a systematic review. Univ. Tor. Med. J. 96 (2), 21–32.

Demetrious, C., Hu, L., Smith, T., Hing, C.B., 2019. Hawthorne effect on surgical studies. ANZ J. Surg. 89 (2), 1567–1576.

Denscombe, M., 2011. The Good Research Guide, fourth ed. Open University Press, Berkshire.

Fry, M., Curtis, K., Considine, J., Shaban, R.Z., 2017. Using observation to collect data in emergency research. Australas. Emerg. Nurs. J. 20 (1), 25–30.

Griffiths, P., Rafferty, A. M., 2010. Outcome measures. In: Gerrish, K., Lacey, A., (eds). The Research Process in Nursing. 6th ed. Wiley-Blackwell, Chichester.

Johnsen, H., Clausen, J., Hvidtjorn, D., Juhl, M., Hegaard, H.K., 2018. Women's experiences of self-reporting health on-line prior to their first midwifery visit: a qualitative study. Women Birth 31 (2), e105–e114. https://doi.org/10.1016/j.wombi.2017.07.013

Newnham, E., McKellar, L., Pincombe, J., 2017. 'It's your body, but…' mixed messages in childbirth education: findings from a hospital ethnography. Midwifery 55, 53–59. https://doi.org/10.1016/j.midw.2017.09.003

Nilsson, C., Olafsdottir, O.A., Lundgren, I., Berg, M., Dellenborg, L., 2019. Midwives' care on a labour ward prior to the introduction of a midwifery model of care: a field of tension. Int. J. Qual. Stud. Health Well-Being 14 (1), 1593037. https://doi.org/10.1080/17482631.2019.1593037

Norris, S., Murphy, F., 2020. A community of practice in a midwifery led unit. How the culture and environment shape the learning experience of student midwives. Midwifery 86, 102685. https://doi.org/10.1016/j.midw.2020.102685

Sosa, G., Crozier, K., Stockl, A., 2018. Midwifery one-to-one support in labour: more than a ratio. Midwifery 62, 230–239. https://doi.org/10.1016/j.midw.2018.04.016

Stellmach, D., Beshar, I., Bedford, J., du Cros, P., Stringer, B., 2018. Anthropology in public health emergencies: what is anthropology good for? BMJ Glob. Health 3 (2), e000534.

Thomas, G., 2017. How to Do Your Research Project: A Guide for Students, third ed. Sage publications, London.

Watson, H., Booth, J., Whyte, R., 2010. Observation. In: Gerrish, K., Lacey, A. (Eds.), The Research Process in Nursing, sixth ed. Wiley-Blackwell, Chichester.

12

EXPERIMENTS

Evidence-based practice has increased the demand for research that can unambiguously demonstrate the best options for clinical care. Experimental design has established itself as the most widely recognised and respected source of such evidence. In medicine, the experiment frequently takes the form of the randomised controlled trial (RCT). This method of collecting research data has become so powerful in determining the effectiveness of treatments that it is widely seen as a gold standard for research against which all other methods are compared. As many clinical procedures in maternity care are influenced by experimental research, it is crucial that midwives can evaluate such studies and not accept them without question.

The purpose of this chapter is to consider the basic principles of experimental design and to recognise the strengths, as well as the limitations, of this approach. As experiments can be designed in a number of ways, this chapter will also outline some of these various forms.

WHY ARE EXPERIMENTS SPECIAL?

Experiments are highly regarded in healthcare and have been traditionally associated with the *scientific method*. This may be due to the belief that they are more accurate or 'objective', than other forms of data collection. This has led to their prominent position in *hierarchies of evidence* (described in Chapter 1) that attempt to indicate the most reliable sources of information. The result is that hierarchies 'privilege', the RCT in a way that makes them the main source of knowledge within medicine (Spiby and Munro, 2010).

Experimental designs use a scientific approach to look for a cause and effect relationship between two variables. The dependent variable (or outcome) is measured, following manipulation of the independent variable (or intervention). For example, in an experimental study to see whether mindfulness decreases anxiety in pregnant women, the outcome that we would want to measure would be anxiety; this would be the dependent variable and mindfulness would be the intervention or independent variable.

Assessing the likelihood of a cause-and-effect relationship also requires statistical calculations. To examine this, it is essential to understand the concept of probability in research. Probability is a number that tells you how likely (or probable) something is to happen. Suppose an experimental study is designed to measure the effect of a particular intervention on length of labour for primiparous women. The women enrolled into the study are placed into one of two groups. One group receives the intervention and the other does not. When the study is complete, the length of labour for all participants is examined. The mean length of labour in the intervention group is shorter than the mean length of labour in the group who did not receive the intervention.

READER ACTIVITY

A question to consider: does the above result prove that the intervention works? We know that length of labour can vary a lot. Is there any possibility that this result could have just happened by chance?

There are a number of reasons why the result does not prove that the intervention reduced the length of labour. To start, we do not know how the women were allocated to each of the two groups. There may have been differences in the way that length of labour was defined and measured. Even if the allocation of women and all other procedures were carried out in accordance with the requirements of an experimental design (these will be explored further on in this chapter), it is possible that the result happened by chance. It would be very difficult to completely rule this out as it may just have been a 'fluke'. Probability is a mathematical calculation to determine the extent to which the results of an experiment could have happened by chance and is indicated by the *p value*. This takes the form of a number less than one, often found in or under a table

of results or in the text of a research article. It is reasonably easy to interpret this when familiar with the basic idea underpinning probability (see Box 12.1).

BOX 12.1
PROBABILITY VALUES

Probability values indicate the extent to which the difference in the results between two groups could have happened by chance. The '*p*' stands for '*probability*'. This translates into how many times out of a hundred, or even a thousand, the difference between two groups of data could happen purely by chance. The smaller the likelihood that a difference could have happened by chance, the more certain we can be that the experiment has demonstrated a cause-and-effect relationship. In other words, the intervention does produce the desired effect.

The value of '*p*' is expressed as a decimal, and it has to be converted to a fraction to work out the element of chance. Take the example of '$p < 0.05$'. We first convert 0.05 to a fraction by drawing a line underneath the numbers so that they become the top line of the fraction; then put a '1' underneath the decimal point, and a '0' underneath every figure after the point. This may sound complicated, but if you write it out for yourself, 0.05 becomes 05/100. In other words, the likelihood of the difference between the results of two groups in the study happening purely by chance is less than 5 in 100 times. Or, put another way, 95 times out of 100 the effect you wanted will be produced by the intervention used in the study.

This figure of $p < 0.05$ is regarded as the minimum value that may suggest a relationship between the dependent and independent variable. Notice that there is still a margin of error. It does not mean that one thing definitely causes the other; the results would have happened purely by chance 5 in 100 times. This means that for 95% of the time you can be satisfied that a cause-and-effect relationship does exist.

The most frequently used values to indicate probability are as follows:

P value	Probability of Difference Happening by Chance
<0.05	Less than 5 in 100
<0.01	Less than 1 in 100
<0.001	Less than 1 in 1000
NS	Non-significant (i.e. the probability that chance is responsible for the result is so large that a '*p*' value is not used).

It is recommended that you consult a statistics book for more information.

CHARACTERISTICS OF EXPERIMENTAL DESIGN

What are the essential features of an experiment? Unlike other methods (apart from action research), the experiment is a form of research where the researcher is active in the situation and not just a gatherer of information. The researcher makes something happen and is responsible for controlling the way that something is introduced into the situation. So a common form of the experiment is where there are two groups of participants and the researcher will introduce an intervention to one group but not the other and then see if those in the experimental group have a different outcome to those in the control group, or not. See Box 12.2 for an example.

According to Daniel (2019), the three elements that confirm a study as a true experiment are:

- Randomisation
- Researcher-controlled manipulation of the independent variable (the experimental variable)
- Researcher control of the experimental situation, including a control or comparison group

Together, these three elements help to rule out alternative ways of explaining a particular outcome to a study other than the variable introduced by the researcher. Each of these elements will now be examined.

Randomisation

Randomisation is a term that may apply to both the sampling procedure used in a study (see Chapter 14) and the allocation of individuals to an experimental group (sometimes called intervention) or control group. Random sampling occurs when every member of a study population (all those with the relevant characteristics, such as those going home from a midwifery-led unit over a 3-month period) has an equal chance of being included in the study. This is not easy to achieve in a total group, as individuals must first agree to take part in a clinical study; it is not simply a case of picking them out of a population and expecting them to accept a form of intervention allocated to them. In most cases, randomisation refers to *random assignment* or *random allocation*. This is the process of allocating participants to either the experimental group or control group in a random manner *once they have agreed to take part in the study*. In other words, an individual entering the study should be allocated to a treatment or intervention group in a way that ensures they have an equal chance of being in either group. The exact method used to randomise those in a study will be explained in Chapter 14. It is a very precise and methodical system and it is not 'haphazard', which is a misunderstanding of the term.

BOX 12.2

EXAMPLE OF A RANDOMISED CONTROL TRIAL: EFFECTIVENESS OF AN ANTENATAL BEHAVIOURAL INTERVENTION BY COMMUNITY MIDWIVES

The aim of this UK study was to investigate the effectiveness of a behavioural brief intervention by midwives (this was the independent variable) in preventing excessive weight gain during pregnancy. The setting was an antenatal clinics in England. Participants were women between 10+0 and 14+6 weeks gestation, not requiring specialist obstetric care. Participants were randomised to usual antenatal care (control group) or usual care plus the intervention (intervention group). The intervention involved community midwives weighing women at antenatal appointments, setting maximum weight gain limits between appointments and providing brief feedback. Women were encouraged to monitor and record their own weight weekly to assess their progress against the maximum limits set by their midwife. Outcome measures were excessive gestational weight gain, depression, anxiety and physical activity (these were the dependent variables). Six hundred and fifty-six women from four maternity centres were recruited: 329 women were randomised to the intervention group and 327 to the control group. The researchers concluded that there was no evidence that the intervention decreased excessive gestational weight gain. There was no significant difference in anxiety or depression scores or in physical activity scores between the groups.

Daley, A., Jolly, K., Jebbh, S.A., Roalfe, A., Mackilllop, L., Lewis, A., et al., 2019. Effectiveness of a behavioural intervention involving regular weighing and feedback by community midwives within routine antenatal care to prevent excessive gestational weight gain: POPS2 randomised controlled trial. BMJ Open. 9 (9), e030174. https://doi.org/10.1136/bmjopen-2019–030174.

The purpose of randomisation is to reduce the possibility of bias where people with certain characteristics that might affect the outcome are unevenly distributed between the two groups in a study. The implication of this is that the groups would initially differ from each other, which would make it impossible to rule out the influence of factors built into the characteristics of those in the two groups. In experimental design, the groups should be similar at the start of the experiment before anything is introduced. If they differ at the end, then it is easier to argue that the difference is due to the experimental variable. Randomisation also ensures that additional factors called 'confounding variables', that may also influence the results, are evenly distributed between the two groups. In other words, randomisation should allow the researcher to compare like with like.

In experimental design, the existence of a comparison group that does not receive the intervention (or independent variable) is crucial. The role of the control group is to act as a comparison by establishing what the typical outcome would be if the experimental variable had not been introduced. In evidence-based practice, this is important in deciding whether an intervention would make any difference to the outcome. The control group theoretically remains the same over the experimental period, as they do not receive the treatment or intervention that forms the independent variable. This allows the investigator to reduce the effect of what has variously been called the 'attention factor', or the 'Hawthorne effect'. This was found in a classic American study on motivation that looked at people working in the Hawthorne plant of an electricity company in Chicago. Although the study set out to examine the effect of heating and lighting and other environmental factors on output, it was found that whether these factors were raised or lowered, productivity increased. It was realised that it was not the heating or lighting that affected the output; it was the result of receiving attention from the researchers that influenced their work level. This gave rise to the term 'Hawthorne effect'. The Hawthorne effect brings about a change in the outcome (dependent variable) due to a feeling of being 'special', which produces a reaction that mimics a real change.

Not all studies have a separate control group. For example, one group can receive two or more interventions in turn, being a conventional approach followed by an experimental approach. In this way, individuals act as their own control. It is also possible for two separate groups to receive the same two interventions but in a different order. Here again, they are acting as their own controls in that they receive both interventions and rule out the possibility that any differences are the result of varying characteristics of those in the two groups. This kind of approach is referred to as a *cross-over design study* (Haseen, 2020).

Manipulation

The second feature of experimental design is manipulation, which means the experimenter manipulates or introduces an intervention or treatment (independent variable) to the experimental group but withholds it from the control group who receive either an alternative or nothing (Polit and Beck, 2018). This can be seen in the example of an RCT by Daley et al. (2019) in Box 12.2. In this RCT, the pregnant participants were randomised into two groups. The intervention group received usual antenatal care and a midwife-led brief intervention and the control group received usual care only.

Control

Control is the final feature of experimental design, where the researcher reduces the possible effect of other variables on the outcome measure of the study. This means that the experimenter must have the ability to control not only the intervention (independent variable) but also other elements within the experimental setting that might make a difference to the outcome (dependent variable). For example, they must ensure that everyone in the study has an equal chance of being in the experimental group (random allocation). If this is achieved, then the researcher can say that they have controlled for extraneous factors that may influence the dependent variable. In the study in Box 12.2, the researchers *controlled* for BMI category (healthy weight/overweight/obese) and recruitment site. That is, they sought to make sure that there was an equal balance between the two groups, in terms of these two characteristics. They achieved this by stratifying participants (in terms of BMI category and recruitment site) and then randomising. This is called *stratified* randomisation.

It is the researcher's ability to achieve maximum control that illustrates the degree of *rigour* in the study.

This includes control over the way any interventions are provided. All procedures must be applied in exactly the same way to each individual so that consistency is achieved, and other possible explanations for differences in outcomes are eliminated. Measurements of the dependent variable should also be under the control of the researcher. The measuring instrument should be accurate and consistent. Where more than one person is involved in the measurement, the researcher should ensure that everyone is measuring in exactly the same way. This is called *inter-rater reliability*.

Taken together, one can see all three features of an experiment make extraordinary demands on the skills and power of the researcher and make experiments a very complex form of research.

Blinding

Before moving on, there is another important aspect of control in an RCT that needs to be highlighted, this is *blinding* (sometimes also called concealment or masking). At the start of a study, as individuals are being allocated to the experimental or control group, it is essential that those carrying out the allocation cannot anticipate the group to which the next person will be allocated. This is so they do not tamper with who goes where, on the basis of their knowledge of what the person might receive. *Blinding* or *masking* means that those in the study do not know the intervention or treatment an individual has received. This is an attempt to maintain the objectivity of the method by protecting the results from the accusation that they are inaccurate as they have been spoilt or compromised by poor design. There are a number of methods for doing this, for example, using specially designed software or sealed envelopes so that it is not possible to anticipate the allocation until the envelope has been opened.

There are three types of blinding: single, double and triple. Single blinding is when one party is blinded to treatment/intervention allocation. This often refers to either the study participants only or the researchers only. Double blinding is when two parties are blinded to treatment allocation. This often refers to study participants and researchers. Lastly, triple blinding is when three parties are blinded to treatment allocation. This usually includes study participants, researchers

and other staff involved in the running of the study (e.g. data collectors, statisticians, etc).

However, there is room for confusion as there are no universally accepted definitions and it is not always clear from a published study which parties are being referred to when stating that the study was double-blinded for example. For this reason, some have called for researchers to explicitly state which parties were blinded and which were not, when publishing their studies (Penić et al., 2020).

Blinding avoids the risk of people acting differently if they know to which group the individual has been allocated, during the course of a clinical trial, thus avoiding the chance of subconscious bias in favour of the experimental intervention. Blinding is an important aspect of clinical RCTs, as it can affect the accuracy of the outcome in trials. In drug trials, it is established practice to ensure that all study participants and those involved in administering the drug (or placebo) are blinded. Usually, an allocated pharmacist will be involved in dispensing the correct medication (or placebo) for each participant. This may be based on a coded list that links to randomisation codes. Alternatively, the active drugs and placebos may be pre-labelled with barcodes by the manufacturer for individual participants. Neither the participants nor those involved in administering the drug know who is having the active drug or who is having the placebo.

Although control is important in midwifery research, blinding is not always sensible or possible. The intervention may be difficult to hide from those receiving it and those involved in the care. For example, it would be impossible to blind participants to an intervention like spending time in water in labour or participation in antenatal yoga. This practical difficulty in blinding is a consequence of variations in the way research is conducted in different healthcare areas, where constraints on the levels of control are inevitable and not necessarily a weakness in design.

This is clear in the example in Box 12.2. Due to the nature of the intervention, it was not possible to blind participants or community midwives to it.

THE HYPOTHESIS

According to Wood and Kerr (2011), the experiment can be categorised as a level-three research question (see Chapter 2 on levels of questions in research). To achieve this level, they suggest that the researcher should be able to predict what will happen (have a hypothesis) and provide a theory based on previous research findings to explain it. One of the chief purposes of the experiment is to test a hypothesis and to establish causality, that is, one variable is capable of causing or bringing about a direct effect on another variable. The researcher should state the hypothesis at the start of the study. This statement can take two forms: *the research or scientific hypothesis* and the *null-hypothesis* (also called a *statistical hypothesis*). The research hypothesis states the predicted difference in outcomes between the two groups. It usually contains words, such as '*more than*', '*higher*', or '*less than*' or '*lower*', whichever indicates a better outcome. The null-hypothesis predicts that there will be no difference between the two groups (see Chapter 7 and also Box 12.3 in this chapter). In other words, the intervention will not affect the outcome. This was the situation in an important study by O'Sullivan et al. (2009), which helped to change women's care in labour. The researchers set out to investigate the effect of feeding during labour on obstetric and neonatal outcomes. They believed that allowing women to have something light to eat during labour would not affect major clinical outcomes, which the study data supported. In this case, the most favourable result would be no difference in outcome between the group who received only water and the group who were allowed light food. It is of note that this study then became one of five studies in a Cochrane systematic review, which led to the conclusion that there is no justification for the restriction

of fluids and food in labour for women at low risk of complications (Singata et al., 2013).

READER ACTIVITY

In the case of the study by O'Sullivan et al. (2009) just mentioned on eating in labour, can you identify the dependent and independent variables?

One helpful method of distinguishing between the two is to identify which comes first chronologically and which come last or is measured last. Items measured last would be the clinical outcomes of the birth; these included spontaneous vaginal birth rate, duration of labour, need for augmentation of labour, instrumental and caesarean birth rates, incidence of vomiting and neonatal outcome. Each of those would be a dependent variable (as an RCT can have more than one dependent variable). What came before them in time was eating the food, so that is the independent variable.

TYPES OF EXPERIMENTS

Experimental design can take a number of alternative forms. Often these variations relate to a second 'control' group and how people are allocated to them, as well as variations in the point at which measurements take place. The classic writers on the subject, Campbell and Stanley (1963), suggested that there were three main variations:

- The pre-test post-test control group
- The post-test only design
- The Solomon four-group design

The Pre-Test Post-Test Control Group

This is the most commonly used and perhaps the best-known design, where subjects are randomly allocated to the experimental or control group. The idea is to have two balanced groups, in terms of the personal attributes, that might make a difference to the outcome. Both groups are measured in relation to an outcome measure (dependent variable) prior to any intervention, and this acts as a base-line measurement. At this point, these measurements should confirm that the two groups are comparable. In the intervention

---

BOX 12.3
HYPOTHESES AND A NULL-HYPOTHESIS

- In the study by Daley et al. (2019) shown in Box 12.2, no **hypothesis** was actually stated, but it could have been stated as follows:
- There will be a lower proportion of women in the intervention group who have gained excessive weight during pregnancy compared to those in the control group receiving usual care only.
- A **null-hypothesis** could be stated as: There will be no difference between the women in the intervention group or the control group, in the proportion of women who have excessive weight gain during pregnancy.

phase, the experimental group receives the new intervention, whilst the control group receives either the current or no intervention/treatment (although they may receive a placebo). Following this phase, both groups are retested or measured again, and a ny differences are subjected to statistical analysis. This calculates the extent to which any differences between the two groups at the end could be due to chance and not the result of the experimental intervention (Fig. 12.1).

This method can be carried out using two different groups measured over the same time period or a single group using a cross-over design (see above). This allows those in the study to act as their own controls. The first approach, using two different groups, is known as an *unrelated, between* or *different subject* design, and the second is known as a *related, within* or *same subject* design. It is worth considering that where one group receives both interventions, there can be a '*carry-over*' effect, where benefits from the first treatment may still influence the individual, once exposed to the second intervention. To reduce this possibility,

the order of the interventions is frequently randomised for those in the group.

Post-Test Only Design

A problem with the pre-test post-test design is that measuring the groups before an intervention is not always possible. There is also the problem that the first measurement may sensitise the subjects in such a way that they perform better on the second occasion because of the experience gained as a result of the first measurement. The post-test only design (Fig. 12.2) is an attempt to reduce this familiarity effect by only measuring the variables at the end of the experiment. The limitation of this design is that it is not possible to say whether the two groups were similar at the start of the study. The difference in measurement could have been due to characteristics that existed within the groups before the intervention.

Solomon Four-Group Design

In order to overcome the disadvantages of both the previous examples, the Solomon four-group design

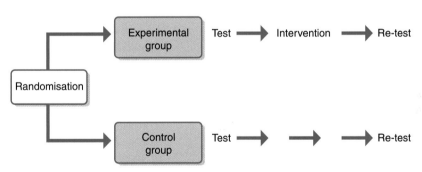

Fig. 12.1 ■ The pre-test, post-test design.

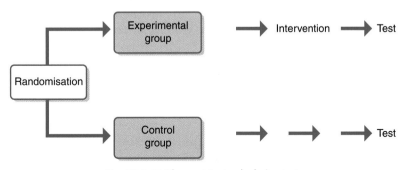

Fig. 12.2 ■ The post-test only design test.

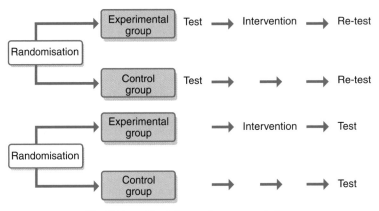

Fig. 12.3 ■ The Solomon four-group design.

has been developed. As can be seen from Fig. 12.3, this is really a combination of both the previous designs. This means that as well as being able to eliminate the disadvantage of an after-only design, the effect of pre-testing can be assessed (Navarro & Siegel, 2018).

The immediate problem is one of gaining a sufficient number of people for all four groups. In addition, the possibility of some people dropping out (*subject mortality* or *subject attrition*) is even greater with this number of participants. The researcher may no longer be comparing like with like if the numbers in some of the groups have changed during the study period. This kind of design is very complex to organise and, naturally, very costly because it is a large-scale design that requires a great deal of time, resources and expertise.

THREATS TO VALIDITY

Although experimental designs are held in high regard, their use does not guarantee accuracy as there are a number of reasons why the results of an experiment may be inaccurate. Threats to validity may relate to problems with the experiment itself which might mean that there are other possible reasons for the results. This is the *internal validity*, and those that relate to the generalisability to other situations is *external validity*.

Internal Threats to Validity

- **Confounding Variables**: This is where another variable other than the intervention has influenced the results. For example, imagine a study on whether extra postnatal support increases breastfeeding rates. Suppose there is a widely publicised health scare on artificial feeds at the same time that the study is being conducted. It could be possible that any increase in breastfeeding rates is due to (or at least influenced by) this. Therefore, it would be a confounding variable.

- **Testing/Observation Effects**: This refers to the consequence of pre-testing on the results of a later retest. For example, a study may be designed, which involves measuring anxiety levels before and after an intervention. The first test may encourage an individual to think about issues that influence how they answer later in the post-test (e.g. accepting screening tests). Here, it is the influence of the first test and not the intervention that has made a difference to the results. In addition to this, the role and behaviour of the researcher may introduce bias if researchers, in their enthusiasm for the study, may subconsciously influence people in non-verbal ways, such as positive nods of the head or smiling when certain answers are given.

- **Instrumentation Issues**: This is when measurement tools or data measurement skills of those involved lead to inaccuracies. This may produce different results that are mistakenly interpreted as due to the independent variable (e.g. variations in weighing scale accuracy).

- **The effects of the passage of time or *maturation*:** This relates to normal physical, psychological and social changes that occur to individuals that are unrelated to the variables in the study. This may result in a change between pre- and post-testing results. For example, during pregnancy, certain physiological changes may be due to the differences in gestation rather than due to an independent variable.
- **Regression**: This is a statistical phenomenon where there is a tendency for extreme scores or measurements in a study to move closer to the mean (average) and is sometimes called *regression to the mean*. It is a problem in studies, involving repeated measurements on the same subject or unit of observation and can be avoided best by good study design in which there is randomisation and a control group (Barnett et al., 2015).
- **Drop-out:** Although an experimental and control group may have been similar at the start of a study, those who decided to drop out of a study may share common characteristics, such as age, parity or being smokers. Consequently, those remaining are no longer quite as similar as those in the other group, so the researcher is no longer comparing like with like.

External Threats to Validity

External validity considers those factors that limit the extent to which findings can be generalised to the wider population and/or to other settings. The main threats that need to be considered are:

- **Selection effects:** This relates to the people selected for inclusion in the study. For example, in some experiments, poor sampling methods may have resulted in women from a particular social class, ethnicity, age group or parity being over-represented in the sample. This would produce results that may not be applicable to all women.
- **Reactive effects:** The factors relating to how people respond within the experiment. Participants may be influenced by feeling special, as in the *Hawthorne effect* mentioned earlier in this chapter, or by a desire to help the experimenter succeed or have positive results. In this situation, the results are not really due to the independent variable and cannot be generalised.
- **Measurement effects:** The effect of measurement techniques on the results. If it is accepted that pre-testing participants' knowledge, mood, or attitudes may influence retesting due to people having an opportunity to reflect on the subject, increasing their self-awareness and even changing behaviour. As a result, testing may reduce the extent to which the results of the study can be applied to others.

Quasi-Experimental Designs

Although experimental design is regarded as one of the strongest methods of establishing cause-and-effect relationships, it is not always possible to apply this approach in every situation. Quasi-experimental designs have some of the features of true experimental design but not all of them. The reasons for this can be practical, such as difficulties in controlling the effect of other independent variables, or ethical where it would not be acceptable to allocate people to an experimental and control group.

READER ACTIVITY

Can you think of potential research studies around maternity care in which it would be unethical to use random allocation? Make a list of the ideas that you have before reading on.

There are many reasons why random allocation may not be possible in maternity-related research. For example, it would not be ethical to allocate some women to a Caesarean section group or a normal birth group, as this would take away choice and could disadvantage them. Similarly, it would not be possible to randomly allocate women to a smoking or non-smoking group to examine the consequence of smoking on the foetus.

Where it is not possible to meet the strict conditions of experiments, the *quasi-experimental design* is an option. This looks very much like an experiment, often with an experimental and control group, and with the researcher introducing an intervention. However, it differs from a true experiment because instead of randomisation, participants are assigned to groups using a non-random method (Siedlecki, 2020).

An example would be women on one maternity ward having sessions on relaxation to measure its effect on stress or anxiety, and those on a second ward being used as a control and not receiving the relaxation. This makes management of the research easier, as all those in one setting will receive the same approach. It also reduces the risk of 'contamination', where individuals may be influenced by what they see happening to those alongside them.

Unfortunately, having all those in one setting receiving the intervention, rather than random allocation, will weaken the extent to which we have compared like with like. Differences between those in the two groups could make a difference to the outcome. In the relaxation example, it could be that some women already practice yoga or meditation, or there could be differences in personality or social circumstances between women on the two wards.

For this reason, quasi-experimental studies are not as persuasive as a true experimental design, as they contain many threats to internal validity (Flannelly et al., 2018; Maciejewski, 2020). It is possible to somewhat strengthen them by taking measurements of both groups prior to the intervention, so that we can see the extent to which they are similar and so accept them as reasonably comparable. In research terms, this approach of two non-randomised groups is referred to as *non-equivalent control group design*. The result is that the studies can best be described as level-two studies (Wood and Kerr, 2011), as they indicate correlation rather than cause and effect.

RETROSPECTIVE STUDIES

In quasi-experimental design, although randomisation is not achieved, the researcher still introduces an independent variable into the situation, exposing the experimental group to the intervention but not the control group. In some situations, not only is it difficult to carry out randomisation, but it can also be difficult to introduce the independent variable. In this situation, the solution is the use of a *retrospective* study. This term means that the difference between the two groups, in relation to the independent variable, has already happened and lies in the past. So, for instance, we might be interested in establishing whether going to antenatal classes has some impact on having a normal birth.

It would be difficult to construct a study and allocate women to the antenatal class attendance group and others to the antenatal class non-attendance group, as it would mean withholding access to facilities to some people who might want to attend classes and for whom they would be beneficial.

A retrospective study would collect data on women who had a normal birth and those that did not and try to establish if there was any pattern as to which group had the highest level of attendance at antenatal classes. In this design, we are looking for associations provided by correlation. This statistical process allows us to identify the extent to which factors seem to go together. Unfortunately, we cannot say that one causes the other, only that they appear to be linked. However, this may be satisfactory in providing the basis for midwifery action or increasing our ability to predict certain events. However, these studies can still play an important role in building evidence.

The strength of both quasi-experimental and retrospective design is their practical nature. They are far more feasible and, because they avoid some of the ethical issues of true experimental designs, are very attractive designs for midwifery research.

CONDUCTING RESEARCH

Experiments are not easy to carry out, so make sure it fits the research aim and then carefully follow the complex demands of this design. Where the purpose of your study is to establish a cause-and-effect relationship, an experimental approach is the method of choice. The key to planning an experimental design is to demonstrate the three aforementioned defining elements of an experiment, namely:

- Randomisation
- Manipulation
- Control

Perhaps one of the most important parts of the design is how random allocation will be managed. This must be done systematically to ensure that everyone has an equal chance of being in the experiment or control group. A major part of the credibility of the study will rest on a convincing management of this aspect.

At an early stage, the researcher must consider the ethical issues raised by an experimental study, particularly in relation to possible harm through an intervention or through withholding a known successful intervention. It is advisable to consult Chapter 8 on ethics to ensure that possible problem areas have been anticipated.

Previous research should be examined carefully, with special attention to design details. In particular, how did the researchers address the threats to internal and external validity? The literature should also provide clues as to the relevant independent variables to be included, and the additional variables that may confound the results (cloud the ability to say that the results have been produced by the independent variable(s) manipulated in the study).

What is the hypothesis that will guide your study design? This should be a clear statement that includes the dependent and independent variable(s). Will the hypothesis be directional and predict that the results of the experimental group will be higher or lower than the control group (referred to as a *one-tailed hypothesis*); non-directional and suggest there will be a difference without saying whether it will be higher or lower in a particular group (referred to as a *two-tailed hypothesis*, as the results could go either way); or a *null-hypothesis*, where it states there would be no difference between the two groups (see Chapter 7)?

Thought should be given to what information will need to be collected in order to test the hypothesis. This will have to be in a numeric form and will be subjected to a statistical test. There are a variety of tests, depending on the form of the experiment and the nature of the numeric values (see Chapter 13). It is at the early design stage that the necessary statistical procedures should be decided. It is recommended that help and advice is sought from someone who is knowledgeable in statistical techniques.

To reduce bias as much as possible, who will collect the data? In some instances, it may be feasible, as well as highly desirable, to have someone not directly involved with the design of the study collect data 'blind', that is, without knowing whether subjects are in the experimental or control group. At the design stage, the necessity and method of blinding the subjects should be considered to produce a 'double-blind', study. Remember that in midwifery, it is not always realistic to expect that those in the study will not know what intervention they have received.

Where several people are collecting data, steps should be taken to ensure they measure, code or collect the information in exactly the same way and with the same degree of accuracy (referred to as *inter-rater* or *inter-observer reliability*). This attention to consistency and accuracy should extend to any equipment used as part of the study or any materials, such as Likert scales or other forms of measurements.

The way the study is carried out must be carefully recorded in sufficient detail so that it can be replicated. A pilot study is essential to familiarise data collectors with the equipment and the procedure.

When conducting the main study, the safety and welfare of the subjects is paramount. This may lead to some individuals being removed from a study if there is any hint of personal danger.

At the end of an experimental study, it is important to base the conclusions only on the statistically tested results. This is not as daunting as it may seem, as most midwives who undertake qualitative research form close links with statisticians who can guide them through the process. For example, midwives undertaking experimental research as part of a masters or PhD programme may be offered support and training through the statistics department at the universities which they are studying. Midwife researchers need a basic working knowledge of statistical methods, but they are not expected to be experts in statistics. They can draw on the knowledge and skills of those who are. The statistical tests will indicate the strength of the relationship between the independent and dependent variables. However, there is always a margin of error in experimental studies. In addition, the sometimes-artificial circumstances and environment of an experiment can make generalisations to practice difficult.

Where it is not possible for practical or ethical reasons, to carry out a true experimental design, the next appropriate design such as quasi-experimental or retrospective designs may be used. The rigour is just as important in these designs as in experimental designs, if not more so. This is because they will be viewed as weaker than an experimental design. Clear attempts should therefore be made to reduce the possibility of the results being explained by factors other than the ones being suggested by the researcher.

All the designs in this section depend on a very clear statistical presentation of the results. It is this aspect of research reports that many midwives can find most demanding. For this reason, the midwifery researcher should explain the statistical procedures as clearly and simply as possible.

CRITIQUING RESEARCH

Critiquing experimental research can be challenging, often because of the reader's unfamiliarity with statistical presentation. Yet a little knowledge and understanding of some of the basic concepts and conventions can clarify the report significantly (see Chapter 13). The first stage is to ensure that the researcher is searching for a cause-and-effect relationship between an independent and a dependent variable. This will usually be evident from the wording of the aim that will suggest the influence of one variable on another. Usually, it will try to answer the question whether one treatment or action is 'more effective', than an alternative. Experimental research should contain a hypothesis, although, unfortunately, this is not present in all reports.

In examining the details of the conduct of the study, the three features of an experiment (*randomisation, manipulation* and *control)* should be present. If randomisation is not present, it is a quasi-experimental study.

Whether experimental or quasi-experimental, consideration should be given to the ethical component and whether the study was approved by an ethics committee. It should be clear to what extent did those in the study give their informed consent and has the avoidance of harm been addressed?

The sample included in the study should be scrutinised in relation to the inclusion and exclusion criteria for those selected for the study. Those in the sample should be typical of those in the larger group they represent. The method of randomisation should be examined to ensure that everyone had an equal chance of being selected for the experimental group. There will often be a diagram showing the flow of people into the different parts or 'arms', of the study and showing how many entered or left the study at different points. This allows you to follow the numbers involved right down to the start of the study and perhaps through to the end of the study period. It should be possible to make a close comparison of those in the final groups to ensure that they are comparable in those factors that might have made a difference to the results. Remember, they should be as similar as possible in all respects, apart from the exposure to the independent variable under investigation.

The researcher should give clear concept and operational definitions for the dependent and independent variables. These definitions should be considered for their adequacy. The intervention should be provided in a standardised way to everyone. Was there a check on this, such as training for those involved in providing the intervention, to ensure consistency? In particular, an assessment should be made of possible inaccuracies in the measurements made following the intervention. Have the issues of reliability and validity been addressed to your satisfaction? In particular, have they measured what they think has been measured? Was this a blind or double-blind study? Are details provided of how these were achieved? If there was no blinding, could this have had an effect on the results?

In the results section, has the researcher used a test of significance to test the probability that any differences between groups could have happened by chance? Here, the size of the p value is important. To what extent has the researcher taken into account the possible threats to internal and external validity? It is worth considering whether the results could be explained by some other factor besides the independent variable.

Depending on the results, what are the implications for practice? What specific recommendations are made in the report? Finally, are you satisfied with the rigour with which the researcher conducted the study? Did the researcher strive for excellence in the way the whole study was designed and carried out?

Above all, do not simply be impressed by the size of the study, its complexity, or the use of statistics. As with any kind of study, it is important that the research holds up to scrutiny. Consider the researcher's attempts to maintain accuracy, avoid bias and to be conscious of the limitations of their study. These will have implications for the extent to which you can generalise the results to your own clinical setting. With all clinical trials, it is wise to look for confirmation from replication studies before adopting a system that may have considerable implications for individual safety and quality of care.

REFLECTIVE PROMPT

Do you think that results from one experimental study would be sufficient evidence to instigate a change practice?

KEY POINTS

- Experimental research, particularly in the form of the RCT, are one of the most respected types of research in evidence-based practice. The reason for this relates to the way that the effectiveness of drugs and treatments have been rigorously tested to reduce the possibility of other explanations for the results.

- Experimental studies are dependent on the three necessary experimental elements of randomisation, control and manipulation. In midwifery, it is not always possible or desirable to achieve these elements. Sometimes it would be unethical or would drastically reduce women's choice or individual midwife's judgement as to what was best in the particular circumstances if strict experimental protocols were followed.

- There are alternatives to a full experimental design, such as quasi-experimental, retrospective and correlation designs. Although these do not produce conclusions that are as 'strong', as experimental designs, they can still inform evidence-based practice.

- Despite the status given to experimental designs, they do have limitations. It is not always possible to control for other factors that might explain the results. In addition, it is sometimes an oversimplification to look for one cause for a phenomenon; sometimes there are several.

- The power of this type of design depends on the use of statistical methods, particularly inferential statistics, which allow inferences to be made about populations based on the study samples. They are also concerned with the role of chance in explaining the difference in the results between groups.

- The effort needed to gain some statistical knowledge and understanding is well worth the reward of being able to read and critique published research, which uses this design. It also enables

midwife researchers to feel confident in using this research approach when appropriate.

REFERENCES

Barnett, A.G., Van Der Pols, J.C., Dobson, A.J., 2015. Correction to: regression to the mean: what it is and how to deal with it. Int. J. Epidemiol. 44 (5), 1748.

Campbell, D.T., Stanley, J.C., 1963. Experimental and Quasi-Experimental Designs for Research. Rand McNally, Chicago, IL.

Daley, A., Jolly, K., Jebbh, S.A., Roalfe, A., Mackilllop, L., Lewis, A., et al., 2019. Effectiveness of a behavioural intervention involving regular weighing and feedback by community midwives within routine antenatal care to prevent excessive gestational weight gain: POPS2 randomised controlled trial. BMJ Open 9 (9). https://doi.org/10.1136/bmjopen-2019-030174 e030174.

Daniel, K.M., 2019. Chapter 2: Introduction to quantitative research. In: Grove, S.K., Gray, J. (Eds.), Understanding Nursing Research: Building an Evidence-Based Practice, seventh ed. Elsevier, St. Louis.

Flannelly, K.J., Flannelly, L.T., Jankowski, K.R.B., 2018. Threats to the internal validity of experimental and quasi-experimental research in healthcare. J. Health Care Chaplain. 24 (3), 107–130. https://doi.org/10.1080/08854726.2017.1421019

Haseen, P., 2020. Crossover trials: what are they and what are their advantages and limitations? https://s4be.cochrane.org/blog/2020/09/07/crossover-trials-what-are-they-and-what-are-their-advantages-and-limitations/ (accessed 18 January 2022).

Maciejewski, M.L., 2020. Quasi-experimental design. Biostat. Epidemiol. 4 (1), 38–47. https://doi.org/10.1080/24709360.2018.1477468

Navarro, M.A., Siegel, J.T., 2018. Solomon four-group design. In: Frey, B.B., (ed). The SAGE Encyclopedia of Educational Research, Measurement, and Evaluation. SAGE Publications Inc. Thousand Oaks, CA. pp. 1553–1554.

O'Sullivan, G., Liu, B., Hart, D., Seed, P., Shennan, A., 2009. Effect of food intake during labour on obstetric outcome: randomised controlled trial. Br. Med. J. 338, b784. https://doi.org/10.1136/bmj.b784 Online.

Penić, A., Begić, D., Balajić, K., Kowalski, M., Marušić, A., Puljak, L., 2020. Definitions of blinding in randomised controlled trials of interventions published in high-impact anaesthesiology journals: a methodological study and survey of authors. BMJ Open 10 (4), e035168.

Polit, D.F., Beck, C.T., 2018. Study Guide for Essentials of Nursing Research Appraising Evidence for Nursing Practice, ninth ed. Walters Kluwer.

Siedlecki, S.L., 2020. Quasi-Experimental Research Designs. Clin. Nurse Spec. 34 (5), 198–202. https://doi.org/10.1097/NUR.0540

Singata, M., Tranmer, J., Gyte, G.M.L., 2013. Restricting oral fluid and food intake during labour. Cochrane Database Syst. Rev. 2013 (8), CD003930. https://doi.org/10.1002/14651858.CD003930.pub3 (accessed 18 January 2022).

Spiby, H., Munro, J. (Eds.), 2010. Evidence Based Midwifery: Applications in Context. Wiley-Blackwell, Chichester, UK.

Wood, M.J., Kerr, J.C., 2011. Basic Steps in Planning Nursing Research: From Question to Proposal, seventh ed. Jones and Bartlett, London.

STATISTICS IN RESEARCH

This is the chapter many readers of research or even researchers may be tempted to skip; however, do not pass on just yet. Understanding the way numbers are presented in research is one of the most important skills that will help readers of research make sense of research articles. It is also an essential chapter if researchers have to present quantitative findings in research or audit. To read research papers in greater depth, every midwife needs to understand some of the key statistical principles that will help in deciding in quantitative research whether the author's conclusions are justified. So, although it is easy to ignore the statistical sections in research, understanding them can have a direct effect on care. If midwives are to integrate evidence-based practice into their care, they must understand research and be able to interpret the data on which it is based (Harvey and Land, 2022).

READER ACTIVITY

Please find a quantitative research paper – what statistical tools do the researchers use to present its data and quantify the research findings?

The aim of this chapter is to explain just some of the common statistical ideas used in quantitative research, the basic principles underpinning them and how to interpret them.

COMMON ATTITUDES TO STATISTICS

Once quantitative researchers have gathered the data from their study, they are faced with transforming the raw results into some kind of order that can be understood. Any summary and presentation of the data will involve numbers and statistical processes, and this is where the problems can start. For many people, the way numbers are presented and the statistical techniques applied to the data creates problems, and this is the point at which some readers decide either to ignore the numbers or put down the article.

Why do statistics make so many people turn cold? Perhaps they remind the reader of unpleasant experiences in school where they felt lost or left behind. For some, the easiest way of coping with these feelings is to give up and pretend statistics do not matter. However, they do matter as statistics help us to identify interesting patterns in data that aid understanding of important clinical research.

This chapter explains just a small selection of some of the statistical procedures met in many research reports. Researchers do not have to learn how to carry out complicated calculations; there are specialised books and courses that will help them know this, and for those carrying out research, there are also people with this expertise to draw on.

If the very word 'statistics' is frightening, let us start by acknowledging that without statistics the results of any study would just be a chaotic jumble of numbers that would provide little meaning. Statistical processes bring order and understanding to all the information that has been collected (Sharples, 2018).

As with research in general, there are some unusual words and symbols to learn and some familiar words that have different meanings (see Table 13.1). One example is the word '*significant*'. This does not mean 'important', but suggests that the difference in the outcomes between two groups in, say, a randomised control trial (RCT), is unlikely to have happened by chance. In other words, the difference between the two groups is more likely to be explained by what the researcher did than by any other explanation. For this reason, when talking or writing about research, unless it is being used it in its statistical sense, it is better to avoid saying something is 'significant'. Similarly, the word '*data*' is plural, so the word '*are*' not '*is*' used, as well as expressions such as 'the data *were* calculated', not '*was*' calculated.

Finally, at the start of this chapter, a common misconception about statistics should be dismissed. It is not true to say '*anything can be proved with statistics*' – rather, some people can misuse them or ignore the rules that affect their use. This is where the reader must have some understanding of statistics in order to ascertain that the results support the conclusions being made. However, most research papers are based on a relatively small number of accepted procedures and assumptions. A reader of research needs to understand the basic principles underpinning its use and can 'read' the symbols and statements used by the researcher (see Table 13.1).

A SIMPLE DIFFERENCE

There are two major categories of statistics used in research: *descriptive* statistics and *inferential* statistics. Descriptive statistics use numbers to paint a picture of features or variables found in a sample as a way of summarising the data in a sample, e.g. measure of location and measure of spread, while inferential statistics are used to test a hypothesis, applying the findings from the sample to the wider population from which it was taken. Inferential statistics are an essential part of RCTs as they indicate the extent to which the intervention introduced by the researcher had an impact on the outcome. Inferential statistics also include the use of *correlation*; this indicates a pattern or association between variables, for example, in a survey. Each of these two categories of statistic are now examined.

DESCRIPTIVE STATISTICS

The aim of descriptive statistics is to summarise the data for a sample so it can be quantified, allowing us to compare groups, for example. Quantitative research is concerned with measuring a variable in a way that produces a numeric value. Some variables such as weight, time and amount of fluid lost have clear operational definitions in the form of standard units of measurement, such as kilograms, minutes and millilitres. For some attributes, such as the physical condition of a baby at birth, scales have been devised in the form of an Apgar score. Other elements such as satisfaction with the birth, or the amount of information received on screening procedures, may have to be turned into numeric values. This is achieved using approximate measures such as Likert scales, where individuals answer a number of statements using options such as 'strongly agree', or 'agree'. The researcher then gives each choice a number, such as:

Strongly agree	Agree	Undecided	Disagree	Strongly disagree
5	4	3	2	1

The basic principle behind all these procedures is to provide the researcher with some form of numeric measurement that can be processed statistically. From these

	TABLE 13.1	
	Common Statistical Symbols and Their Meaning	
Symbol	Meaning	Use
$\sum$	Greek symbol meaning add together what follows	As part of a formula providing instructions, e.g. $\sum x$, which means add together each value for the variable collected
$<$	Less than	Indicates set value, e.g. $P < .05$ means that the value of P is below or smaller than .05
$>$	Greater than	Indicates the opposite of the above as in $P > .05$, which means that the value is greater than .05 *NB: the open end of the symbol means greater than, and the closed end means less than reading from the left hand side of the symbol*
$\geq$	Equal to or greater than	To indicate a condition to be met during a calculation
$\pm$	Plus and minus the figure that follows	Used for example in standard deviation (sd) where the figure that follows the symbol is taken away from the mean and then added to the mean to give the range between which the majority of values in the data set will fall
χ^2	Symbol for the chi-squared test (pronounced 'ki-squared') as in kite	This test indicates the chances that any differences between the groups in the study could have happened by chance. The test is used with 'nominal data' (i.e. falling into one category or another, such as yes or no) and compares the actual results with what might have been expected if there was no difference between the groups
$P < .05$	Used as part of statistical tests to indicate the level of probability of being wrong if a real difference between the groups involved was assumed	This is the minimum level set for tests of significance to indicate that the results are unlikely to have happened purely by chance. Roughly, it means you would be wrong 5 times in 100 if you said there was a real difference between the groups involved. Other values showing a progressively more statistically significant result include $P < .01$ (1 in 100), and $P < .001$ (1 in a 1000)
NS	Not significant	This abbreviation suggests that there was not a statistical difference between the outcomes of an experimental and control group. Testing has failed to reach the level $P < .05$; therefore the study has failed to demonstrate a real difference between the groups concerned
r_s	The symbol for Spearman's rho (pronounced 'row')	Used to indicate a correlation between two variables measured at least at the ordinal level. The strength of this will be somewhere between $+1$ and -1
r	The symbol for the Pearson Product-moment (usually referred to as Pearson r)	The same as the above only this is used where both variables are measured at either interval or ratio level. This falls into the category of parametric statistics as it indicates features (parameters) of the population from which the sample is taken
t	The t-test symbol	This parametric test examines the difference in the means of two groups to see if they are statistically different. There are two versions, the t-test for independent samples, i.e. two different groups, and the t-test for matched or paired groups, i.e. the same group before and after an intervention
CI	Confidence Interval	This is an upper and lower figure between which the value measured in the sample is estimated to lie in the population as a whole

examples, it can be seen that some numbers express quantities that are more precise and exact, while others are a more general statement of quantity. Time and volume can be checked and agreed objectively as accurate. Other measurements are less precise and objective, for example, an estimation of blood loss or dilatation of the cervix. This is an important observation, as some researchers will claim a greater degree of objectivity and accuracy for their data than is possible. For some studies, numbers have been produced more as a convenience to allow statistical procedures to take place than as a precise measurement.

Levels of Measurement

These are equally as important to inferential statistics as which statistical tests can be used is partly determined by whether the data are categorical or scale (interval or ratio in the definition). All numbers look the same. It is possible to construct any combination of numbers using the numbers 0 to 9. In statistical theory, numbers are used to represent different ideas depending on the characteristics of the number. One simple, but very important categorisation, is the following four *levels of measurement*:

1. Nominal Level (or Categorical Level)

This is the most basic level. It places or 'nominates' a variable into a particular category that is mutually exclusive (it can only be put into one category) and uses a number as a label for that category. So midwives working only in the community may be categorised under the heading '1', midwives working only in the hospital setting could be categorised as '2', while those working in both might be '3'. This means that those in the category '1' are the same or equivalent; it does not mean that it takes two community midwives to make one hospital midwife; it just provides a label that happens to be a number, it is not a measurement of quantity. They could just as easily have been labelled using a letter of the alphabet, as in the case of blood groups, colours or anything else.

2. Ordinal Level

The data are categorical but the categories have an order to them, e.g. age groups. As they go up each level, the higher category has the characteristics of the level below but has extra, more advanced, qualities. So, numbers in this second group not only label a category but also indicate sequence or rank order. For example, arrivals at a

clinical area might be given the sequential numeric values 1, 2, 3, 4 to indicate the order in which they entered that area. This would indicate that number 3 was two behind number 1, and one ahead of number 4. However, the researcher cannot do much more with the numbers. They do not know how much later each person was behind the one in front. There may have been a split second between numbers 1 and 2 and several hours before number 3 entered and a day before number 4 entered.

The relevance of this category of measurement is that it takes the same form of the numbers used in a Likert scale or Apgar score. Although the parts of the scale can be labelled 1 to 5, as in the case of a Likert scale, there is no indication of the precise distance between each point. The distance between 'agree' and 'strongly agree', may not be the same as that between 'disagree' and 'strongly disagree'. All that can be said is that the numbers indicate sequence or rank order along a continuum.

Both nominal and ordinal levels of measurement form a single subcategory in the levels of measurement called *categorical data* – they put things in categories that are identified by a number. They both possess very basic properties that restrict the statistical procedures that can be carried out on them. However, it depends on the statistical procedures to allow the researcher to have a dependent variable that is categorical. These are non-parametric tests, e.g. chi-squares test and therefore less statistically powerful than parametric tests. The researcher can still get descriptive statistics from categorical data, e.g. percentage of people choosing a particular option on a Likert scale. The next two categories are far more sophisticated and provide more useful information.

3. Interval Level

This level produces numbers that allocate units to a category, indicate sequence, but this time, the distances between the different points are the same. This means that they can be 'averaged', and have other procedures carried out on them. Along with the next category, the interval level indicates 'true numbers' that measure amounts and does not simply use numbers as a label.

4. Ratio Level

This is the final, and highest, level of measurement. It is very much like the interval level except for one crucial factor, and that is there is an absolute zero point in the measurement scale below which it is impossible to record a value. For example, temperature readings in Fahrenheit or centigrade are interval level because it is possible to have a minus figure, such as minus five degrees centigrade. This is because zero in Fahrenheit and centigrade are arbitrary points, not an absolute zero. Height, age and weight are all ratio level as it is impossible to have less than a zero amount of any of them.

The importance of the last two levels of measurement is that they quantify something, and they are always measured in units of some kind, such as kilograms, hours, minutes, and centimetres. It is this property that makes them suitable for statistical procedures in that the other levels of nominal and ordinal do not measure the quantity of anything but simply categorise by using numbers to label the categories or in the case of ordinal data by placing them in sequence. For this reason, the interval and ratio levels are classed as numeric levels and the nominal and ordinal levels are seen as categorical levels. The key characteristics of these four levels of measurement are summarised in Table 13.2.

Space has been devoted to the explanation of these levels as many of the principles of statistical analysis are based on this categorisation system; therefore, their importance to understanding statistics should not be underestimated. In the next section, the problem of making descriptive statistics meaningful to the reader is explored.

Summarising Descriptive Data: Measures of Central Tendency

Analysing the results of a study can be one of the most exciting parts of a study for the researcher, but this can be one of the most challenging aspects for the reader of a research report. Yet, the reason for processing data is to make them easier to understand. It is no use presenting results in terms of each person's answers to a questionnaire or physical assessment expressed in the numeric values for each answer, as in the following:

It would mean very little, as it is not clear what the numbers relate to, and there is no pattern visible that makes sense between the two respondents. The answer is to use summary statistics that allow us to convey meaning by summarising quite large collections of

TABLE 13.2		
Properties and Characteristics of Each Level of Measurement		
Level	Properties	Characteristics
Nominal	Most basic of all	Names, categorises variables
Ordinal	Basic non-measurement	Numbers used to categorise into sequence or 'rank order'
Interval	Measures properties of variable	Equal distance between units; no absolute zero
		Sophisticated statistical procedures possible
Ratio	Highest level	Absolute zero, equal distance between units
		Suited to sophisticated statistical procedures

numbers. This is the aim of descriptive statistics, summarising the data for a sample so it can be quantified.

An important form of summary statistic is the *measure of central tendency*. This is a clumsy way of saying the number that appears typical in the group, or the number that represents the central value found in the entire collection of a frequency distribution. If this sounds like the 'average', this would be right, but in statistics, there are a number of different ways of calculating 'the average', each known by a different name.

Mean

This is what is commonly call the 'average'. For instance, it may be referred to as *'on average, I take half an hour to get home from work'*, or that *'on average, people watch television for four hours a day'*. It does not mean that the figure is exact; sometimes it may be more, while sometimes it may be less; but when things even out, it is reasonably typical.

It is not difficult to calculate the 'average' or 'mean' of something. If a researcher had to work out the average length of time that 10 members of staff in the clinical area had been qualified, researchers would ask each one how long they had been qualified, add them all together and divide by the total number of people.

Respondent A:	21	2	29	17	2	55	34	23	7	81	64	34	3	29	46	50
Respondent B:	18	37	4	21	31	8	30	15	1	2	57	41	75	4	7	47

Easy! To write down that process so others could repeat it, the statistician would symbolise each stage to produce the following formula:

$$\frac{\sum X}{N}$$

The symbols translate as:

$\sum$ = Add together each of the following

X = The numeric value of the item the researcher is interested in from each person

— = The sign for 'divide by' used in a fraction

N = The total number in the group.

The formula looks baffling but understanding the symbols and the sequence in which to carry out the procedures makes it clearer. This is how even the most complicated formulae work; each symbol is translated into an instruction that is carried out in a set sequence.

The mean can only be calculated if the level of data is either interval or ratio, that is, where the numbers reach a numeric level of measurement and are actually measuring something in recognisable units of quantity. It does not work for categorical data such as calculating the average star sign of people in a group where Aquarius = 1, Pisces = 2, etc. Neither does it really work with ordinal data, although the reader will see an average figure for Likert scale values calculated.

There is one big drawback in using the mean, and that is it is influenced by untypical numbers that are much higher or much lower than the majority of other numbers in the group or 'data set'. These more extreme values are called 'outliers' because when individual results are plotted on a graph, they are the ones that stand out because they are out of line with the main results. The result would be an untypical value of what is typical in the group and can sometimes mislead the mean for a group of results because there may be a small number of untypical results pulling the mean up or down. This is illustrated in Box 13.1.

Median

The median is a useful calculation of central tendency, as it is not influenced by extreme values. The median is calculated by taking every single figure in the set of numbers, such as length of second stage of labour for 20 women. They are all then put in rank order from the smallest to the biggest. The median is the value of the unit in the middle of this row or *distribution* of numbers.

Let's take an example to illustrate the advantage of the median over the mean. Imagine nine children have been booked for a birthday party at a restaurant. Unfortunately, the only information the restaurant has to prepare for the type of party is the name of the person who made the booking. They need to know whether to provide a children's jelly and blancmange type party or a fairly wild alcoholic affair. The solution is to telephone and ask for the average (mean) age of those attending.

If the set of ages (values) in line a) in Box 13.1 were used to supply the mean, the figure communicated would be 8.6 or, corrected up to the nearest whole figure, 9 years. The median could be calculated once each item in the data set had been put in rank order from the smallest to the biggest (which has already been done) by identifying the 'middle' value. This would be the fifth number, as there would be four numbers on either side of it. In this example, the median would also be 9 years.

Now what if the two 11-year-olds felt they were too old for such a 'childish' celebration and decided to back out, leaving Grandma and her twin sister Elsie, both 72, to accompany the children instead? If the restaurant rang up this time to be told the average age in the party was 22.2, or 22 to the nearest whole figure, they may lay on a very alcoholic adult type of birthday party. However, if they had asked for the median, the value would have still been 9 because it is the position

---

BOX 13.1
AGES OF THOSE ATTENDING A PARTY

a) *Ages of a group of children going to a birthday party:*
   6 6 8 8 **9 9** 10 11 11
   median = 9/mean = 8.6

b) *Ages of children plus Grandma and her twin sister Elsie going to a birthday party:*
   6 6 8 8 **9 9** 10 72 72
   median = 9/mean = 22.2
   NB: The median is a more stable calculation, as outliers (untypical large or small figures) do not influence it; the mean is influenced by outliers and can produce an unrepresentative figure.

in the rank order that is used to calculate the answer, not the combined values.

How is the median calculated where there is an even number of items in the data set, as in the set below?

6 6 8 8 9 9 10 11

The answer is to first identify the midpoint again. This time it would be a line drawn between 8 and 9, as there would be four values on each side of the line. Simply adding the values of the numbers on either side of the line together and dividing by two would produce the median of 8.5 (8 + 9 = 17 ÷ 2 = 8.5) years. In other words, it is the mean of the combined values of the numbers on either side of the line that splits the ranked sequence of numbers into two halves.

A good way of remembering what is achieved through calculating the median is that it provides a cut-off point along a ranked order of numbers so that half of all the values are below that cut-off point; the median value, and the remaining half are above it.

One disadvantage of the median is that it could only uses a couple of numbers to calculate and can provide an 'average' value that is not contained in the data set. It also becomes very unwieldy to calculate if there is a very large set of values in the data set, as each one has to be placed in rank order to locate the middle value. However, knowing both the mean and the median will give the reader insight into whether there are outliers in the distribution. The closer the two values are together, the less likely there are to be outliers affecting the mean.

Mode

The final method of calculating an average is the mode. This is the most frequently appearing value in the data set. Returning to the set of values in (b) in Box 13.1 and adjusting it slightly to make it the following:

c) Adjusted distribution of ages:
6 6 6 8 8 9 9 10 72 72

The mode would be 6, as that is the number that appears the greatest number of times. However, if there were three 6-year-olds and three 9-year-olds, then there would be two modes, 6 and 9. This is referred to as a *bimodal distribution*. Just to complicate things,

if there had been three 8-year-olds as well as three 6-year-olds and three 9-year-olds, it would have been *multimodal*.

This is not a very useful way of saying what is typical in the group, as the mode can change drastically as a result of one number that can shift the mode anywhere in the distribution. This can be confirmed by taking c) above and changing the first and last digit as follows:

d) Final adjustment of ages:
6 6 8 8 9 9 10 72 72 72

The mode has now swung from one end of the line to the other end by just changing two numbers. This illustrates the point that each statistical calculation has its own special characteristics, and it is necessary to know something about these in order to know when they can be misleading. When painting a picture of what is typical in a group of results (or data set), or what is around the middle value, the researcher has to be very careful which method of calculation they choose, as they can alter the result radically by using a different calculation. The mode can be useful for categorical data and if the data are words (qualitative), e.g. favourite pet of a group of 5-year-olds.

The Standard Deviation

This is a measure of spread, i.e. a measure of the variability in a data set. It is very much linked to the measure of central tendency and is a way of quantifying how well the measure of central tendency represents the data. The final statistical method in this section allows us to go back to the mean and make it more useful by using the mean in combination with the *standard deviation*.

The standard deviation (abbreviated to 'sd') is a measurement derived by working out the average distance of each item in a data set from the mean. If the height of 30 women was measured, the mean might be 1.62 m. The standard deviation, when calculated to establish the mean distance of each woman's height from the overall mean, might work out at 8 cm. The value of the standard deviation is then added to the mean (1.62 m + 8 cm) to give 1.70 m as an upper value and is then taken away from the mean (1.62 m − 8 cm) to give 1.54 m as a lower value. Where there is an even pattern in the variable concerned (explained in the following section under the heading 'normal distribution'), the majority of people (around 68%) will lie in this range between the mean and plus and minus one standard deviation (± 1 sd).

The smaller the standard deviation in relation to the mean, the closer all the values will be to the mean. This would suggest that the mean is reasonably typical of the values in the group. The larger the standard deviation, the more spread out the values will be, as there will be a large variation between the values above and below the mean (the mean plus and minus the standard deviation). In this case, this indicates that the mean is not very helpful in gaining an idea of what is typical in the group.

The standard deviation is also used to identify if the attributes of those in two groups, for example in an RCT, are closely matched, or whether they are different, and if so, how different. This is achieved by comparing the mean and standard deviation in the two groups. The researcher would not expect the results to be identical but would want to feel they were reasonably close and that any discrepancies did not suggest clinically significant variations that might make a difference to the interpretation of the results. Standard deviation cannot be used with a median as it is calculated using the deviation of each point from the mean value. Researchers use an interquartile range as a measure of spread in combination with the median.

Normal Distribution

In looking at the way individual values are spread around the mean, there is one particular pattern they can take that is important to the statistician, and this is called the *normal distribution*. Normal distribution is a theoretical concept that has a major influence on a number of important statistical decisions, including those in inferential statistics, discussed below. It relates to interval and ratio data and can be outlined as follows. If the frequency distribution of characteristics such as height or blood pressure from a large number of people was plotted on a graph, they would form a very distinctive shape. This is because in a large sample the numbers of very tall people and the numbers of very short people appear in about the same ratio with the majority of people being fairly close to the mean height. The curve on the graph would look like the outline of a church bell, where the majority of people

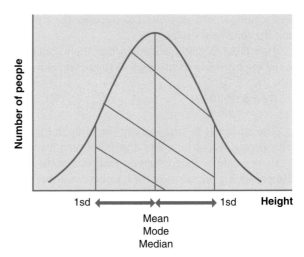

Fig. 13.1 ■ Normal distribution curve.

would be in the mid-section and the slope of the curve of the bell shape would come down to the small number of people, on either side of the majority, who were either very tall or very short (see Fig. 13.1).

The distinctive characteristic of such distribution is that the mean, mode and median would all hit the same value. This would appear on a graph as one line passing from the very apex of the bell (the tallest point on the curve) to the baseline of the graph. The shape is said to be symmetrical, in that if the shape was cut out of the page on which it appeared and folded down the midline formed by the mean, each side would touch perfectly like a mirror image, without any overlaps.

This kind of a shape has a mathematical property whereby if one standard deviation on either side of this midline was measured, then the area under the curve inside the lines formed by the upper and lower standard deviation points would include the values from about 68% of all the individuals in the study. This is a constant result for all variables that have a normal distribution.

The usefulness of this is that if a variable is reasonably normally distributed and if the mean was known, by calculating the standard deviation and working out one standard deviation above and below the mean, it can be assured that the majority of people in the sample (68%) will measure somewhere between this upper and lower level of measurement. This can be extended to two standard deviations (± 2 sd) to give an upper and lower level between which about 95% of all the values will fall. However, most studies use one standard deviation to give a picture of the majority of measurements.

It is worth ending by saying that this idea of a normal distribution is part of statistical theory. Distributions in reality rarely exactly fit the normal distribution. Nevertheless, it is taken as providing a reasonably useful guide to producing meaningful statistical interpretations of results.

Presentation of Descriptive Results

Having looked at some of the basic principles of descriptive statistics, it is important to look at common diagrammatical ways of presenting results and how readers and researchers can make sense of them. Although researchers describe the results in words in the main body or text of their report, they frequently use some visual displays to help the reader 'see' the results. This visual presentation can take a number of forms, as shown in Table 13.4. These can include summary tables, which present the major numerical findings, and graphical figures such as bar charts, histograms, pie charts and line graphs.

Each of these can convey complex information more efficiently than words because of the visual representation of a large amount of numbers. An examination of a visual display also allows the reader to observe the overall pattern or trend of the results, which is more difficult to understand when presented in the form of words. However, the researcher must choose the right format for the information, and the reader must understand the principles and shorthand used by the writer. Any form of visual display must also be presented in such a way that they do not mislead the reader in interpreting the results (Walters and Freeman, 2010).

Although Table 13.3 outlines a range of common data presentation forms, for many people reading research reports, the tables, charts and diagrams can become like holes in the page; they do not really exist. It is necessary for readers of research and researchers understand how to read tables and diagrams. The next section is an attempt to overcome this with the help of some guidelines.

How to Read Tables?

Tables form the most popular choice for presenting numeric data in research as they allow the results of a variety of variables to be presented side by side to give a clear overview. In this way, the purpose of a table is

TABLE 13.3
Common Data Presentation Forms

Type	Description
Tables	Labelled columns and rows of numbers. Can take the form of frequency tables, where just one variable is examined, or cross-tabulations where two or more variables are shown. One variable can then be displayed in terms of another variable (intention to breast feed or formula feed by parity).
Bar Charts	A block diagram used to show amounts of a discrete (cannot be broken down into smaller units) variable, such as male/female. The blocks, or 'bars', do not touch. They can be shown in a vertical format or horizontal format. They can be 'stacked' bar charts, where each bar totals 100% and is divided within its length into subgroups by proportion.
Histograms	As above, but shows a continuous (can be broken down into smaller units of measurement) variable. The blocks will touch to show they are on a continuous scale.
Pie Charts	This is a circle divided into appropriate 'slices' to show the quantity of different categories. The result must add up to 100%. These work well when there are between three and six slices providing the majority of slices are not too 'thin'.
Line Graphs	Lines that join points plotted on a graph to show trends in the data.

to create a kind of numeric photograph of a situation from a distance but at the same time allow the reader to zoom in to close-up by examining particular squares, or 'cells', in the table (Denscombe, 2011).

Tables come in two different kinds: a *frequency table* and a *cross-tabulation* or *contingency* table. A frequency table looks at how often (frequently) categories of one variable occurred in the data. For example, Table 13.4 illustrates a frequency table for age of a sample of women in a survey.

The second type of table takes the frequency table and looks for possible patterns by introducing another variable, such as parity, so that the first variable is broken down into another variable. This is called a *cross-tabulation* or *contingency table*, where one factor is 'contingent', that is, conditional or dependent, on another. An illustration of this type of table is shown in

Table 13.5 where parity is cross-tabulated with age in a second survey of women.

When reading a table, the first task is to examine the layout and headings. Start by reading the following and look at a cross-tabulation from an article at the same time. Start by establishing from the title what the table represents. Is there just one variable, which would indicate a frequency table, or is it a cross-tabulation with two or more variables? This will help anticipate what kind of a pattern it may contain. Then, look at the columns and rows. Each should be clearly labelled at the top of the columns and to the left of the rows. This helps to 'read' the table in terms of what the numbers 'stand for' or represent.

A useful starting point for exploring a summary table is to look down each column for the highest numbers to get a feel for which item or category was the largest. Ask yourself, 'Is that what I would have expected?' How close in value are the other items to the highest? Again, is that what could have expected,

or is this an unexpected, clinically relevant finding? Also, consider the reverse of this by identifying which categories have the smallest values. Could it have anticipated that or is it unusual? Look too at the relative size or pattern in the values of all the numbers. This will give some idea of the rank order of the items in terms of which is the highest, the next highest, and so on. Some tables may present the order of the rows in rank order as part of the format. Do these numbers go down gradually in size, or are there some items with large values followed by a sudden drop down to the next value? This will tell if there is some consistency in the distribution, or whether most responses fell into a small number of categories that were mentioned by, or typical of, most people in the study.

Where there are a number of columns in the table, it is useful to make comparisons across each item indicated by the row headings to see if the value of the number in each column is similar or different. If different, are the differences small or large? Once patterns are starting to emerge amongst the results, ask the following questions:

- What does this suggest?
- Is this what would be expected or not?
- So what?

This type of reflection and analysis will provide opinions about the findings and how they relate to the study aim. What could be the 'story' or explanation behind the findings? Answers can then be compared with the researcher's comments on each table. Examine the tables and then read the researcher's comments rather than simply accepting what is said unquestioningly.

TABLE 13.4		
Example of a Frequency Table		
Age Group	Number	Percentage
<18	23	10.3
18 – 21	47	21.2
22 – 26	53	23.9
27 – 30	42	18.9
31 – 34	35	15.8
>35	22	9.9
Total	**222**	**100**

TABLE 13.5				
Example of a Cross-Tabulation Table				
	Primigravida		Multigravida	
Age Group	Number	Percentage	Number	Percentage
<18	32	17.5	2	1.0
18 – 21	40	21.9	31	15.3
22 – 26	42	23.0	47	23.1
27 – 30	34	18.5	54	26.6
31 – 34	23	12.6	40	19.7
>35	12	6.5	29	14.3
Total	183	100	203	100

These points are also useful when constructing tables. The first point is to establish if the information will be easier to communicate in the form of a summary table. If the answer is 'yes', then the researcher will need to identify how much information is needed to put in each table. Avoid overloading the reader with too much information. However, sometimes it is easier to compare two situations, such as Caesarean section rate between primigravida and multigravida women by putting them in the same table to make comparisons and contrasts more evident.

Tables From Randomised Control Trials

Where the table represents the results from an RCT, there are certain conventions the researcher should observe. These include which variables are shown as columns or rows. The convention is that column headings are used to display the independent variable, and the row headings indicate the dependent variable. The purpose is to allow the researcher to see any patterns in the data.

To help answer the question of what the table shows, the researcher will indicate if they have used inferential statistics on the table and what was found. This is indicated either underneath the table or as a column in the table, where the researcher should indicate the statistical test used, the result, and the '*P*' value, which indicates whether the differences could have happened purely by chance (see Chapter 12).

Making Sense of Bar Charts and Pie Charts

Although tables provide an overall view of data and allow readers to zoom in on specific parts, it is important to be able to interpret and keep track of a lot of ideas at once. This means it is necessary to be able to visualise differences in size between quantities. Bar charts, histograms and pie charts are different, as they provide instant visual comparisons.

Bar charts contain a series of rectangles or 'blocks' presented either vertically or horizontally and represent the values or scores for a number of categories. They are an ideal way of highlighting comparisons between variables. This can be between two or more variables where the height or length of the bars will draw attention to differences between them. Good bar charts are presented in size order from the largest down to the smallest. This helps the eye and brain follow the relative differences in size easier.

Histograms are used for one variable to look at the frequency distribution of the continuous data being interpreted and can also be used to see if the data are normally distributed, as the histogram will be bell shaped if it is. They are similar in appearance to bar charts, but each block touches those on either side of them as the data they represent are on a continuous scale ranging from zero upwards. In most bar charts, the order of the blocks does not matter, as they are separate (discrete) items and could be reordered without changing the meaning, for example reasons given for giving up breastfeeding (McDonald et al., 2010). These are separate categories and could be moved around depending on the numbers choosing each category. In histograms, this would be impossible, as with variables such as height, weight, or number of weeks' breastfeeding, the order of the blocks cannot be rearranged without destroying the natural sequence.

Making sense of bar charts, and histograms, is a matter of comparison between blocks and establishing the overall pattern on display. The essential question to answer is: 'How does this relate to the research aim?' Is the pattern important to the research, and is it clinically relevant? In examining such charts, look carefully at the size of the scale used, as the author or publishers can make a small difference between two outcomes seem quite large merely by making the scale of the diagram bigger. It is always wise, therefore, to consider the question: 'Is the difference really remarkable, or does the scale of the figure exaggerate the relative differences?'

Pie charts are another common form of graphic presentation of results. A pie chart is a circle 'sliced-up' to represent the relative proportion of each of the categories in a response. Pie charts work well with nominal or categorical levels of measurement, where all the items added together make up a total of 100% (so people cannot choose or fall into more than one category). Although these are really helpful to compare one variable in proportion to another as part of the whole, they do not work well once the number of 'slices' exceeds five (Walters and Freeman, 2010).

Line graphs are often used to display change over time – it is portrayed as a series of data points connected by straight line segments on two axes. It encourages the reviewer to ascertain the relationship between two sets of values. Line graphs are drawn so that the independent data are on the horizontal x-axis (e.g. time) and the dependent data are on the vertical y-axis. They are useful in that they show data variables and trends very clearly and can help to make predictions about the results of data not yet recorded, as seen regularly as a way to present Covid information during the pandemic (BBC, 2022).

All the data presentation methods described in this section serve the same purpose, that is, to convey the results of data analysis quickly, clearly and meaningfully. The problem for the researcher is to show the results in a way that is easily assimilated by the reader and makes the interpretation of the data clear and interesting. When reading research reports, all forms of presenting the data should be carefully examined and not overlooked; remember, 'every picture tells a story'.

INFERENTIAL STATISTICS

So far, this chapter has considered descriptive statistics in depth and mentioned inferential statistics only in passing. This last category is more complex than the previous one, and so, as the aim of this book is to act as an introduction to key ideas in research, this section will be somewhat restricted, and simplified. More in-depth details can be gained from some of the many statistical texts available or statistics chapters in more advanced research books.

In simple terms, inferential statistics are used in two main ways. The first use is to estimate the probability that characteristics found in a sample accurately reflect those that may exist in the population as a whole. This will be returned to this in Chapter 14 on sampling; here, the point is that one of the basic assumptions of inferential statistics is that the sample has been drawn using probability sampling methods. This means the sample was chosen in such a way as to ensure it is reasonably representative of the larger group. If this has been achieved, then the sample should be found in a similar pattern in the larger population from which they have been drawn. The use of inferential statistics allows the researcher to indicate the probability that this match is true, within reasonable limits known as a confidence interval (CI). This is similar to the use of standard deviation, which is used in its construction, and gives upper and lower limits between which the attribute or variable might lie within in the larger population.

The second main use of inferential statistics is to help the researcher decide if the results of an experiment support the hypothesis that there is a difference between the experimental and control groups. This is achieved by being able to take an alternative hypothesis, i.e. that if there is a difference between the experimental and control groups it is more likely to be due to the intervention rather than simply due to chance or some other explanation. This is known as the alternative hypothesis as statistical tests examine the null hypothesis that suggests that any differences between the experimental and control groups, for example, are due to chance. This seems a very complicated procedure, but one that follows statistical logic and conventions. The hesitant language is due to the difficulty of designing the perfect and conclusive research study. Statistical procedures allow us to provide some reassurance to support conclusions from well-designed experimental studies.

There are two types of inferential statistics: *parametric* and *non-parametric tests*. Parametric tests relate to the existence of real differences between experimental and control groups or the likelihood of characteristics in the sample being found in the wider population. However, they require a number of strict conditions to be met before they can be used. These include the following:

- The level of measurement applied to the variable must be interval or ratio (this is why understanding the levels of measurement is important).
- The distribution (spread) of the variable must be close to a normal distribution (spread evenly on either side of the mean to form a bell-shaped curve if plotted on a graph).
- The spread of the measurements should be uniformly close to the mean and not include a large number of 'outliers' – this condition is referred to as 'homogeneity of variance.'

Despite these guidelines, the rules are sometimes broken on the assumption that these constraints are open to a certain amount of leeway. The advice for the novice, however, is that where there is any doubt about the features of the data, use non-parametric tests. For each parametric test, there is a non-parametric equivalent so that the same calculation can be made; however, the strength of the relationship indicated by the test may be different.

A further distinction can be made regarding inferential statistics that can be divided into two main categories: first, those that seek to establish a consistent pattern or *correlation* between two variables, and second, *tests of significance*, and the latter of which are used to support or reject hypotheses.

Correlation

'Caution: correlation does not indicate cause'
(Denscombe, 2011: 259)

This statistical calculation explores the relationship between two variables collected from each person or item in a sample (e.g. width of pelvis and length of labour) and attempts to assess if they are related. It is important to stress it does not attempt to say that one causes the other, only that some kind of pattern or association exists between them. Correlation is an attempt to answer the question to what extent are two variables related to each other in terms of *strength* – how closely are they related, and *direction* – whether they are positively related, that is, do measurements of both variables go up together or down together, or whether they are negatively related, that is, as one variable goes up the other goes down.

The strength of the relationship in correlation is measured by a *correlation coefficient*. This is a single number that is the product of a calculation that provides a measure of how closely the two variables are related. The correlation coefficient is measured on a scale between plus one (+1), which is a perfect *positive* correlation, and minus one (−1), a perfect *negative* correlation. When the calculation reveals that there is no relationship between two variables, the coefficient (the number that indicates the strength of the relationship) will be zero. In other words, this is a scale that looks something like Fig. 13.2.

An illustration will clarify the way in which all correlations lie somewhere on the line in Fig. 13.2. A perfect positive correlation between personal income and an individual's expenditure on clothes would mean that a 10% increase in income would result in an extra 10% increase in the amount spent on clothes. In the case of a negative correlation, it would mean that as measurements of one variable go up, for instance cost of travelling by train per kilometre, there would be a corresponding decrease in the number of rail passengers. A perfect negative correlation of −1 would be indicated when a 14% increase in the cost of rail fares per kilometre would result in a 14% drop in the number of passengers. If a researcher wants to predict a value of y based on a given value of x then researchers use a *regression*. The regression model is a statistical procedure that allows a researcher to estimate the linear, or straight line, relationship that relates two or more variables. This linear relationship summarises the amount of change in one variable that is associated with the change in another variable or variables. Regression can also be tested for statistical significance to test whether the observed linear relationship could have emerged by chance or not.

The important point about correlation is that it measures *similarities*, whereas tests of significance, which are used in RCTs, measure *differences*. This is a key principle in understanding the different purposes of these two statistical techniques. The usefulness of knowing a correlation exists is that it allows us to plan or make broad predictions that will be reasonably accurate depending on the strength of the correlation. So, for instance, it is known that there is a reasonably strong positive relationship between social class and the number of mothers who breastfeed. This means that if geographical areas are compared using a scale of social class, it can be expected that the demand for

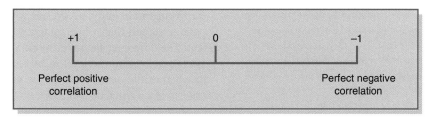

Fig. 13.2 ■ Scale used to indicate correlation coefficient.

support for breastfeeding will be higher in those areas with a higher social class distribution. This kind of information is crucial in planning modern health care delivery.

As there is rarely a perfect correlation between variables, a strong relationship will be anything from a value of 0.5 up to 0.8. A medium relationship will be around 0.3 to 0.4. A strong negative relationship, where the value of one variable goes up while another measure goes down, would be from −0.5 to −0.8. A useful checklist of correlation levels and their meanings is shown in Table 13.6.

Calculating Correlation

There are two main methods of calculating correlation depending on the type of data being examined. Where one of the variables is measured using an ordinal level of measurement, such as a Likert scale, or similar scale such as an Apgar score, where the precise difference between points on a scale is not known, then Spearman's rho (pronounced 'row') is used. This is indicated by the symbol r_s. If the measurements for both variables in a correlation are at interval or ratio level and if they comply to a number of other stringent criteria, then a more accurate method called the Pearson product moment, usually referred to as Pearson r (or sometimes more informally as Pearson's r) is used.

Both measures use the same scale of between +1 and −1 to show the strength of the relationship between the two sets of measurements. Although Pearson r is a more accurate measurement, the nature

TABLE 13.6
Interpreting Correlation

Where the correlation coefficient is:

0.9 to +1	A very strong to perfect positive correlation
0.5 up to 0.8	A good to strong positive relationship
0.3 or 0.4	A reasonable positive relationship
0 to 0.2	No to little evidence of a positive relationship
0 to −0.2	No to little evidence of a negative or inverse relationship
−0.3 or −0.4	A reasonable negative or inverse relationship
−0.5 to −0.8	A good to strong negative or inverse relationship
−0.9 to −1	A very strong to perfect negative or inverse correlation

of the measurements used in midwifery means that Spearman's rho may be more common.

Multiple Regression

Before leaving correlation, it is worth mentioning a natural development of the technique, which is multiple regression. Whereas correlation works on the relationship between two variables, multiple regression takes the same idea but extends it to take into account at the same time a larger number of interval or ratio variables that might be related to a particular outcome. Technically, a researcher could include categorical variables in a multiple regression, but if there were more than two groups, then this is quite a complicated procedure that involves making dummy variables.

Tests of Significance

Tests of significance are crucial in clinical trials where researchers attempt to demonstrate that the intervention they introduced (the independent or predictor variable) had an effect on a dependent variable (outcome). In choosing a test of significance, researchers must ensure that the requirements for using the test are met by the data collected. Tests of significance can be either parametric or non-parametric. As indicated earlier, parametric tests provide the greatest degree of accuracy. A favourable statistical result using a parametric test indicates an important finding. However, the stringent conditions relating to the level of measurement and distribution of the data within the sample must be fulfilled before they can be accepted with confidence.

The conditions for using non-parametric tests are a lot easier to meet, and they can be used with much smaller data sets compared to parametric tests, but the degree of accuracy is less certain. Non-parametric tests tend to be less statistically powerful as they are less able to detect marginal but real differences between groups. In other words, the chances of being wrong in saying that real differences have been found between the groups in a study are greater when using a non-parametric test than when using a parametric equivalent. The difference between the data that can be used is again related to the level of measurement and also to whether the distribution of the variable meets the criteria of a normal distribution.

Some of the commonly encountered tests of significance are outlined in Table 13.7. Further details of these can be found in many of the statistics and research texts.

CONDUCTING RESEARCH

One of the inevitable demands on the quantitative researcher is to demonstrate an understanding of statistical techniques and the ability to use the right tests for the data collected. The method of analysis has to be considered at the design stage. As each item in the tool of data collection is chosen, the researcher should consider the level of measurement that will be required. The basic principle is to collect data at the highest level practical, for example, specific age should be collected rather than grouped data (ordinal) or even nominal level, e.g. below 21, or 21 to 25, unless it is known for sure that calculations such as mean, median or standard deviation will not be required. Collecting data at the highest level ensures a greater choice in data presentation and analysis and greater accuracy of the results.

Consulting other researchers' findings is helpful in deciding how to present information, such as in the form of a table or other visual display. Consider whether some variables need to be cross-tabulated with other items of information. It may be useful to construct 'dummy' tables at this point to explore the different ways data might be displayed. Decide which variables will be shown as columns and which in rows as well as the direction in which percentages will be calculated (row percentages or column percentages). The appropriate statistical calculations or tests can also be written alongside the dummy tables to remind the researcher at a later stage.

The level of measurement will influence the options available for presentation, especially where graphical presentations are concerned. So, for instance, nominal- and ordinal-level data can be shown as a table but are often clearer as a bar chart or pie chart. Interval- and ratio-level data can be displayed as a histogram, but not as a bar chart, as they are suitable for continuous data. Line graphs can also be used for interval and ratio data.

At the data input stage, the data from the raw questionnaires, observation checklists, etc. are entered on the computer. Quality control of data inputting should be built into the process, especially where more than

TABLE 13.7
Common Statistical Tests and Procedures

Name of Test	Type	Description
t-test Independent t-test Dependent t-test	Parametric test used on interval and ratio data.	The independent t-test is used to compare the means of two separate groups. The dependent t-test measures two means in the same group, using a 'before and after/pre-test post-test' design.
Mann–Whitney U test	Non-parametric equivalent of the t-test.	Used to compare the means of two groups with ordinal data, where data are not normally distributed.
Wilcoxon test	The non-parametric equivalent of the dependent t-test.	Used where scores are in pairs, such as pre-test post-test design, but where data are not normally distributed.
Chi-squared test (χ^2)	Non-parametric test The simple χ^2 uses nominal data, the complex χ^2 is used where there are three or more sets of data.	Looks at whether the difference between two groups was as expected. Are the groups the same or different? Applies to nominal or ordinal data.
Pearson coefficient (Pearson r)	Parametric test that establishes the relationship between two interval or ratio variables.	The size of the relationship is indicated on a scale between +1 and −1. Strong relationships are usually around 0.5 – 0.8 positive or negative.
Spearman's coefficient Spearman's rho ('row') r	This is the non-parametric version of the above and is used with nominal or ordinal data.	As above.

one person is involved in entering the data. The random checking of data entered is worthwhile to confirm the accuracy and pick up errors. Unfortunately, there is nothing similar to a spell checker to pick up errors in typing numbers; they all have to be checked against the originals.

One of the first tasks of the data analysis stage is to summarise the data ready for statistical processing. Summarising can be as simple as counting how many times options were chosen or occurred in a frequency distribution. This is carried out on the characteristics of the sample, such as age, parity, grade of staff, or whatever sample characteristics have been collected. At the planning stage, the grouping or banding of some data might need to take place, so, for instance, lengths of time or age may be grouped (remembering the points made earlier on levels of measurement). The size of the bandings can be determined from previous research, but it is worth noting that too small a banding can lead to information overload and hide broader patterns; too large a banding will lose the sensitivity of some data in highlighting differences amongst smaller groupings. It is good practice to determine the descriptive statistics before doing any inferential statistics.

One major error to avoid in grouping categories is overlapping the groups. Taking the example of age, there is no point in having one group 20 to 25 and then the next group 25 to 30, as 25 appears twice. It should be 20 to 25 then 26 to 30 and so on.

Once the data have been processed they can be selectively turned into visual displays. Most computers are now capable of producing tables and, through spreadsheet programmes such as Excel, can present their content in a number of appropriate forms such as bar charts and pie charts. As with other aspects of the research process, it is important to pay attention to detail. Look at this aspect of the research as a crucial part of getting key points across. Unless the statistical elements in the research have been carried out professionally and to a high standard, the credibility of the results will suffer.

CRITIQUING RESEARCH

The purpose of this chapter has been to help the reader become more familiar with a small number of the basic ideas behind statistical analysis and forms of data presentation. These are most commonly encountered in the results sections of research papers or presentations. The immediate reaction of many people confronted by statistics is to panic. This is an emotional response that can be controlled. The information in this chapter has hopefully helped the reader to realise there is a logic and order to statistics that can be appreciated and understood, and it is not necessary to know it all.

When faced with a quantitative research paper, the first thing to do is to look very carefully at the labels attached to the tables and figures. What do they show? Then look at how this information is presented to you, and begin to read the story it reveals. Look at tables or figures and ask yourself, 'Are these descriptive or inferential statistics?' If they are descriptive, then examine the size of categories. How big was the study, is there a pattern to the frequencies across the categories (which categories have the biggest numbers attached to them, which have the smallest)? Would the size of these have been anticipated? Look at the relative size between the categories. Is there a slow step down in size or are there one or two large categories, and then a big drop in size before the next categories?

Whether it is a table or diagram, is it clear to read and see what is going on? What does it suggest to you? Are there questions raised as a result of the pattern being presented? Where inferential statistics are used, look in or below the table, where there should be additional information such as the tests that have been carried out and the 'P' values that have been produced. This may even be in the methods sections under 'statistical analysis', or where the results are described. What does the size of these values suggest to you? The closer the 'P' value is to 1, the more likely the null hypothesis is to be correct and there is no difference between groups or variables; the closer it is to zero (starting from a value of $P < .05$ and getting smaller) the more likely the alternative hypothesis of a real difference between the groups produced by the independent variable is to be true.

In the case of an RCT, has the author demonstrated statistically that the groups were comparable to start? If not, is there anything about the differences that could play a part in interpreting the results? Similarly, in the case of an RCT, could the numbers dropping out of any of the groups have made a difference to the meaningful comparisons between the groups?

Once the figures and tables have been scrutinised for meaning, read through the text to see what the writer makes of all this. Do they talk through the tables and point out things that may not have been noticed, or explained what the results suggested to them? Where the data raised questions, do the authors answer those questions for you? Where there are unfamiliar statistical elements or things that may have been forgotten, check them out in this chapter or in a more advanced statistics reference book. Depending on where the article is published, the reader may feel questions such as whether the authors have used appropriate statistical procedures or tests should have been established by the journal.

Do not ignore tables and figures. Do try and get something out of them. Each time a reader of research does this thorough analysis, they will learn a little bit more, and become more relaxed about reading the statistical elements in a study.

READER ACTIVITY

Please find a quantitative research paper outlining an RCT:
- Do you understand the statistics presented in the paper?
- Are the statistics presented correctly?
- Do they support the findings of the study?

KEY POINTS

- Collecting quantitative data means that statistical processes will be involved in the analysis stage. Understanding the principles behind these processes is important in correctly interpreting the findings of research.
- Research findings are presented following certain conventions and use presentation methods such as tables, bar charts, line graphs, histograms and pie charts. Every picture tells a story, so these should never be overlooked.
- Statistics fall into two main categories of descriptive and inferential. Users of research need to know the principles and assumptions on which these are based as well as those relating to parametric and non-parametric tests.
- The level of measurement of the data will influence many of the decisions made in the research process. An understanding of these levels is crucial to understanding why certain decisions are made in the choice of statistical techniques
- The type of data, e.g. is it scale or categorical, is really important when deciding what statistical test should be used.
- Although the jargon and symbols used in statistics may look intimidating, in reality, a basic understanding is not difficult to achieve. Competency in understanding basic statistical principles is essential to applying research to evidence-based practice.

REFERENCES

BBC News., 2022. Covid-19 in the UK: How many coronavirus cases are there in my area https://www.bbc.co.uk/news/uk-51768274.

Denscombe, M., 2011. The Good Research Guide for Small-Scale Social Research Projects, fourth ed. Open University Press McGraw-Hill Education, Maidenhead, Berkshire.

Harvey, M., Land, L., 2022. Research Methods for Nurses and Midwives: theory and practice, second ed. Sage Publishers, London.

McDonald, S.J., Henderson, J.J., Faulkner, S., Evans, S.F., Hagan, R., 2010. Effect of an extended midwifery postnatal support programme on the duration of breast feeding: a randomised controlled trial. Midwifery, 26 (1), pp. 88–100.

Sharples, L., 2018. The Role of Statistics in the Era of Big Data: Electronic Health Records for Healthcare Research. Stat. Prob. Lett. 136, 105–110. https://doi.org/10.1016/j.spl.2018.02.044

Walters, S., Freeman, J., 2010. Descriptive analysis of quantitative data. In: Gerrish, K., Lacey, A. (Eds.), The Research Process in Nursing, sixth ed. Wiley-Blackwell, Chichester.

14

SAMPLING METHODS

CHAPTER OUTLINE

WHY SAMPLE?

Sampling is important because it is rarely possible to collect information from an entire group. For example, we cannot send a questionnaire to every pregnant woman in Britain as many would have given birth before we found out who should be included. It can also be extremely expensive to gather information from a total group, and it may not always be that much more accurate than a well-selected sample. The solution is to select a sample from the population in such a way that the process creates the minimum of bias and represents the characteristics of those in the population as closely as possible. A biased sample would consist of people, events or things that were very different from those in the total group. Suppose that the aim of a study was to understand women's infant feeding intentions during pregnancy. Imagine that just for convenience, a group of pregnant midwives were selected as the study sample and are asked how they intended feeding their baby. This would be a biased sample as it would not be representative of the target population. We would expect there to be a difference between this sample and the total population of pregnant women. This would make conclusions and practice decisions based on the results unreliable. They can only be generalised if the sample has been selected to exclude or minimise bias.

The outcome of any research project is dependent on both the reliability and validity of the data collection method used and the type and quality of the sample on which the results are based. Sampling is an area of research that contains a number of specialised words and ideas that require attention. In this chapter, the issues relating to who or what is included in the sample, and the alternative methods for choosing the sample, known as sampling strategies, will be examined.

It is useful to clarify the difference between a 'population' and 'sample' as these are two common terms used in sampling. There is a clear difference between them. The population is the total group of people, things or events the researcher is interested in saying something about, e.g. midwives who have a higher degree or women who have a home birth. The sample is a section of those from the population who are accessed to provide data to answer the study question or aim. The main issue is to select the sample so that they resemble the *target population* closely enough to provide similar results to those that would have been produced by the wider group. The method of selecting the sample is a key methodological issue in research. This selection method is called the *sampling strategy* and describes the process of choosing individuals, events or behaviours for participation in a study. There are a number of ways of arriving at a sample. The choice will vary depending on whether the research approach is:

- Experimental
- Survey
- Qualitative

The choice of sampling strategy will be influenced by how far the researcher wants to generalise, that is, apply the findings to the wider population. The more important it is to achieve a close fit between the sample and the population, the more complex the sampling strategy used. Whatever the purpose of the study, the researcher is faced with three vital questions:

- *Who* or what will make up the sample?
- *How* will they be chosen?
- *How many* will be chosen?

The remainder of the chapter will illustrate the way in which these questions are answered.

INCLUSION/EXCLUSION CRITERIA

Before we select our sample we need to define our target population accurately. This is achieved by specifying *inclusion* and *exclusion criteria*. Inclusion criteria are the characteristics we want those in our sample to possess. Examples of inclusion criteria would be women who have a normal vaginal birth at term, or women in certain age groups with no complications of pregnancy. In other words, it is the characteristics they *must* possess to allow them to stand for the general group we want to say something about.

Exclusion criteria consist of those characteristics we do not want those in our sample to possess because it may make them untypical and so bias the results. There may be other reasons for excluding some people from a study, such as the risk of harm for those with a certain medical condition or characteristics.

The researcher must consider the inclusion and exclusion criteria at the planning stage, as these will form part of the detail put into a *research proposal* or outline of an intended piece of research. These details will also be included in any final report and allow the reader to consider whether the criteria could lead to some limitations in applying the results to other groups. Clear examples of inclusion and exclusion criteria are found in randomised control trials (RCTs) that are very sensitive to bias.

So, for example, the following inclusion and exclusion criteria appear in a published RCT by Ayerle et al. (2018), which looked at the effects of the birthing room environment on vaginal births and other outcomes:

Inclusion Criteria: Primiparae and multiparae of all ages with a singleton pregnancy in cephalic presentation, between 37 + 0 weeks to 41 + 6 weeks pregnant on admission to the OU, in active first stage and intending to have a VB are eligible to participate in the study. Pregnant minors will be included if their legal guardian agrees with their participation.

Exclusion Criteria: Pregnant women will be excluded if they are in the active second stage, want a water birth or have limited ability to understand essential oral and written information about the trial. Women will also be excluded if an evidence-based risk exists for the woman or her baby, i.e. pathological cardiotocography on admission (based on the International Federation of Gynaecology and Obstetrics's FIGO score), if it is an emergency admission or if there is an indication for CS according to the clinical guidelines of the UK's 'National Institute for Health and Care Excellence.'

In the presented example, note how specific the criteria are and how clear definitions are used.

SAMPLING METHODS

Different research approaches will require different sampling methods, although some methods can be used in a variety of approaches. In any situation, the researcher must try to draw the sample in such a way as to:

- Reduce sampling bias
- Increase representativeness

Sampling bias refers to the systematic enrolment of participants who either overrepresent or underrepresent a subgroup or segment of the population, and it is a weakness in study design (Knechel, 2019). Where sampling bias is avoided, or minimised, there is a greater chance that the results can be applied to situations other than the one in which the data were gathered. In other words, it is easier to generalise from the results.

Bias is reduced if the researcher can increase the representativeness of those chosen for the sample. They should match the population they represent as closely as possible in the ways that might influence the outcome of the study. This would include variables such as parity, social class, age, ethnicity and education level. The researcher should establish the distribution of such variables in the population and then demonstrate statistically that the sample does not differ significantly from the total group in the possession of those characteristics.

Table 14.1 outlines the main sampling strategies linked to the various broad research approaches, as there are some clear differences in sampling methods and sample sizes between quantitative and qualitative approaches.

EXPERIMENTAL SAMPLING APPROACHES

As we saw in Chapter 12, experiments play a key role in establishing the presence of cause-and-effect relationships between variables. To achieve this, sampling must be carried out in a very meticulous way so that an accurate conclusion can be deduced from the results. The method of sampling is drawn from a number of options grouped under the heading of random sampling methods. These options form what are called probability sampling methods. Using this approach, every unit in the population, whether it is people, things or events, should have an equal chance of being selected. If this criterion is achieved, it means that some of the more sophisticated statistical tests can be applied to the results. These allow the accuracy of statements made about the results to be calculated. Some examples of sampling methods in experimental design are:

- Simple random sample
- Stratified sample
- Proportionate sampling

TABLE 14.1
Sampling Method by Broad Research Approach

Research Approach	Sampling Method
Experimental	Simple random Stratified sampling Proportionate random
Quasi-experimental and ex post facto	Comparative groups Systematic random
Survey	Simple random Stratified random Proportionate random Systematic random Opportunity/convenience/accidental Quota
Qualitative	Purposive Opportunity/convenience/ accidental Snowball/network/chain/ nominated Theoretical

Simple Random Sample

In random sampling, a sample is selected randomly but it does not mean that this is a haphazard, casual or indiscriminate way of selecting people for a study.

One essential distinction is between a *random sample* and *random allocation*. In a random sample, those eligible to be included in the study are identified from the larger population and are selected for inclusion in the research. This does not mean they have agreed to be included in the study or that they will willingly take part. In the view of some researchers, findings can only be generalised if random sampling has taken place.

Random allocation is frequently used in health service experimental research; it is the system by which individuals who have agreed to take part in a study are allocated to either the experimental or control group so that there is minimum bias surrounding who ends up in which group. There is no guarantee that those who agree to take part in a random allocation research project are similar to the wider population. In fact, those who agree to take part in research may be very different from the general population.

In order to achieve a random sample, the researcher must have a complete list, or *sampling frame*, of all those who could be accessed to take part in the study, that is, the *study population*. Fig. 14.1 depicts the relationship between the study population – the sampling frame and the sample. A sampling frame can be defined as a list of the study population who meet the inclusion and exclusion criteria of the study. The study population should naturally mirror the target population as closely as possible. So women who have had a previous caesarean section may be the target population, and those who have had a previous caesarean section in one local maternity unit in the last 5 years will be the study population. Once the frame is constructed, individuals are consecutively given a number to identify them for the purposes of sample selection. Individuals are then randomly selected for inclusion in the study, or not. This can be done in a number of different ways. One way is to use a specially constructed table of random numbers. Another is to use a list of computer-generated random numbers or software that is designed to support random allocation. Whichever way it is done, the people in the sampling frame should be allocated into the intervention group or the control/placebo group at

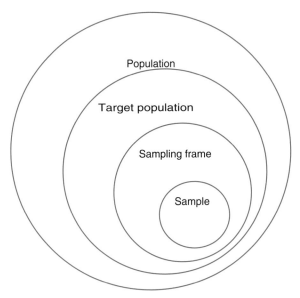

Fig. 14.1 ■ Diagram depicting the sample in relation to the population.

random. In an RCT where a sampling frame cannot be constructed, for example, if people were to be selected for a prospective study as they entered the system, say at a booking clinic, the researcher might use sealed envelopes. So if the researcher wished to use two groups of 25 women, the following method could be set up:

A pack of envelopes would be numbered from 1 to 50. In those envelopes whose number corresponded with 1 of the 25 numbers drawn from the random table, there would be a slip of paper in the envelope saying 'Group A' that would indicate the experimental group. All the other envelopes would have a slip indicating 'Group B' that would be the control group. The envelopes would then be placed in number sequence from 1 to 50. As each person who had agreed to take part entered the study, the researcher would open the next envelope in sequence and follow the instructions. As long as the researcher was not involved in setting up the envelopes, the use of 'A' or 'B' would 'blind' both the participant and the researcher to which group the individual had been allocated (see Chapter 12 for more on blinding in experimental studies).

Stratified Sample

The basic principle of a simple random sample is that everyone has an equal chance of being allocated to either the experimental or control group. There are cases, however, where this method may result in an over-representation of certain characteristics in one of the groups. So, for instance, it could still just turn out that the experimental group has mainly primigravida women and the control group mainly multigravida women, and this may have a distorting effect on the outcome measure, as labour for primigravid and multigravid women can be different.

To avoid this, the researcher can first stratify the sample into parity and then sample each parity group appropriately. In the case of a prospective experimental design, the researcher could use numbered envelopes for each parity group. Once it is established whether the individual agreeing to take part in the study is primigravida or multigravida, the next envelope in the appropriate pile is opened. This way there should be an even spread of each parity group in both the experimental and control group. This can be done for many characteristics like age group, socioeconomic status or ethnicity.

Proportionate Sampling

This is a type of stratified sampling in which the number of participants are selected in proportion to their occurrence in the population. So, with the example of parity, it might be considered important that each experimental and control group reflects the proportion of primigravida to multigravida women. So for example, if there were a proportion of 60% multigravida and 40% primigravida women birthing in a particular clinical area, then a proportional sample would provide a sample with the same ratio.

QUASI-EXPERIMENTAL AND RETROSPECTIVE DESIGNS

Chapter 12 discussed a number of alternatives to RCTs, such as quasi-experimental and retrospective designs. Quasi-experimental designs are used where it is not possible, usually for reasons such as ethical difficulties or practical constraints, to randomly allocate people to experimental and control groups. In these circumstances, groups already formed are used. Examples would be women on two different wards, or couples attending two different locations for antenatal education. One location is used for the experimental group,

and the other for the control group, and the results from both groups are compared.

READER ACTIVITY

Can you identify any weaknesses with this type of allocation?

There may be important differences between the groups that may influence the outcome following an experimental intervention. Although this is a fundamental sampling weakness, in many cases, this choice of design is the only one available. In these circumstances, the researcher will attempt to illustrate the comparability between the two groups by identifying and describing key demographic characteristics, such as age, parity, socioeconomic status.

As there is an unequal difference in the chance of people ending up in the experimental as opposed to the control group (everyone on one ward would have a 100% chance and those on the comparison or control ward would have 0% chance), this is known as a non-probability sampling method. This is not as accurate a means of detecting true differences between groups as a probability sampling method, and for this reason, non-probability sampling methods are less respected than probability methods. However, a non-probability sampling method has the advantage of being practical and often the best that can be done under the circumstances.

Retrospective studies, also discussed in Chapter 12, are very similar to the quasi-experimental approach in the sampling methods used. Because the retrospective study examines people or situations after they have happened, the formation of groups will have already taken place before the start of the study. The researcher cannot introduce a variable, but searches for groups or individuals who share a common identity or characteristic, such as smoking, mode of birth or infant feeding behaviour such as deciding to breastfeed. Again, this is a non-probability method, and we cannot generalise the findings to other situations with the same confidence as we can with probability sampling methods.

SURVEY METHODS

Although experimental designs are important to support evidence-based practice, a far more frequently used approach to research in midwifery is that of the survey. Here, some of the sampling methods already mentioned can be used and fall into both the probability and non-probability sampling methods.

Simple Random Sampling

Surveys are very powerful where they are based on a simple random sample. Here, everyone from the study population has an equal chance of being included in the survey. The method has been described under experiments, where a sampling frame containing everyone fitting the inclusion criteria is constructed; a table of random numbers or computer software is then used to pick out the appropriate number of individuals for inclusion in the survey.

The advantage of using this method is that it is possible to make generalisations concerning the wider population on the basis of a random sample. This is because it falls into the category of probability sampling methods. One disadvantage of this method, however, is the difficulty of constructing a suitable sampling frame where there are a large number of eligible individuals in the target population or where no list of likely individuals exists.

Stratified Sampling

The process of simple random sampling in surveys can be refined further by dividing those eligible to be included in the sample into appropriate strata and then sampling from within each of the groups created. Examples of this would include grouping women by parity, or in the case of midwives, grade, or length of experience.

The advantage of a stratified sample is that it ensures that those from relevant subgroups are included in the study. The disadvantages include the difficulty of predicting which subgroups might make a difference to the outcome and then the problem of dividing the sampling frame into those characteristics. For instance, if it was thought that women with high self-esteem were more likely to breastfeed in relation to those with medium or low self-esteem, it would be difficult first to divide the target group into strata by level of self-confidence without the prior use of a scale measuring self-esteem.

Proportionate Sampling

Proportionate sampling is a type of stratified sampling, and, as with experimental approaches, in a sur-

vey, there would be an attempt to construct subgroups within the sample that were similar in proportion to the broader population. The aim would be to ensure that an unrepresentative proportion in one group did not produce a biased result. An example would be a survey of midwives' views on a particular aspect of midwifery. To ensure that the influence of the midwife's grade was kept constant, the population would first be stratified according to grade; then, the numbers selected from each group would mirror the proportion of each grade in the population. Again, this example would use a sampling frame and table of random numbers, or computer-generated random numbers. The advantage of this approach is a greater chance of accuracy and reduction in bias. The problems are similar to stratified sampling, and that is the difficulty of having prior knowledge of the size and location of some of the subgroups.

Systematic Sampling

In some surveys where individuals or objects are being selected for inclusion from a very large study population, systematic sampling is used in order to gain elements across the entire population. This is achieved by numbering all those who fit the inclusion criteria and then using a table of random numbers. The first number is selected randomly, and then the subsequent individuals would be selected following a predetermined frequency, such as every 5th, 10th or, with very long lists, every, 20th, 50th or even 100th person or object.

The *sampling interval*, that is, the distance between each unit in the sample, can be determined by first deciding on the total number required in the sample and then dividing that into the total number in the group. An example would be a questionnaire given to a sample of women who had delivered in a particular unit over a 1-year period. If it was decided that the sample size required should be 100, and there were 3000 deliveries, then $3000 \div 100 = 30$. Therefore, the sampling interval would be every 30th person. However, remember that in survey studies the response rate may be low (see Chapter 9), and this will need to be considered when planning sample size.

Cluster Sampling

Cluster sampling is a multistage approach in which clusters of participants that represent the target population are identified. It is used for two reasons (Grove and Gray, 2019):

1. To obtain a geographically dispersed sample that is manageable (in clusters) rather than completely spread across the country, or in the case of international research, across the world.
2. Where the individual elements making up a population are unknown a multistage cluster sampling approach can be used.

Imagine a national survey of the opinions of general practitioners (GPs) regarding how they perceived the role of the midwife in providing care for women in the community. A sampling frame of all GPs would be a tall order; instead, the researchers may first produce a sampling frame of all health regions within Britain, and randomly select, say, a sample of 10 regions. For each region, they could then construct a sampling frame of districts. From this, a total of three districts from each area might be chosen. The final sampling frame might be a list of all GP practices within the districts randomly chosen. From this, a final total of 20 GP practices could be randomly chosen and every GPs in those practices sent questionnaires.

It is clear from this example why it is called *multistage sampling*. At each stage, a sampling frame is constructed, and a simple random sample selected. Each level consists of the construction of the next sampling frame until the size of the units is manageable, at which point everyone in the group is included. The advantage of this system is that it can achieve an accessible sample from an almost impossible total population. This reduces costs, as those included are found close together, making access and communication easier and also making a probability method possible where a sampling frame with each person listed is not realistic. The disadvantage is that the number of layers to the sampling process increases the danger of not arriving at a truly representative sample.

Convenience/Opportunity/Accidental Sampling

These three terms are often used to describe the same approach to sampling where the researcher includes in the study those people to whom they have easy access, and who happen to be in the right place at the right time. Here, the researcher selects the most easily accessible people from the population. This is the method used by market researchers where people are stopped in the street and asked to answer questions. It is this method that people frequently mistake for a random sample.

Along with the next two following methods described, this approach falls into the category of a non-probability sampling method, as everyone does not have the same chance of being included. There is no way of knowing whether those in this type of sample are representative of the larger group. The ability to generalise from the findings is consequently restricted. Nevertheless, these approaches continue to be very popular because they are very pragmatic in gaining quick and easy access to a sample and provide an indication of possible responses to questions.

Examples of convenience samples might be women attending a particular antenatal clinic on a certain day, or midwives attending a study day who might be asked their opinions on some midwifery issue. The relevance of terms such as convenience or opportunity can be clearly seen from these examples.

One further example of a convenience sample is the self-selecting sample, who are people who volunteer to take part in a study, for example, by returning a questionnaire or responding to a poster or advertisement to take part in a survey. Examples can be found in both magazines and professional journals. With this method, there is little the researcher can do to ensure that those returning questionnaires are typical and so there is always the possibility of bias.

In summary, the advantage of the convenience sampling approach is that it is simple, cheap, and quick and does not require the construction of elaborate sampling frames. The main disadvantage is sampling bias, in that those who happen to be around a particular location or in one particular group may not be typical of the wider population they represent. The same is true for those who self-select themselves into a survey because this will not necessarily produce a sample that is representative of the target population, as some segments of the population are likely to be systematically under-represented.

Quota Sampling

This method is a refinement of convenience sampling and attempts to produce a sample that is similar in certain key characteristics to the total population. The market researcher will use quota sampling by selecting so many people in certain age groups or occupation groups in order to argue that the sample is 'similar in structure' to the total population. In midwifery, there may be a similar attempt to include quotas such as so many women who are primigravida and so many multigravida, or in various age groups, or have experienced certain types of labour.

In many respects, quota sampling is similar in purpose to stratified sampling, but it differs from a stratified sample in that the participants are not randomly selected from each strata. The advantage of quota sampling is that the researcher is in a stronger position to say that because the sample is similar to the total population, then the results may be reasonably representative. The disadvantages are similar to stratified sampling, in that there is an assumption that the subgroupings that may make a difference to the results are already known and that the size of each of the groups is also known so that the size of the quotas can be calculated. It also depends on the information that allocates respondents to either one quota or another being easily ascertained from potential respondents.

Surveys, then, can be based on a variety of sampling methods. Some of these will result in statistical precision where probability sampling methods have been used. Where these are employed, reasonably large samples may be sought and chosen from the wider population using random sampling approaches based on accurate sampling frames. The aim of this kind of survey is to be able to generalise the results to the wider population. Other approaches based on non-probability sampling methods are less precise but a lot easier to conduct. Although it is difficult to judge their accuracy, they can provide useful 'snapshots' of situations that can be used as the basis for action.

QUALITATIVE APPROACHES

As qualitative research differs in so many respects from quantitative research, it is no surprise that the approach to sampling is also different. Because the aim is not to achieve a large representative sample from which generalisations can be made, sampling is not based on probability methods. The aim is rather to gather information from people who can provide inside information on specific kinds of experiences or who are part of a particular culture or subgroup. In terms of inclusion criteria, the most important factor is that they have knowledge or experience of the topic or phenomenon under examination. Those who are part of a qualitative study do not 'stand for' the larger population, in the same way as in quantitative research; they are included on the basis that they are members of an appropriate group. However, there is an attempt in many studies to get a cross-section of representative people.

The main choices of sampling methods in qualitative research include:

- Purposive
- Convenience
- Snowball/network/chain/nominated sample
- Theoretical

Purposive Sampling

Purposive sampling, also known as *judgemental sampling*, involves the researcher handpicking those in the sample on the basis of the researcher's knowledge of characteristics they know the individual possesses. It can also refer to the location or setting of the study. Although this seems likely to result in a biased sample, its aim is to achieve the opposite by ensuring that a range of opinions or experiences is included.

The advantages of this method are that the sample is known to possess key characteristics that should be included in the survey; it is very practical and efficient in terms of time and money. The disadvantage is clearly that we are dependent on the researcher's judgement, which cannot be checked.

Convenience Sample

Just as the purposive sample provides the researcher with relevant information, so the convenience sample within qualitative research is relevant as long as those at hand have the necessary information or experience relevant to the purpose of the study. The convenience sample can be used in both phenomenological studies and ethnographic research where the researcher draws on the experiences and activities of those who just happen to be in the setting being observed or under study. The appropriateness of this method again illustrates the flexibility in this approach to data collection.

Snowball Sampling (Also Called Network, Chain or Nominated Sampling)

All of these terms describe the situation where the researcher identifies individuals with the necessary characteristics or experiences and then asks them to suggest others who may be willing to participate in the study. This kind of sampling method is used where the researcher finds it difficult to identify useful informants. The advantage of this method is that 'nominated' contacts tend to have characteristics in common, and therefore, it is a good way to collect a sample of people who share the characteristic under study. It is particularly useful in recruiting participants from socially devalued populations and the hard-to-reach (Grove and Gray, 2019). This may include those individuals who cannot be easily contacted due to homelessness or because they do not own a phone or computer. It may also include those who hide characteristics for fear that an undesirable label may be attached to them, e.g. mothers who take illegal drugs. In many of these cases, sampling frames just do not exist.

In a study by Feeley and Thompson in 2016 on why women choose to freebirth, a combination of purposive and snowballing was used to find their sample participants. They used purposive sampling via social media freebirth support groups and then a snowball technique was used in that they asked participants to forward the study information to anyone else who matched the inclusion criteria.

It is clear to see why these methods were appropriate and effective in reaching women who had chosen to birth outside the conventional systems and therefore midwives and other healthcare professionals were unlikely to be able to identify or reach. However, there is potential for bias with this sampling procedure, as subjects are not independent of each other. Another potential weakness is that the method may still miss those who are isolated from a social network and therefore such views may be missing from the data and consequently unable to contribute to developing the evidence.

Theoretical Sampling

Theoretical sampling is frequently used in grounded theory (see Chapter 4) as a way of selecting the sample and as a way of guiding the decision to stop data gathering. This is based on the principle that those in the sample can provide examples and insights into the concepts or theoretical issues that underpin the study. This helps to determine who will be included in the sample and if further individuals may help shed light on the issues pursued and contribute to completing the theory being developed. Codes are generated from the rich data to develop theories and concepts. Data collection continues until no new insights are gained, and there is a repetition of information already gained (Grove and Gray, 2019). This is called *theoretical saturation*. At this point, data collection can stop and no further participants are required.

SAMPLE SIZE

One of the most difficult tasks for the researcher at the planning stage is to estimate how many people, things or events are going to be included in the sample. As the type of study, to a large extent, influences the size of a sample, it is useful to consider the question of size under each of the headings already used in this chapter.

Experimental Designs

As experimental designs are concerned with accuracy, there are some statistical guidelines the researcher can use in choosing a suitable sample size. The important factor is the size of the difference the researcher is looking for between the results of the experimental group and the control group before it can be said that an intervention has been successful. Unfortunately, for many conditions or situations, the difference between one group and another when measured on physiological outcomes may be quite small. This would mean that for differences to appear, the study would have to include quite a large number of people before that difference was clearly visible and statistically relevant. This is why, in medical research, the size of the sample can run into hundreds and sometimes even thousands.

The statistical procedure of *power analysis* should be used to estimate the total size of the sample needed given an anticipated difference in the results between two groups. *Power* in this context means the ability of a study to detect differences in a population that actually exist (Grove and Gray, 2019). Therefore, the assumptions and mathematical calculations involved will provide an estimate of how many participants will be required in a study. The results of power analysis calculations should be included within the information on sample size. In an RCT by Maycock et al. (2015) that aimed to evaluate the effect of three breastfeeding promotion interventions aimed at male partners, they described how they decided on a sample size as follows:

> 'It is assumed that at 26 weeks, there is at least a 10% difference in the proportion of mothers' breastfeeding between any two of the groups. A sample size of 300 participants (fathers) is required in each of the 3 intervention groups and control group to be able to detect the difference at 80% power and 5% level of significance, using a Log-rank survival test. Assuming a loss to follow-up of 25% in each group, a total of 400 participants for each group will be recruited (Total n recruited = 1600 couples, total n required = 1200)'.

The concept of 80% power in the example presented means that the number of participants has been calculated to detect an 80% chance of the test having significant results. Midwife researchers need not fear the statistical terminology and techniques described. It is perfectly acceptable to seek support from statisticians to carry out such calculations. An awareness of the need for power calculations and some basic understanding of the process is useful when reading about sample size in experimental studies, but a midwife is not expected to be an expert on this statistical method. Moreover, in midwifery, the number of experimental studies is relatively small, and some of those undertaken can be quite modest in sample size. In many studies, practical considerations such as time and resources play a big part in dictating the size of experimental groups. Closely examining the literature for the size of previous studies can be a great help to the researcher in estimating possible sample size. It is important to think consider both the total number of people admitted to a trial and the size of the subgroups used in the analysis of the results. Where the sample is divided into different subgroups such as parity or age, the size of the groups can be quite small, even though at the start the overall sample might have been quite large.

One problem in experimental designs is the dropout rate from the study. This is referred to as *sample mortality* or *attrition*. Although the size of the sample can seem large to start, if the study is carried out over a long time period, or consists of several periods of testing and data collection, there can be a number of people who leave the study. This can have consequences where there is a larger proportion dropping out of one of the groups, as it can lead to an imbalance in the characteristics of the experimental and control group members so that they may no longer be comparable. The best the researcher can do is to try to make the size of the groups as large as is practical and to ensure that the size is reasonably in line with any previous research.

Surveys

The optimum sample size in surveys is variable, as it relates to the size of the total population. In surveys where the aim is to be able to generalise quite accurately to the total population, the sample size might be in the hundreds, but in other studies, where the total population itself is quite small, such as the number of male midwives, the sample is also likely to be small. In choosing the sample size, the larger the sample the better is generally advocated (Glasper and Rees, 2017). This is on the grounds that the larger the sample, the more representative it is likely to be. However, there is also agreement that a large sample does not compensate for poor sampling methods. The ultimate criterion for assessing is the extent to which those include are clearly representative of the target sample group. In other words, the researcher should be concerned with the quality of the sampling method and the extent to which it avoids bias rather than simply including as large a number as possible.

The researcher should also consider the extent to which the variables included in the survey vary in the population. The more something varies, the larger the sample needed to gather a range of responses. The less something varies, the easier it is to capture the range of experience or opinion with a smaller sample.

As with experimental studies, it is often practical considerations that influence sample size. These include time, money and the availability of subjects. Another practicality is that sometimes response rates to surveys are low (see Chapter 9), and therefore estimations of expected response rates may need to be taken into consideration when making decisions about the sample size needed.

Qualitative Research

As we have seen throughout this and other chapters, qualitative research is so different from quantitative research that different considerations exist in almost all elements of the study, including sample size. Holloway and Galvin (2017: 151) note that sample size in qualitative research is not an indicator of the importance of the study or the quality of the findings and point out that generally qualitative samples consist of fairly small numbers with anything from 4 to 50 participants. Although larger numbers are possible, they are not common. It is more usual to find much smaller numbers such as the five participants in a study by Meegan and Martin (2020) that explored the experience of student midwives completing the theory and practice aspects of the Newborn Infant Physical Examination within their pre-registration midwifery programme. In this study, Interpretive Phenomenological Analysis (IPA) was used; a methodology that typically uses a small number of participants to concentrate on the uniqueness of each case and elicit depth and detail around participants' experiences (see Chapter 4 for more details on this). A somewhat larger study by Nuzum et al. (2018) that explored the impact of stillbirth on bereaved parents interviewed 12 participants. Although both of these studies would appear too small within a quantitative paradigm, within the qualitative paradigm, the sample size is wholly appropriate as long as it leads to rich, thick data and enlightening findings.

CONSIDERATIONS WHEN CONDUCTING RESEARCH

In conducting a research project, some important decisions have to be made about the sample. One of the first considerations is to be clear on who or what will comprise the sample. For this to be achieved, unambiguous inclusion and exclusion criteria must be decided. This can be developed through reflection, discussion and by considering similar published research.

The type of study to be conducted and the research approach will influence both the size and the method of selecting the sample.

READER ACTIVITY

1. In a study that seeks to understand the experience of parents who have triplets, what sort of sampling methods could be considered?

What sample size do you think would be appropriate?
2. In a study to find out if a new antenatal course for parents-to-be increases breastfeeding uptake, what sort of sampling methods could be considered?
What sample size do you think would be appropriate?

In the case of an experimental approach, a probability sampling method should be used with a reasonable sample size in each of the experimental and control groups, again guided by the experiences of similar studies. If ethical or practical constraints prevent random allocation, then a quasi-experimental or retrospective approach may be used.

In survey designs, the important decision is the extent to which there is a need to generalise further than the sample group. This will influence the choice between probability and non-probability sampling methods. Where probability sampling methods are required, a sampling frame of all possible candidates for the study is required. This should be as complete as possible to avoid bias.

In surveys that are more exploratory and do not require generalisations to be made to the larger population and for qualitative studies, non-probability methods can be chosen. These are far more flexible and do not require a sampling frame of individuals.

In terms of sample size, the approach used will dictate whether a large sample of 100 or above will be required or whether smaller numbers of 10 or even less will be adequate.

When writing up a research report, the researcher should clearly specify the details of the sample in the methods section. This should include the rationale behind the inclusion and exclusion criteria, the sampling approach and the choice of sample size. Any changes to the sample size during the study should also be indicated along with an examination of the possible impact this may have had on the study outcomes.

CONSIDERATIONS WHEN CRITIQUING RESEARCH

In critiquing research, the reader should consider whether the sampling method is aligned. This means they need to consider if the sampling method is an appropriate one given the research question, approach and design.

One important area to consider is the extent to which the inclusion and exclusion criteria may reduce or increase bias. What is the rationale given by the researcher for the choice of criteria? Using your own professional judgement, do those included seem more or less representative as a result of the selection criteria?

Was the appropriate sampling method used in the study? There should be a clear rationale for the choice of sampling method and clear details concerning the process of selecting the sample. This should be examined carefully to ensure that the correct procedures are evident. For example, if the researcher says a random sample was used, can we be sure they do not mean a convenience sample? If it is truly a random sample, there should be mention of a sampling frame and table of random numbers or other device.

A common error is for the researcher to generalise further than the sampling criteria would allow. For instance, statements may be made about all women in pregnancy or labour when the sample consisted of only primigravida women or excluded those of a certain age, social class or other social characteristics. Similarly, attempts may be made to generalise to all midwives when the study only included hospital-based midwives and excluded those working in community settings.

The influence of sample size should also be assessed. Does the researcher justify the size of the sample selected? In an experimental design, was there any problem with the number of individuals dropping out of the study (subject attrition) that may have affected the extent to which the groups were comparable at the end of the study? All participants at the commencement of the study should be accounted for at the end.

If the researcher is using a qualitative design, we should expect small numbers and not criticise them for a small sample but instead consider the depth and richness of the data as this should be the benefit with a small sample. However, we should still expect some detail on the sample characteristics so that we can judge whether they were in a position to provide information on the phenomenon that forms the focus of the study. If demographic details are provided on the sample, it is possible to *situate the sample*. This is not so that any generalisations can be made, as in qualitative research this is not a justifiable aim (see Chapter 4). However,

it increases awareness of the participants' characteristics. This assists in assessing whether the sample was appropriate and sufficient to justify the findings (Gill, 2020) and to make judgements about how *applicable* or *transferable* the study findings might be to other people in other settings.

KEY POINTS

- Usually, research is conducted on a sample taken as representative of a larger group. A sample can consist of people, objects or events.
- A sample should be defined in terms of inclusion and exclusion criteria.
- Sampling methods vary according to research approach. Sampling methods, or strategies, can be divided into probability and non-probability methods.
- Probability sampling allows generalisations to be made from the findings to the larger target population. Other options under this heading include simple random sampling, systematic random sampling, stratified random sampling, proportionate random sampling and cluster sampling. In experimental designs, random allocation is more usual and it means that individuals are allocated to the experimental and control groups at random.
- Non-probability sampling methods include opportunity or convenience sampling, quota sampling, snowball sampling and purposive sampling. These are usually used in qualitative methods, and they may also be used in surveys.
- In non-probability sampling methods, it is not possible to say whether the findings are generalisable. In the case of qualitative research, it is not the intention to generalise to a wider population, only to say that findings may be relevant and applicable when considering the topic or issue.
- Sample size is influenced by the nature of the study, the availability of subjects about, e.g. midwives and factors such as response rate. Experimental studies may be modest in size ranging from 25 to 40 in each group, to quite large numbers such as 100 to 200 or considerably more in each group. Similarly, surveys can range from around 20 to several 100 s. Qualitative research can be anything

from under 10 to more usually around 12 to 20. These numbers provide a very rough guide only.

REFERENCES

Ayerle, G.M., Schäfers, R., Mattern, E., Striebich, S., Haastert, B., Vomhof, M., et al., 2018. Effects of the birthing room environment on vaginal births and client-centred outcomes for women at term planning a vaginal birth: BE-UP, a multicentre randomised controlled trial. Trials 19 (1), 641. https://go.exlibris.link/8DmkLxw6

Feeley, C., Thomson, G., 2016. Why do some women choose to freebirth in the UK? An interpretative phenomenological study. BMC Pregnancy Childbirth 16 (1), 59.

Gill, S.L., 2020. Qualitative sampling methods. J. Hum Lact 36 (4), 579–581.

Glasper, E.A., Rees, C., 2017. Nursing and Healthcare Research at a Glance. Wiley Blackwell, Chichester.

Grove, S.K., Gray, J., 2019. Understanding Nursing Research: Building an Evidence-based Practice, seventh ed. Elsevier, St. Louis, MO.

Holloway, I., Galvin, K.T., 2017. Qualitative Research in Nursing and Healthcare, fourth ed. Wiley Blackwell, Chichester.

Knechel, N., 2019. What's in a sample? Why selecting the right research participants matters. J. Emerg Nurs. 45 (3), 332–334.

Maycock, B.R., Scott, J.A., Hauck, Y.L., Burns, S.K., Robinson, S., Giglia, R., et al., 2015. A study to prolong breastfeeding duration: design and rationale of the Parent Infant Feeding Initiative (PIFI) randomised controlled trial. BMC Pregnancy Childbirth 15 (1), 159.

Meegan, S., Martin, T., 2020. Exploring the experiences of student midwives completing the newborn infant physical examination. Br. J. Midwifery 28 (2), 115–119.

Nuzum, D., Meaney, S., O'Donoghue, K., 2018. The impact of stillbirth on bereaved parents: a qualitative study. PloS One 13 (1), e0191635.

15

WRITING AN UNDERGRADUATE DISSERTATION

Many undergraduate midwifery programmes have a dissertation module in the final year of the course. This may seem to be daunting task, but it can be an exciting opportunity to explore an area of midwifery practice in more depth. Usually, there is limited opportunity for primary research in an undergraduate degree course, often due to time constraints, although there may be more scope within four-year masters-level pre-registration programmes. Therefore, most dissertations are built around a literature review and may be around 6,000 to 10,000 words in length.

Dissertations are original pieces of work, but good dissertations are much more; the concept is that it is more than just reviewing the evidence, it is combining it in an original and innovative way. For instance, the literature on obesity and water births is limited, but a good dissertation would combine the evidence on obesity with the benefits of water for birth to create new insights. Sometimes dissertations encompass change management and leadership strategies, often with a safety focus, where students are encouraged to think critically about how to implement a maternity service improvement.

AIMS OF AN UNDERGRADUATE DISSERTATION

- To produce a large-scale piece of academic writing towards the end of an undergraduate degree.
- To ask a research question and strive to answer it by utilising and analysing the literature.
- To demonstrate the ability to conduct a literature review, seeking literature and evidence from a wide range of sources.
- To demonstrate the ability to critically evaluate different sources of evidence.
- To facilitate a critical application of findings from the literature review to midwifery care and practice.

CHOOSING A DISSERTATION TOPIC

- Is there an area of practice you feel passionate about?
- Is this an area of practice that you would like to explore in more depth?
- Will the knowledge gained be useful to your role on qualification?

- Is this an area where you might be interested in practising in or developing further in the future?

While no topics relating to midwifery or women's health are strictly off-limits, it is not advisable to choose a topic where there is very little research, or one that is outside the remit of the midwife, for instance.

Once the area of focus for the dissertation has been decided, the next step is to formulate the area of interest into a research question. This may be straightforward, but if the topic is very broad, it may also help to narrow down the focus to one that is more manageable for an undergraduate dissertation. The research question needs to be answerable, i.e. there needs to be some research available, even if there are gaps (Fig. 15.1).

UNDERSTANDING THE MODULE

How is the module structured? Details will be outlined in the module guide and discussed when the module is launched. It is important to know how the module is planned, and understanding the module is often reflected in the outcome.

What input will there be from the wider university? Often, university library services will provide support in accessing literature and academic writing, so if you have not accessed their services before, this is the time to do so.

There may be group tutorials, alongside one-to-one supervisory meetings, where aspects of the dissertation are explored and debated. Formative presentations are also embedded into some dissertations where students outline their research and share initial findings;

through the debate that often occurs, this often helps them focus on the direction of travel of the dissertation by asking '*What does the literature suggest from your reading so far?*'

WORKING WITH A SUPERVISOR

Students are usually allocated a supervisor to guide them through the stages of the dissertation. Often, this is an academic who shares an interest or has expertise in the area of focus. It is typically the student's responsibility to arrange and attend regular, normally monthly, meetings with their supervisor. The supervisor will not generally chase a student who is not engaging, as they will expect a senior student midwife to be self-motivated and organised as an independent autonomous learner. Within the supervisory process, it is useful if the student develops an action plan with specific aims and negotiates with the supervisor what they will review and discuss and at what time. As the process unfolds, the supervisor will also be able to review drafts of chapters and provide feedback to help develop the argument and debate, etc. However, ensure that any work for review and discussion is sent to the supervisor in a timely manner beforehand, allowing them sufficient time to read it.

UNDERTAKING A LITERATURE REVIEW

The role of the literature review in research is detailed in Chapter 3. In an undergraduate dissertation, the literature review used is usually traditional or narrative. It is an in-depth review of all sources of information available on a topic, which has already been critically analysed, provided a summary of key landmark findings, identified gaps and unresolved issues. Importantly, the research question needs to be sufficiently focused to enable the student to find relevant literature. The university library will be able to help with literature searching using databases, and the subject librarian will be able to offer guidance and support by advising on key words and suggesting suitable databases.

READER ACTIVITY

Read some published literature reviews:
- How are they structured?
- How could this influence your literature review?

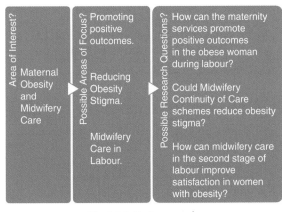

Fig. 15.1 ▪ An example.

STRUCTURE OF A DISSERTATION

The structure of an undergraduate dissertation will be decided by the module leader and their teaching team, so ensure the module guide is perused and questions/queries directed to the module leader. However, this section provides a broad overview of the content and a typical layout and structure (Table 15.1). A discussion on each aspect will help clarify the individual components of the dissertation.

Consider the dissertation as the detailing of a journey, where the narrative details how a research question was developed and answered through the undertaking of a literature review. It should take the reader from the beginning with a rationale for the chosen topic through the literature searching technique to how the literature was critiqued. Themes should be identified and discussed from the literature and key concepts applied to midwifery practice through the creation of recommendations (Greetham, 2019; Williams, 2018).

A Typical Dissertation

- Has a clear choice of research question – *INTRODUCTION*
- Demonstrates a methodical approach to searching, organising and analysing the literature – *RESEARCH METHODOLOGY CHAPTER*

TABLE 15.1

A Typical Dissertation Structure

Please refer to the University's Module Guide for the definitive requirements, but here is a suggested format:

- Cover Page
- Acknowledgements
- List of Contents
- List of Tables and Figures
- Glossary
- Title
- Abstract
- Introduction
- Methodology Chapter
- Findings or Themes Chapter
- Discussion Chapter
- Conclusion
- References
- Appendices

- Provides a consistent and comprehensive critical appraisal of the evidence presented as themes – *FINDINGS CHAPTERS*
- Can critically evaluate key areas relating to the evidence and apply these to midwifery practice – *DISCUSSION CHAPTER*
- Brings the discussion to a conclusion, identifying gaps in the evidence, etc., and answers the research question – *CONCLUSION* (Table 15.1)

What To Include in Each Section

Cover Page: this is usually provided in template form, which requires a name, title and course details, plus a statement which testifies that the dissertation is the students' own work.

Acknowledgements: it is polite to mention and recognise any help and support that may have been received during the creation of the dissertation. This may be the dissertation supervisor, an outside agency or an expert in the field, or even a family member who provided moral or practical support, for example, proofreading.

List of Contents: this is important and provides structure to the dissertation, with chapters and sub-divisions, including appendices. Microsoft Word can help in this respect by providing headings and page numbers to create a professional looking contents page.

List of Tables and Figures: it shows an attention to detail and looks professional to list tables and figures by linking them to the relevant part of the text, for example the first figure in Chapter 4 would be numbered 'Figure 4.1', with the second as 'Figure 4.2' and so on.

Glossary: a glossary of terms and any abbreviations used may be a useful addition and help with clarity, etc., for the reader.

Title: this is usually phrased as a research question.

Abstract: most research papers have an abstract. This provides a brief summary of the research, and in the case of a dissertation, this would provide a brief summary of the dissertation. It is usually only 300 to 500 words in length and often has sub-headings. It outlines the background of the dissertation, the main methods used, the main results and the main conclusions and recommendations.

Introduction: this is the first main content section of the dissertation. It can be quite descriptive, but usually provides the background of the topic focus, the justification for choice of topic, including the reasons, which may be anecdotal, for choosing the topic. There should be a clear identification for the research question.

Methodology: this is where the underpinning methodology and methods used to conduct the literature review are discussed, identifying the types of evidence that was considered within the dissertation. It provides detail of how literature was accessed, including inclusion and exclusion criteria, and the critical framework used to review the literature. This detail then shows how themes were developed and provides a smooth link to the next chapter, i.e. the 'findings chapter'.

Findings or Themes Chapter: this is where there is a review and critical discussion of the literature and evidence relating to the research question. The length of the dissertation reflects the number of 'themes' to be discussed, usually under sub-headings. Evidence of critical appraisal of the literature is also included in this chapter; however, this is not a summary of each article selected for the review; it is an explanation of what the review says when the selected literature is considered as a whole. Again, a link to the next chapter is a useful addition here.

Discussion Chapter: this is a very important part of any dissertation. It provides a summary of the main themes, but more crucially, it provides a synthesis of the main themes, i.e. it asks *'What's new?'* Can the themes that have been identified be drawn together to reframe the discussion as in 'So what?' i.e. how can it be applied to midwifery practice?

Conclusion: as its name suggests, this is where the discussion is brought to a close. What recommendations for practice are there? What are the limitations of the study or evidence? Are there gaps in the evidence or other questions that need answers?

References: these must be comprehensive and accurately presented and must reflect the referencing guidelines of the university. There are some online tools that may help with referencing, for example, Cite This For Me, Endnote and RefWorks, and many are licensed by universities for use by students, so check with the Library as to what is available.

Appendices: this is where all relevant supporting information is placed and referred to in the text. Examples include tables detailing the literature searching technique, i.e. databases searched, keywords used, Boolean phrases used and 'hits' received and how it was narrowed down to a usable amount of literature. It would also include the critical framework that was used to critique the research.

Post-Dissertation

By this stage, feedback and a mark will have been received, and so the question is 'what now?' Once completed, the undergraduate midwifery dissertation may be of the standard that deserves to be shared with others. Assessor feedback will identify whether the dissertation is worthy of publication, and if it is, consider communicating the findings of the dissertation by means of conference papers, posters or published articles. It will need some further work, as the dissertation will need to be adjusted to meet the requirements of publishers, etc. Most dissertation supervisors will usually be very happy to support a student to do this, although often students may want to leave this until they have qualified – either way, it will look very impressive to have a publication or conference presentation on a curriculum vitae.

Students should also be prepared to discuss their dissertation at an interview for their first position as a midwife on completion of the programme. All senior midwives are looking at service improvements and would be interested in dissertation findings. It may lead along a career pathway into a specialist midwife role or being able to undertake primary research to further understand the issue and enhance midwifery care and practice.

Good Luck!

REFLECTIVE PROMPT

- What key points will you take from this chapter when preparing and writing your undergraduate dissertation?

KEY POINTS

- Midwifery research and evidence has entered a new era on its evolutionary journey, and now, emphasis must be placed on developing a supportive midwifery research culture
- More midwives are developing the practical skills of undertaking research
- There is no shortage of clinical problems that need examining, and new developments that need evaluation
- This starts at the undergraduate level, where students are expected to undertake a dissertation as part of their pre-registration midwifery programme
- This then leads to more midwives undertaking Masters, PhDs and other doctoral-level courses to prepare them to become independent researchers who can make an original contribution to midwifery knowledge
- Midwifery research influences midwifery practice and develops maternity services, promoting

safe and effective care (NMC, 2019). Therefore, a dissertation is an important component of a pre-registration programme and is more than just academic exercise. Many employers ask newly qualified students about their dissertation topics at interviews for newly qualified midwife posts, so it is always worth considering this aspect when choosing a focus. An undergraduate dissertation may also be the stepping stone to becoming involved in further research or a specialist midwife post or lead into masters and doctoral studies.

REFERENCES

Greetham, B., 2019. How To Write Your Undergraduate Dissertation, third ed. Springer Nature Press, London.

NMC, 2019. Standards of Proficiency for Midwives. https://www.nmc.org.uk/globalassets/sitedocuments/standards/standards-of-proficiency-for-midwives.pdf.

Williams, K., 2018. Planning Your Dissertation, second ed. Red Globe Press, Springer Nature Limited, London.

16

THE CHALLENGE FOR THE FUTURE

The last chapter of a novel usually reveals all and brings the plot to a resolution. It often has a happy or at least intriguing ending, so that the reader puts down the book with a feeling of contentment, perhaps mixed with a tinge of regret that the characters will no longer be a feature of their life. Non-fiction books are not like that. The aim of this chapter is to emphasise that what has gone before in the previous chapters is only the beginning.

This chapter challenges the reader to continue absorbing and applying the information in this book on an increasingly regular basis as part of an individual's clinical practice. It will also encourage the reader to make a vital contribution to evidence-based practice by helping to perpetuate the research culture in midwifery. This is the last chapter, but it is not goodbye.

The future of maternity care is likely to be demanding as well as challenging for the midwife as time moves further into the 21st century. The UK birth rate has fallen steadily since 2012 and is now at 1.58 children per woman (Office of National Statistics, 2020). There are multifactorial reasons for and this situation has been exacerbated by the coronavirus pandemic

(2020–2022 and possibly well into the future…?), which has caused increasing anxiety over job insecurity, financial hardship and the extra pressures on women juggling childcare, home schooling and work. Narrators tell of a society where the financial and emotional costs of bringing up children present obstacles to developing a career while parenting. This results in many women deciding against motherhood. This is layered on the changing demographic profile of childbearing women, which has changed significantly over the past couple of decades, resulting in additional care from the multi-agency team (Box 16.1).

Such changes will require an even greater emphasis on an efficient and safe midwifery service in order to cope with the complexity of demands. The direction of travel currently undertaken in midwifery and the maternity services is maternity continuity of care(r) (MCoC). MCoC is part of the Maternity Transformation Programme in the UK and is a model of care provided by midwives, who are organised into teams of eight or fewer (Cumberledge, 2016; NHS, 2021). Each full-time midwife in the team will provide

BOX 16.1

DEMOGRAPHIC PROFILE OF CHILDBEARING IN THE UK

- The age of new mothers has risen to 30 years of age, with just over 50% choosing marriage in which to raise a family
- There is an increased number of mothers with co-morbidities, with higher rates of complications requiring investigation, management, and intervention
- The rates of obesity in childbearing-age women is increasing, with an associated increased rate of co-morbidities present and an increased rate of complications
- An increasing social and ethnic diversity, leading to communication difficulties and significant clinical challenges for maternity care
- There is a rising operative birth rate, which is connected to all of the above

BOX 16.2

ENHANCED OUTCOMES FROM AN MCOC MODEL

PHYSICAL OUTCOMES

- 24% less likely to experience preterm birth (Medley et al., 2018)
- 16% less likely to experience a pregnancy loss overall and 19% less likely to experience a pregnancy loss before 24 weeks (Ota et al., 2020)
- 15% less likely to experience regional analgesia
- 16% less likely to have an episiotomy
- 10% less likely to experience instrumental vaginal birth
- 7 times more likely to be attended at birth by a known midwife (Sandall et al., 2015)
- Improves outcomes for Black and Asian Women by helping to avoid unconscious bias (Homer et al., 2017; Rayment-Jones et al., 2015; 2019; 2020; 2021)

RELATIONAL OUTCOMES

- Relational midwifery care improves women's experience and increases their perceptions of trust, safety in the quality care they receive (Sandall et al., 2015)
- Women also reported a higher level of satisfaction with information giving, advice and explanations
- Helps women make informed decisions about place of birth, preparation for labour and birth, and decisions about intrapartum analgesia and feeling in control during labour and birth (Sandall et al., 2015)
- Enhances the relationship between midwife and woman (Fenwick et al., 2018; Perriman and Davis, 2018)
- Improves effectiveness of the workforce through better team-working (Fenwick et al., 2018; West and Lyubovnikova, 2013)

MCoC, Maternity continuity of care.

antenatal, intrapartum and postnatal midwifery care to around 36 women per year, with support from the interdisciplinary team. The evidence for its benefits is clearly based on models employing continuity across antenatal, intrapartum, and postnatal care (Box 16.2). MCoC models promote better outcomes for women and their babies and foster a better birth experience for women:

It ... sets out a vision for safe and personalised maternity services in England: one that puts the needs of the woman, her baby and family at the heart of care; with staff who are supported to deliver high quality – and continuously improving – care. NHS (2021: 33)

This lends itself to future research investigation foci where MCoC schemes will be evaluated and analysed.

OUR RESEARCH

I suppose no textbook on research would be complete without some discussion on the editor's research and research interests. We both have had varied and interesting careers in midwifery spanning several decades and have seen midwifery develop significantly as a profession. Just in its pre-registration education, it has gone from apprentice-style training to a minimum of a degree level education in the last three to four decades.

Rowena's doctoral focus was on obesity and childbearing, and her thesis was entitled: "*An Interpretive Exploration of the Experiences of Mothers with Obesity*

and Midwives who Care for the Obese Mother during Childbearing" (Doughty, 2019).

The aim of the study was to generate data that facilitated an exploration and interpretation of the experiences of obese mothers during childbearing and the perspectives of midwives who have experienced the provision of care for obese mothers during childbearing. The study had several objectives: first, the study would capture the experiences of obese mothers. The study would generate data on the mother's experiences of obesity and provide an understanding of the experiences of obese mothers during childbearing and their experiences of the maternity services. Second, the study would capture the views and experiences of midwives who care for obese mothers during childbearing and provide an understanding of their experiences. Third, through the analysis of the data generated, the researcher would be able to contribute to theoretical and practice debates within academic and professional arenas. Implications for policy, including midwifery practice, would be identified and may influence the future provision of maternity services and the practice of midwifery. Lastly, the study would identify areas worthy of further research (Fig. 16.1).

An interpretivist qualitative approach using in-depth semi-structured interviews was chosen. The study was designed to facilitate the recruitment of mothers' post-birth and obtain their experiences retrospectively and women were recruited through Slimming World. Professionals with experience of caring for mothers with obesity during childbearing were also recruited.

Following thematic analysis three themes were identified:

- **The Reductionist Approach to Maternity Care:** this theme focused on obesity and BMI, maternal obesity and the impact on maternal choice, and maternal obesity and midwifery care.
- **The Lost Opportunities for Health Promotion:** this theme focused on the mother–midwife relationship and the impact of obesity on communication and the minimalisation of excessive gestational weight gain during pregnancy.
- **The Experiences and Everyday Theories of Obesity:** this theme focused on weight stigma, the normalisation of obesity and women's lay theory through their own weight journey.

Diane's interests have focused on the way that midwives make evidence-based decisions in practice. Although evidence-based healthcare was first described by Sackett (1996), there had been very little guidance on how Sackett's model, which was originally described in relation to medical care, should be adapted for midwifery care. This led to two, linked journal papers about evidence-based decision-making in midwifery. In paper one evidence-based decision-making was explored and its place in midwifery established (Menage, 2016a). In paper two, a model of evidence-based midwifery care was proposed.

Decision-making was explored, and its place in midwifery was established (Ménage, 2016a). In paper two, a

model of evidence-based midwifery care for midwifery was proposed (Ménage, 2016b). The model places evidence from research alongside evidence from the woman herself, the midwife, and takes into account evidence about resources available. The partnership between a woman and midwife is central to the decision-making. All four aspects of the sources of evidence (research, resources, the woman, and the midwife) are set in the context of the physical, social, legal, cultural and professional environment where the decision-making takes place. MCoC lends itself to this model of decision-making as it allows the midwife/woman partnership to remain central. The model is shown in Fig. 16.2.

Publication of the model was a milestone for evidence-based midwifery. However, midwifery is continually evolving. In 2019, Ashforth and Kitson-Reynolds proposed a model that acknowledged and built on the Ménage (2016b) model, but with added emphasis on the interactions between the different types of research. This is how concepts and frameworks are developed and adapted and add to the body of dynamic knowledge that is midwifery. Models such as these can be tested as part of studies to understand their use by midwives and student midwives during clinical decision-making (Ashforth and Kitson-Reynolds, 2019).

Compassionate Midwifery

Diane's PhD research study aimed to develop a deep understanding of compassionate midwifery from the woman's perspective in order to inform practice, education and service provision and guide future research in this area (Ménage et al., 2020). Compassion is held up as an important aspect of healthcare and yet there was a lack of research into compassion related to midwifery care. The study addressed that omission by analysing what is meant by *compassionate midwifery* and by examining women's lived experience of receiving compassion from midwives.

The key objectives were:

- To identify women who believe they have personally experienced compassionate midwifery care.
- To identify the ways in which women experience compassion in midwifery.
- To explore women's thoughts and feelings about compassionate midwifery care.
- To gain an understanding of the impact of compassionate midwifery on women.

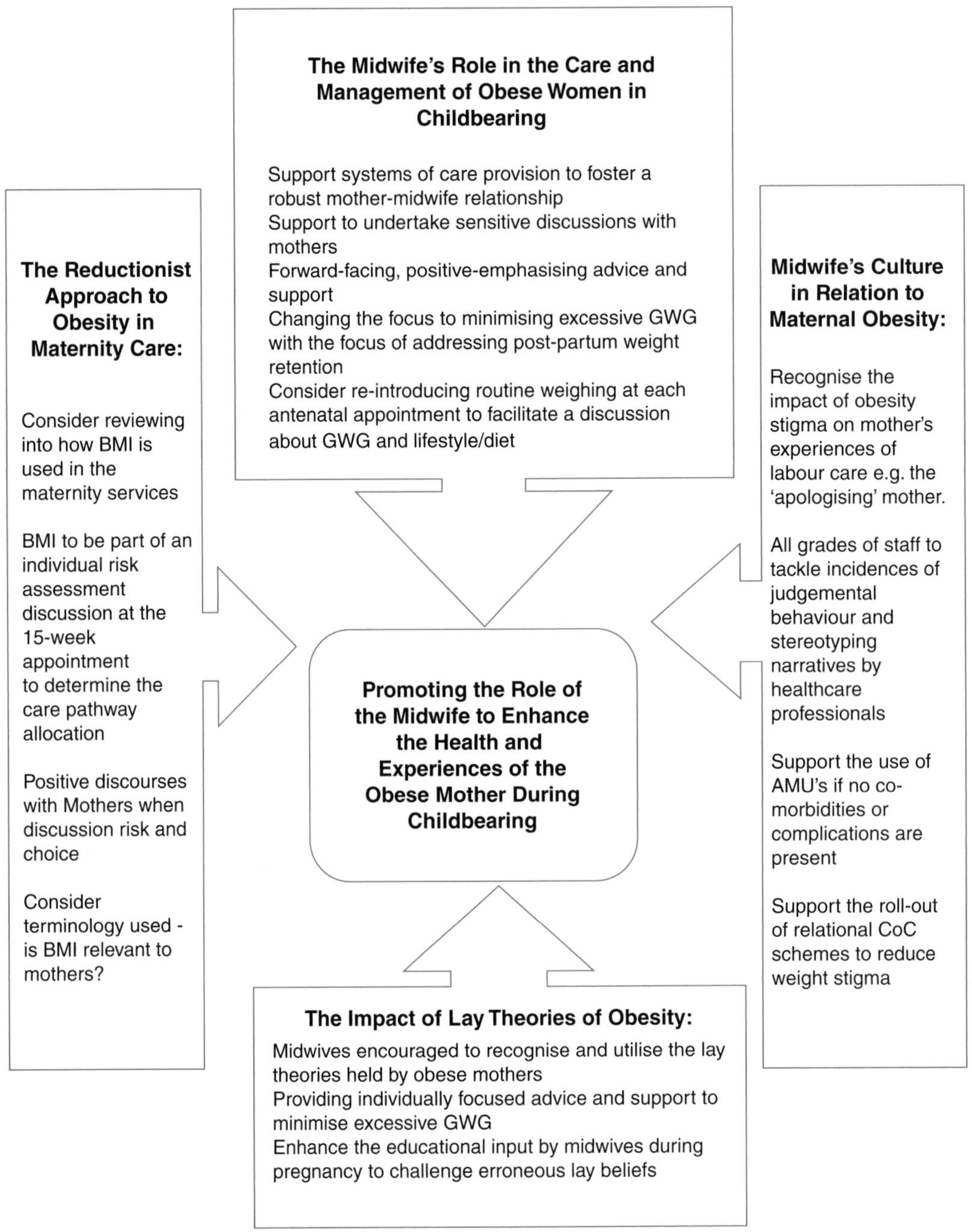

The Midwife's Role in the Care and Management of Obese Women in Childbearing

Support systems of care provision to foster a robust mother-midwife relationship
Support to undertake sensitive discussions with mothers
Forward-facing, positive-emphasising advice and support
Changing the focus to minimising excessive GWG with the focus of addressing post-partum weight retention
Consider re-introducing routine weighing at each antenatal appointment to facilitate a discussion about GWG and lifestyle/diet

The Reductionist Approach to Obesity in Maternity Care:

Consider reviewing into how BMI is used in the maternity services

BMI to be part of an individual risk assessment discussion at the 15-week appointment to determine the care pathway allocation

Positive discourses with Mothers when discussion risk and choice

Consider terminology used - is BMI relevant to mothers?

Midwife's Culture in Relation to Maternal Obesity:

Recognise the impact of obesity stigma on mother's experiences of labour care e.g. the 'apologising' mother.

All grades of staff to tackle incidences of judgemental behaviour and stereotyping narratives by healthcare professionals

Support the use of AMU's if no co-morbidities or complications are present

Support the roll-out of relational CoC schemes to reduce weight stigma

Promoting the Role of the Midwife to Enhance the Health and Experiences of the Obese Mother During Childbearing

The Impact of Lay Theories of Obesity:
Midwives encouraged to recognise and utilise the lay theories held by obese mothers
Providing individually focused advice and support to minimise excessive GWG
Enhance the educational input by midwives during pregnancy to challenge erroneous lay beliefs

Fig. 16.1 ■ The original contribution (Doughty, 2019).

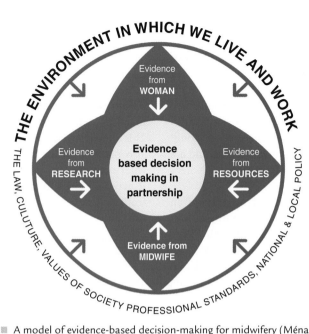

Fig. 16.2 ▪ A model of evidence-based decision-making for midwifery (Ménage, 2016b).

A qualitative study was conducted with 17 women participants who identified themselves as having received compassionate midwifery. Women's rich accounts of their care were analysed using the principles of interpretive phenomenological analysis (IPA) (see Chapter 4). The findings revealed that the women participants set their experiences of compassion from midwives within the context of their individual *Need for Compassion* at the time. Women's need for compassion related to their anxiety, vulnerability, physical or emotional pain, and the transition to motherhood. Compassionate midwifery made a difference to women by making them feel safer and more able to cope. Three major themes represented how women experienced compassion through a sense of the midwife:

- *Being with them.* This was something that women very quickly recognised in midwives.
- *Being in a relationship* with them.
- Being treated in ways that made them feel more *empowered.*

A dynamic model of *Compassionate Midwifery in Balance* was proposed based on the study findings, depicting the key features of compassionate midwifery. The findings offer a resource on compassion in midwifery that is both research based and informed by women service users and has been used to inform practice and education.

EVOLVING THE DYNAMIC RESEARCH CULTURE IN MIDWIFERY

The way ahead lies in midwifery students developing research skills during their pre-registration education to ensure all midwives are able to critically analyse published work. This is embedded in the Nursing and Midwifery Council (NMC) standards for the Future Midwife (NMC, 2019) and will see all students, at the point of graduation and on entering the NMC register as a midwife, armed with the skills to be able to critique the evidence that underpins midwifery practice as they start their midwifery career.

At the point of registration, the midwife will be able to: "*demonstrate the knowledge, skills and ability to identify, critically analyse, and interpret research evidence…*" (Outcome 1.4) (NMC, 2019: 14).

Increasingly, midwives are expected to be involved in research as part of the day job. It is anticipated that senior midwives, consultant midwives and midwifery lecturers will carry out research as part of their substantive role. At the same time, all midwives could be expected to participate in multidisciplinary research; this ensures that midwifery also influences the research and practice of other professional groups. This kind of activity is a sign of a mature profession.

It is not a case of taking midwives out of clinical practice; it is enhancing that practice through informed researchers. As a career option, more midwifery graduates are becoming midwifery researchers, often alongside master's and doctorate-level qualifications, and are producing high-quality research to inform midwifery practice.

This book has already attempted to provide an understanding of the ways in which midwives can become critical readers of research. Although this is a useful quality for the individual, it becomes even more valuable where it contributes to a research culture. This means sharing the results of critiquing with others, first, on a small informal basis with colleagues who may also be developing this skill and then with a larger group of midwives. This can be as part of a small research appreciation group, as a journal club or through blogs and tweets that provide the opportunity to reflect on practice and be open to change and ways of achieving it. The idea of journal clubs, blogs and tweets has been supported as a way of promoting and disseminating the use of research findings in practice by keeping up to date with the latest research and improving the quality of care provided.

THE IMPORTANCE OF RESEARCH EVIDENCE IN CHANGE MANAGEMENT AND LEADERSHIP

The NMC expects midwives to *"promote safe and effective care, drawing on best available evidence"* (NMC, 2019: 13). The NMC also expects midwives to be able to not only use research to keep updated and to inform their practice but to develop practice (Outcome 5B) through scholarship, change management and leadership (NMC, 2019). Any change management process requires the development team to consider the research evidence. Being able to access and understand the research evidence is a vital part of change process; it may be expected that midwives present their case for change to a Trust Board, for example, as well as disseminating the evidence in a useable format to all those

impacted by the change. These skills go hand-in-hand with sound leadership skills.

Critical reviews of the literature can also be undertaken by small groups of midwives as a basis for establishing clinical standards, as a way of solving clinical problems, or simply exploring new techniques and practices (Amelink-Verburg et al., 2010; Shallow, 2010). This should not only improve the use of research but also place it within the context of professional midwifery practice and the needs and wishes of women. It may also identify topics and foci that could benefit from a clearer evidence base.

SUPPORT WHEN CONDUCTING RESEARCH

To carry out research successfully, it is important to have support from professional, educational and managerial colleagues. The researcher must possess a good level of research knowledge through undergraduate-level study and should be able to call upon an experienced researcher or research supervisor to provide guidance. If the research is part of a master's or doctorate-level programme, the research student will have access to a university library with librarians and databases. They will also be allocated a research supervisor(s) who will have experience in supporting research students and may have expertise in the topic area being investigated. This will help make the research process a truly fruitful and fulfilling activity. A good experience may encourage involvement in further research activities.

DISSEMINATION RESEARCH FINDINGS

Once the study is complete, it must be communicated. Who to disseminate this to will depend on the research focus and findings. It will include the research team and/or department and Trust managers who may have funded it. It should also, where possible, include those who may have taken part, even if this takes the form of a one-page summary, to let them know that their participation contributed to something tangible. Subsequently, a clear attempt should be made to disseminate it widely, namely:

- a conference poster
- a conference paper
- a journal article, i.e. publication
- a blog or tweet

Each has its own format and audience and serves a different function. Poster presentations are a good introduction to research presentations, as they expose the researcher to the minimum of intimidation. These depend on visual impact and gaining the viewer's attention. Attending a conference that has a wide variety of posters helps with generating ideas. It is a good idea to include the researcher's name and email address on the poster so people can get in touch for more information. Often conference organisers will provide abstract and summaries from all presentations and posters that will also include name and contact details. For both conference and poster presentations, business cards will be extremely useful and can be given out to interested attendees. Posters are an ideal way to 'sell' the key research findings directly to those who are interested in them. As posters are so portable and have impact, they can also be used to great effect in the clinical area.

A conference paper requires verbal and visual presentation skills, good voice projection, enthusiasm, and a willingness/ability to share the work with a group. PowerPoint presentations can support the conference paper by emphasising key points and words and easy to assimilate tables that are neither too small to see nor too crowded with information. Many healthcare organisations hold local conferences that are an ideal means of communicating findings to a large and often mixed group of health professionals.

A journal article is one of the best ways to communicate research to a wide audience. Journal articles differ depending on the journal, as each has its target audience and journal style. It is not good practice to submit to more than one journal at a time. However, it is acceptable to rework an article, once published, for another journal as long as it is not simply a rehash; focus instead on a slightly different theme by considering the target audience. Do not try to condense a whole dissertation or a long assignment into a four thousand words or less article, just concentrate on two or three of the main themes. Make the article interesting by thinking of it from the reader's point of view.

When writing articles seek the advice of someone who has already published. Co-authorship is also an alternative where you enlist the skills of someone with publishing experience but always insist on the primary contributor/author's name going first. It is however common practice to include the PhD or master's supervisors on the finished research papers.

The usual structure for conference papers, posters or articles is as follows:

- Introduction to the topic (what was the problem?).
- What does the literature say about it (literature review)?
- What was the research aim (research question)?
- How did you go about it (methods and sample)?
- What did you find (results)?
- What does it all mean (discussion)?
- What do you recommend?

Blogs and tweets are short and snappy headlines of research dissemination using social media platforms. These can be the stepping stones for information-sharing and networking, which may lead to further projects and research.

Whichever medium is chosen, remember the audience and the message that is being communicated. Do not perpetuate the myth that research is written in jargon by using over-elaborate 'scientific' language and research terms and concepts that require a great deal of prior knowledge from the reader. Where technical terms are used, make sure that their meaning is clear to the novice. Remember, the aim is to clarify not mystify.

THREATS TO EVIDENCE

In Chapter 1, the nature of evidence was explored and the advantages of evidence built from high-quality research studies were discussed. In Chapter 2, research was defined as the systematic collection of information using carefully designed and controlled methods that answer specific questions objectively and as accurately as possible. With a belief in evidence-based care, it is difficult to see how this could be seriously challenged and yet it has never been more under threat. As a society, this is an information age in which Googling the answer to questions is now second nature. Social media, online videos, blogs and websites are generally how individuals find answers. While this is incredibly useful in some circumstances, it is important to go back to basics and remember that all information is not equal. The danger is that people are lulled into a false sense of security and begin to assume what people are reading and sharing is reliable information. It is not easy because there has been an increasing trend in published articles of health-related misinformation, and social media now plays a major role in its propagation (Snyder et al., 2020; Wang et al., 2019). As midwives, it is important to remember that many of the women and families midwives care for are also being exposed to this.

Midwives must tread a fine line by respecting individual women's needs, views and decisions while at the same time sensitively providing evidence-based information. To do this, midwives need to be discerning about where information comes from and how it was compiled. The ability to *question* has been emphasised throughout this book, and in this final chapter, the editors would be negligent if they did not remind readers of the need to keep questioning and continue seeking to understand what constitutes good evidence and what is not. This book has provided a comprehensive range of tools to differentiate between the best available evidence based on high-quality research and questionable evidence based on poor-quality research. However, it is also increasingly important to differentiate between best available evidence and opinion, journalism, and misinformation. An inability or unwillingness to do this is perhaps the biggest threat to evidence-based care (Pulido et al., 2020). It has never been more important to be aware that it is a midwife's professional responsibility to practise evidence-based midwifery.

CONCLUSION

Throughout this book, the emphasis has been placed on the acquisition of research-based knowledge and skills to enable the reader to become skilled at critiquing research. This is a prerequisite for moving the culture and practice of professional midwifery forward, and it is supported by the NMC (2019). It is more than understanding research; however, it is about applying the literature carefully to the individual situation and woman. This is embedded in professional reflection where continuous self-reflection, alongside intuitive thinking, is an essential part of being an accountable, autonomous, independent, professional midwife (NMC, 2019) who is able to justify their clinical decisions (Jefford et al., 2017).

REFLECTION PROMPTS

Do you think you have the skills to use evidence and research to underpin your practice as a midwife?
What areas do you need to develop?
How could you develop your research skills and abilities?

KEY POINTS

- Midwifery research and evidence is fundamental to develop the profession, and increasingly midwives are undertaking research either as full-time midwifery researcher or as research midwives or as a part of their role, e.g. specialist and consultant midwives.
- Research is embedded into midwifery care and maternity service provision and underpins all innovation and practice development
- The role of the midwife as a colleague, scholar and leader is firmly embedded into the Future Midwife Standards (NMC, 2019).
- More midwives are undertaking MSc-level study at entry level (pre-registration) and post-registration which lead to PhD studies and other doctoral-level courses which prepare them to become independent researchers who can make an original contribution to midwifery knowledge.
- Once complete, midwifery research should be communicated by means of conference papers, blogs, tweets, posters and published articles and is an integral part of the research process.
- Graduate midwives are taught to critique research and contribute to critical reviews of the literature; these activities contribute to the wider research culture of the clinical area and inform midwifery practice and maternity policy and guidelines.

REFERENCES

Amelink-Verburg, M., Herschderfer, K., Offerhaus, P., Buitendijk, S., 2010. The development of evidence based midwifery in the Netherlands: the journey from midwifery knowledge to midwifery research to midwifery standards of practice. In: Spiby, H., Munro, J. (Eds.), Evidence-Based Midwifery: Applications in Context. Wiley-Blackwell, Chichester.

Ashforth, E., Kitson-Reynolds, E., 2019. Decision-making: Do existing models reflect the complex and multifaceted nature of women-centred contemporary midwifery practice? Pract. Midwife. 22 (1).

Cumberledge, J., 2016. Better Births: The National Maternity Review. england.maternityreview@nhs.net www.england.nhs.uk/ourwork/futurenhs/mat-review.

Doughty, R., 2019. An Interpretive Exploration of the Experiences of Mothers with Obesity and Midwives who Care for the Obese Mother during Childbearing. Unpublished PhD Thesis. De Montfort University, Leicester.

Fenwick, J., Sidebotham, M., Gamble, J., Creedy, D.K., 2018. The emotional and professional wellbeing of Australian midwives: a comparison between those providing continuity of midwifery care and those not providing continuity. Women Birth. 31 (1), 38–43.

Homer, C.S., Leap, N., Edwards, N., Sandall, J., 2017. Midwifery continuity of carer in an area of high socio-economic disadvantage in London: a retrospective analysis of Albany Midwifery Practice outcomes using routine data (1997–2009). Midwifery 48, 1–10.

Jefford, E., Jomeen, J., Martin, C., 2017. Enhanced decision-making assessment in midwifery. Midwifery 20 (2), 39.

Medley, N., Vogel, J.P., Care, A., Alfirevic, Z., 2018. Interventions during pregnancy to prevent preterm birth: an overview of Cochrane systematic reviews. Cochrane Database Syst. Rev. 11 (11), CD012505.

Ménage, D., 2016a. Part 2: a model for evidence-based decision-making in midwifery care. Brit. J. Midwifery 24 (2), 137–143.

Ménage, D., 2016b. Part 1: a model for evidence-based decision-making in midwifery care. Brit. J. Midwifery 24 (1), 44–49.

Menage, D., Bailey, E., Lees, S., Coad, J., 2020. Women's lived experience of compassionate midwifery: human and professional. Midwifery 85, 102662. https://doi.org/10.1016/j.midw.2020.102662

NHS, 2021. Delivering Midwifery Continuity of Carer at full scale; Guidance on planning, implementation and monitoring 2021/22. https://www.england.nhs.uk/wp-content/uploads/2021/10/B0961_Delivering-midwifery-continuity-of-carer-at-full-scale.pdf

NMC., 2019. Standards framework for nursing and midwifery education. [online] Available at: https://www.nmc.org.uk/standards-for-education-and-training/standards-framework-for-nursing-and-midwifery-education/

Office of National Statistics., 2020. Available at: https://www.ons.gov.uk/

Ota, E., da Silva Lopes, K., Middleton, P., Flenady, V., et al., 2020. Antenatal interventions for preventing stillbirth, fetal loss and perinatal death: an overview of Cochrane systematic reviews. Cochrane Database Syst. Rev. 12 (12), CD009599.

Perriman, N., Davis, D.L., Ferguson, S., 2018. What women value in the midwifery continuity of care model: a systematic review with meta-synthesis. Midwifery 62, 220–229.

Pulido, C.M., Ruiz-Eugenio, L., Redondo-Sama, G., Villarejo-Carballido, B., 2020. A new application of social impact in social media for overcoming fake news in health. Int. J. Environ. Res. Public Health 17 (7), 2430. https://doi.org/10.3390/ijerph17072430

Rayment-Jones, H., Murrells, T., Sandall, J., 2015. An investigation of the relationship between the caseload model of midwifery for socially disadvantaged women and childbirth outcomes using routine data – a retrospective, observational study. Midwifery 31 (4), 409–417.

Rayment-Jones, H., Harris, J., Harden, A., Khan, Z., Sandall, J., 2019. How do women with social risk factors experience United Kingdom maternity care? A realist synthesis. Birth 46 (3), 461–474.

Rayment-Jones, H., Silverio, S.A., Harris, J., Harden, A., Sandall, J., 2020. Project 20: midwives' insight into continuity of care models for women with social risk factors: What works, for whom, in what circumstances, and how. Midwifery 84, 1026–1054.

Rayment-Jones, H., Dalrymple, K., Harris, J., Harden, A., Parslow, E., Georgi, T., Sandall, J., 2021. Project 20: does continuity of care and community-based antenatal care improve maternal and neonatal birth outcomes for women with social risk factors? A prospective, observational study. PLoS One 16 (5), e0250947.

Sackett, D.L., Rosenberg, W.M., Gray, J.A., Haynes, R.B., Richardson, W.S., 1996. Evidence based medicine: what it is and what it isn't. BMJ 312 (7023), 71–72. https://doi.org/10.1136/bmj.312.7023.71

Sandall, J., Soltani, H., Gates, S., Shennan, A., Devane, D., 2015. Midwife-led continuity models versus other models of care for childbearing women. Cochrane Database Syst. Rev. 4. Art. No.: CD004667.

Shallow, H., 2010. Guidelines and the Consultant Midwife: the challenges of the interdisciplinary guideline group. In: Spiby, H., Munro, J. (Eds.), Evidence-Based Midwifery: Applications in Context. Wiley-Blackwell, Chichester.

Snyder, K., Pelster, A.K., Dinkel, D., 2020. Healthy eating and physical activity among breastfeeding women: the role of misinformation. BMC Pregnancy Childbirth 20 (1) 470–470. https://doi.org/10.1186/s12884-020-03153-x

Wang, Y., McKee, M., Torbica, A., Stuckler, D., 2019. Systematic literature review on the spread of health-related misinformation on social media. Soc. Sci. Med. 240 112552–112552. https://doi.org/10.1016/j.socscimed.2019.112552

West, M.A., Lyubovnikova, J., 2013. Illusions of team working in health care. J. Health. Organ. Manag. 27 (1), 134–142.

GLOSSARY OF COMMON RESEARCH TERMS

Abstract: Published reports and dissertations usually begin with an abstract. This is one or more paragraphs giving a brief, but succinct, overview of the study. If you read this, you should be able to establish if the study is relevant to you.

Accidental sampling/sample: *See Convenience sampling.*

Action research: A broad term for practice based research that involves the introduction and evaluation of change. There is no control group, meaning that it would be wrong to make generalisations based on an action research study. However, something is introduced that might make a positive difference to the setting. All those in the setting participate in deciding what should take place and how. The implementation and the research go on simultaneously. It has a great potential in midwifery and it is steadily gaining popularity.

After-only design: Form of experimental design where there is only one measurement taken following the introduction of an intervention. This has the advantage of not building on previous exposure to information or measurements. However, the disadvantage is that there is no baseline available to know if there has been any improvement from a previous level. An alternative is the pre-test post-test design where measurements are made both before and after the intervention.

ANCOVA: Abbreviation of **AN**alysis of **COVA**riance. This is a statistical procedure used to test mean differences among groups on a dependent variable and tries to ensure that other variables (or covariates) are not influencing the apparent relationship.

Anonymity: An essential principle of ethics that protects the identity of individuals who have taken part in a study. Achieved by avoiding the use of personal names or identifying details about the individual or setting.

ANOVA: Similar to the above and stands for **AN**alysis **Of VA**riance. In this statistical procedure, the mean difference between three or more groups and compares how much variability there is within the groups as well as between them. It is used to determine if these are *significantly* different from each other.

Applicability: In qualitative research, which is not generalisable, applicability should be considered. This is how well the study findings might apply (or not) to other groups in other settings. The terms *transferability* and *fittingness* are also used in a similar way.

Applied research: Research that seeks to solve a practical problem rather than simply add to our knowledge on a topic or concept.

Attention factor: Explanation for changes in behaviour due to participants reacting to being in a study. See also: *Hawthorne effect.*

Auditability: In qualitative research, the judgement that the researcher has provided sufficient detail to allow the reader to follow an audit trial and confirm the researcher's conclusions.

Audit trail: In qualitative research, the detail that indicates the way the researcher moved from individual quotes, or observations, to key categories used to make sense of the findings. This contributes to the credibility of the research.

Authenticity: Part of the criteria for assessing the soundness of qualitative research. It demonstrates what attempts were made to check the accuracy of the findings, e.g. member's check where participants confirm the accuracy of what was recorded. A further method is the use of 'thick' or rich descriptions of the way in which the study was conducted and the environments and incidents encountered. These should allow readers to feel almost as though they are there.

Autonomous or Autonomy: This means 'self-governing' and relates to the basic ethical principles of the right of individuals to make decisions about themselves and whether to take part in a study.

Back chaining: In searching or sourcing the literature, a method of finding further studies by consulting the references in a particular publication. See also: *forward chaining*.

Bar graph: A way of illustrating the results of quantitative research in the form of blocks that help the reader to see differences between variables and groups. They differ from histograms, as bar graphs have a space between each bar since the data are discrete, such as primigravida and multigravida, and not continuous data such as height or weight.

Baseline measurements: These are measurements made before a change or intervention takes place. This acts as a comparison for later measurements. Used in experimental studies as part of the 'before' measurement.

Basic research: The opposite of applied research. The purpose is to add to knowledge or theory on a topic or concept.

Before and after designs: A type of experimental design, also known as a pre-test and post-test design, where measurements are taken before an intervention and after. This has the advantage of establishing changes from a baseline measure. In some situations, however, it can be a disadvantage as people are sensitised to issues or abilities that may influence the performance on the 'after' part of the measurement. An alternative is the after-only design.

Beneficence: In ethics, relates to the principle of doing only good and avoiding harm. This principle ensures that the researcher considers how the study will be of benefit.

Bias: Anything that distorts or affects the study in a way that will alter or influence the accuracy of the findings. Usually relates to an untypical or unrepresentative sample but can relate to other elements. It is not always easy to spot bias: you need to ask whether there is anything about the way the study was conducted that could have had an adverse influence on the accuracy of the findings.

Bimodal distribution: A statistical description of the distribution of a variable where the data indicate there are two values that occur with equal frequency. Plotted on a graph, a bimodal distribution would be indicated by two peaks.

Blinding: Also called '**masking**'. The procedure involved in hiding from those involved in a randomised control trial (RCT) who is receiving which intervention. It is used to reduce the possibility that subjects will behave differently if they believe they are receiving a beneficial treatment. A single-blind study is where the subjects are unaware of which intervention they are receiving, and double-blind is where both the subjects and those measuring outcomes or providing care are unaware of an individual's group membership. This is taken as an element of rigour in RCTs and is sometimes a criterion for the inclusion of studies in a systematic review of the literature. Blinding is not possible in all interventions (e.g. episiotomies) when an intervention is clearly apparent.

Blind review: This does not relate to the conduct of a study, but to the process of publication. It is a system whereby those asked to evaluate the suitability of an article for publication are not given the names of the authors. This reduces the accusation that only certain people's work appears in print. It is designed to ensure fair publishing opportunities where work is chosen on merit, not on the name of the author.

Bracketing: In qualitative research, researchers are encouraged to identify their own experiences or expectations that may influence their preconceived ideas about the study and put aside or 'bracket' these so that they do not unduly influence interpretations of the findings. There is controversy over the extent to which this is possible.

Case study: This is an in-depth study of a single individual or location, such as a clinical area, used to develop insights. The generalisability of the results is low as it depends on how representative the individual or location is of their kind.

Causal relationship: The objective of experimental designs is to establish evidence of a causal relationship between an independent variable (the cause) and a dependent variable (the effect). It is confirmed by the statistical relationship between the two variables.

Cell: Tables displaying the results of research are often divided into a number of segments or boxes. These are referred to as cells. One of the most frequently encountered tables is the 2×2 table that has four cells, e.g. male, female, yes and no.

Chi-squared test (χ^2): (Pronounced 'ki-squared'): In statistics, a non-parametric test that seeks to establish if the difference between the observed results of a categorical variable (e.g. male, female) is statistically different from the expected value and is unlikely to have happened by chance.

CINAHL: An abbreviation for the database Cumulative Index Nursing and Allied Health Literature. Used in the process of reviewing the literature.

Clinical trial: Research approach that tests the effectiveness of a particular clinical intervention in an experimental design. Statistical analysis is used to establish the extent to which differences between treatments could be due to chance factors.

Closed questions: Used in questionnaires or interviews where the respondent is only provided with certain options from which to choose. This makes analysis an easy counting job but may not accurately represent the respondent's true answer.

Coding: Method of analysing qualitative data where an identifying name or category heading is given to recurring items or themes running through the findings.

Cohort: In sampling, a total group with some shared characteristics or experience from whom data are collected

Concept definition: The meaning or definition of a concept used by the researcher in the study. This is stated to clarify the meaning and avoid confusion with competing definitions.

Confirmability: Used in qualitative research as part of ensuring the researcher has demonstrated that the findings are accurate, genuine, and a true representation of the processes involved. If the researcher has met the criteria of *auditability*, *credibility* and *fittingness*, then confirmability is achieved.

Confounding variable: A variable, often in an experimental study, that may influence (confound or cloud) the outcome and get in the way of a clear explanation of the results.

Consent form: Used as part of ethical principles to ensure the researcher can demonstrate that informed consent has been given. Those taking part in the study, or someone acting on their behalf if this is not possible, should sign this. A witness to the signature who is not a health professional may also be required.

Constant comparative method: This is a method of analysing qualitative data where comparisons are made with previously noted items or categories to ensure consistency in the method of analysis. It is particularly associated with *grounded theory* (see grounded theory).

Constructionist research: Qualitative research based on the theory that people *construct* their reality on the basis of their interpretation and the meaning they give to important elements in their life. Using this theory, the role of the researcher is not simply to describe but to gain an understanding of individuals' ideas and constructions around their experiences.

Continuous data: A form of data where the measurements flow along a single scale incrementally, such as height, blood pressure and age. The opposite is discrete data, where items fall into one category or another and do not flow along a numeric scale, e.g. male, female.

Control: An essential feature of experimental design where the researcher has control over the design, particularly in regard to variables that might influence the findings of the study.

Control group: In an experimental design, the subjects who receive the usual treatment, or placebo, and not the intervention or form of the independent variable being tested. The results of measurements from the control group are compared with those of an *experimental group* to establish the existence of a cause-and-effect relationship.

Convenience sampling: Also called **opportunity or accidental sampling**. A non-probability sampling method that uses those who are in the right place at the right time and are willing to participate in a study. The limitation is there is little to guarantee they are representative of the total group. However, it is an inexpensive, quick way of recruiting a sample.

Correlation: A statistical technique that searches for a relationship between two variables in a study. A positive correlation means that as one variable increases, so does the other (e.g. height and weight);

a negative correlation is where as one variable goes up, the other goes down (e.g. outdoor temperature and weight of clothing). The strength of a correlation is indicated by a *correlation coefficient* that indicates how certain we can be that a clear pattern exists.

Correlation studies: The aim of these is to reveal a clear pattern of association. It does not imply a cause-and-effect relationship, only that there is a consistent pattern between two variables. An example would be a correlation between breastfeeding mothers and social class. Social class does not cause women to breastfeed; it is merely a pattern or association that is seen to exist between the two. Although the pattern may be reasonably stable, it does not happen in all cases.

Covert observation: Where those in an observation study are unaware they are being observed. The opposite is overt observation where observation is carried out as a visible activity. Covert observations can raise ethical concerns, as informed consent may not have been given.

Credibility: Used in qualitative research to ensure that the findings are a true representation of what was said, seen or heard. One method of achieving this is to give informants transcripts of interviews or conversations to confirm as accurate. This is called *respondent validation* or *member checking*. Another method is to use more than one person to independently analyse the data and then compare for convergence or different perspectives.

Critique: A balanced assessment of a research study that considers not only the findings but also how it was conducted and its strengths and limitations.

Crossover design study: Form of experimental design where a group receives first one intervention, is measured, and then receives a second intervention and is re-measured. This can be done with a single group or more than one group. Individuals receive both interventions and act as their own control. The biggest problem is the carry-over effect, where the benefits of the first intervention may affect the evaluation of the second. Interventions are frequently randomly allocated to individuals to reduce this problem.

Cross-sectional study: A survey that looks at a situation at one point in time by including different aspects of one group rather than following the same group over time (a longitudinal study), e.g. women at different points of pregnancy. This is more cost effective than a longitudinal study but may come up with different findings than following the same group through time.

Cross-tabulation: One form of presenting a table of results where one variable, such as age, is broken down by another variable, e.g. parity.

Cultural strangeness: Technique used in qualitative research, especially ethnographic research, where researchers attempt to distance themselves from a familiar environment in order to see things through a stranger's eyes. The aim is to question taken-for-granted assumptions and activities.

Data: Information collected in a study.

Data saturation: *See Saturation.*

Deductive reasoning: This is a method of analysis that starts from general theories or propositions and then examines the specific results that may support these general statements. This approach characterises quantitative research, particularly experimental designs.

Dependability: Part of the criteria used to assess the authenticity of qualitative research. The researcher must demonstrate that the findings are credible through such mechanisms as prolonged and in-depth data gathering. If *credibility* is established, then dependability is said to have been achieved.

Dependent variable: In experimental design, the variable that forms the outcome measured in the study, or the 'effect'. The independent variable is the presumed 'cause'. So in a study examining the relationship between information-giving and feelings of control during a birth, the feelings of control during the birth would be the dependent variable or effect, and the information would be the independent variable, or cause.

Descriptive research: A research approach that seeks to paint a picture of a situation either in numbers, as in quantitative research, or words, as in qualitative research.

Descriptive statistics: One of the two main forms of statistical analysis that attempts to describe a situation in numbers. The second main form of statistics is *inferential statistics* that allow inferences to be made about the wider population from which the sample is taken.

Design: This is the plan of action followed by the researcher to achieve the goals of the research, e.g. survey design and experimental design.

Directional hypothesis: Also called the research hypothesis, where a clear prediction is made of the expected outcome between two groups in an experimental setting. This form of hypothesis is indicated by the use of such terms as 'greater than', 'smaller than', or 'more often than', in relation to the measurements between the experimental and control groups. Other forms of hypotheses include *non-directional* and *null-hypothesis*.

Discrete data: Also called discontinuous data. A form of data where the measurements fall into clearly different categories, such as male and female. The opposite is continuous data where the measurements flow from one value to another on one scale incrementally, such as height, blood pressure and age.

Emic perspective: In qualitative research, this looks at things from the perspective of those experiencing it using their own words. The opposite is the *etic* perspective, that is, the outsider or researcher's perspective, found in quantitative research.

Empirical evidence: The collection of data in the real world involving the senses of sight, touch and hearing, rather than through assumption or abstract development of an argument. Health service research is largely empirical. Empirical evidence is concrete information that has been gathered in the real world to answer a specific question.

Ethics: A code of research practices and principles considered correct. When planning research involving human subjects, the researcher must consider ethical principles including informed consent, anonymity, an estimation of any possible harm and justice, that is, treating everyone fairly. These provide high-quality research and are part of research governance.

Ethnography: A type of qualitative research that attempts to uncover the social world of a cultural group, clients or health staff, from the perspective of those in the situation. It has its roots in anthropology and uses observation and interviews over a reasonable time period.

Etic: In qualitative research, the perspective of the researcher, or outsider. The opposite is the *emic* perspective, which is the insider view of things, in their own words.

Evidence-based practice: A philosophy of basing clinical activity on sound research evidence. Decisions about practice must take into account the service-user's perspective and the clinicians' experience, skills and resources. The aim is to follow best practices for each person receiving health care support.

Experimental design: A classic approach to quantitative research that aims to establish cause-and-effect relationships. It usually consists of two groups where an independent variable in the form of an intervention is contrasted with either usual procedures or a placebo. Accurate measurements are made of the dependent variable to establish statistically if any changes could have happened by chance, or whether the changes are due to the independent variable.

Experimental group: In an experimental design, those who receive the independent variable or intervention form the experimental group. The results are compared with a *control group*.

Experimental intervention: This is the form of the independent variable introduced into the experimental group in experimental design and not to those in the control group. It is this that is presumed to be the 'cause' in the cause-and-effect relationship that is the subject of the experiment.

Ex post facto: A research approach used where an experimental approach involving manipulation of the independent variable by the researcher is not possible. It consists of examining groups where the independent variable is already present in those forming one of the groups, e.g. smoking. Ex post facto literally means 'after the fact'. As it lacks manipulation and control, it is not as strong at indicating causal relationships as the experimental design, as the findings may be explained by other factors.

Face validity: A 'face value' judgement, often made by an expert, on the likelihood that a method of measurement will produce accurate results. Frequently used in relation to questionnaires and assessment scales.

Feminist research: A research approach that high-lights the disadvantages facing women because they are women, with the intention of improving the situation. Feminist researchers seek to understand women's experiences, address power imbalances and improve women's lives.

Fieldwork: In qualitative research, data collection that takes place in the natural environment or setting in which those involved in the study are usually found. This is usually carried out for long periods of time in order to observe this group under a range of circumstances. It is the opposite of 'laboratory research' in quantitative research, which is an artificially constructed or controlled environment.

Fieldwork notes/diary: Part of data collection in qualitative research. These describe the details and personal thoughts kept by the researcher whilst engaged in a study and will be used as part of the study findings.

Findings: Often used as the qualitative equivalent to the quantitative term 'results' in quantitative studies, meaning the product of data gathering and analysis.

Fittingness: Used in qualitative research to assess how well the study findings can fit with or apply to other situations. This is not the same as generalisability in qualitative research though.

Fixed alternative questions: In questionnaire design, where respondents are given a list of alternatives from which to choose. The opposite is open questions.

Focus groups: Interview design that uses a small group of individuals to talk about their experiences, feelings or views.

Focused interviews: Where the interviewer uses a flexible and informal approach that centres on a broad list of topics or subject headings with a respondent.

Follow-up study: Used to return to respondents after an initial study to discover any changes or outcomes that have developed. This is a separate study from a previous one and not the same as a 'before and after' study.

Forced choice: *See Fixed alternative questions.*

Forward chaining: Similar to *back chaining* but instead of using one article's references to seek previous studies, it entails the identification of relevant articles in databases where the option 'cited by' is offered. This will take the searcher forward in time to more recent articles that have drawn on or made reference to a previous study.

Frequency distribution: In descriptive statistical presentations, the numbers falling into each of the categories used in the analysis of a question. Often shown in a table.

Gatekeeper: In qualitative research, used to refer to those in a setting who can control or limit the researcher's access to subjects, settings or events.

Generalisability: In quantitative research, the ability to apply the results of a study to the population (see population).

Grounded theory: A type of qualitative research where the aim is to produce an explanation or theory that is 'grounded' in the findings and arises inductively through the researcher's interpretation and analysis. Developed by Barney Glaser and Anselm Strauss.

Hawthorne effect: Where the behaviour of individuals in a study may be influenced by the knowledge of their involvement or participation in a study. Similar to the placebo effect, this is an attention factor that is a threat to the validity of a study. The name is taken from an American study on worker motivation set in the Hawthorne electrical plant in Chicago.

Histogram: Line drawing used to display numeric results in the shape of a series of blocks. Histograms differ from bar graphs in that the blocks touch, as they use continuous rather than discrete data.

Historical research: A research design that looks systematically at past situations or problems, using historical records, objects, diaries and verbal or visual accounts produced by those who witnessed them.

Hypothesis: In experimental designs, this is the researcher's prediction of what they might find if the theory being tested can be supported. It outlines the relationship between the independent and dependent variables in the study. It can take a number of different forms such as directional, non-directional and 'null'.

Inclusion and exclusion criteria: In sampling, the characteristics that help to identify those who qualify to take part in the study (inclusion criteria) and those who may introduce bias and be unrepresentative, or who may be put at risk by participation (exclusion criteria).

Independent variable: In experimental research, this is the cause or intervention that is believed to influence an outcome or dependent variable.

Inductive reasoning or approach: This form of analysis starts with a group of observations or data that are used to formulate general principles that might explain the patterns or relationships apparent in the findings. This form of reasoning is a feature of qualitative research. It is the opposite of *deductive reasoning*, which starts with general principles, and then examines the data to confirm the explanation.

Inferential statistics: One of the two main categories of statistical analysis that use the numerical results of a study as the basis of inferences to a wider group. The second main form of statistics is *descriptive statistics*, which provides a numeric picture of a situation found in a study.

Informant: In qualitative research, the name given to those in the sample who provide information relevant to the aim of the study. The term *participant* is often preferred.

Informed consent: Also called *valid consent*. An ethical requirement to gain permission from an individual invited to take part in research based on a full understanding of what will happen, possible advantages and disadvantages, and other relevant details. It is expected that this should be gained in writing.

Institutional review board (IRB): The American equivalent of a local research ethics committee (LREC). Its role is to provide ethical approval for studies.

Instrument: The tool used to collect data in a study such as a questionnaire or assessment scale.

Internal validity: The ability of the research design to measure the true effect of the intervention rather than the effect of influences outside the study (see confounding variables).

Inter-rater reliability: The extent to which more than one data collector in a study assesses the same outcome, situation or result in an identical way.

Interval measurement: Level of measurement that produces numerical values. Differs from the higher category of ratio level in that it does not have an absolute zero.

Interview guide: Used in in-depth interviews as a way of providing a broad structure and direction. Takes the form of loosely formed questions, topics or subjects that can be referred to in a flexible way. Differs from an interview schedule that is more structured and fixed.

Interview: Method of collecting data through face-to-face, telephone or interactive method (e.g. on-line). Can be on a one-to-one or focus group basis. Interviews vary in structure and depth.

Interview schedule: Fixed list of questions similar to a questionnaire used in interviews to produce standardised results. Differs from interview guide, which is more flexible.

Item: In a Likert scale, used to describe a statement to which the respondent may choose options ranging from 'strongly agree' or to 'strongly disagree'.

Judgemental sample: More commonly known as a purposive sample. This is a non-probability sampling strategy where those in the study are picked on the basis of the researcher's knowledge of their characteristics that will contribute to a balanced or representative sample.

Justice: The ethical principle that all those involved in research should be treated fairly and equally as human beings.

Key informant: In qualitative research, someone who has a special position in the setting or who has valuable information. Key informants provide the researcher with major insights or details crucial to the study.

Key word: In reviewing the literature, this is the word(s) entered into the database in order to discover what has been published under the topic investigated. Care is needed, as words commonly used may not be the same as those under which suitable articles are stored. American spellings can also be problematic.

Level of significance: The 'P' or probability level in a study that indicates the extent to which the results could have happened by chance. The minimum level is usually set at '$P < .05$', which means that, statistically, there is less than five in a hundred chance of being wrong if the researcher maintained there was a relationship between the independent and dependent variables in the study.

Levels of measurement: A categorisation of the different properties of numbers. Includes nominal, ordinal, interval and ratio levels. These play an important part in determining the appropriate statistical tests that may be used with the data collected.

Likert scale: A method of measuring opinion or attitude by asking respondents to 'strongly agree' to 'strongly disagree' with a list of statements or 'items' in an interview or questionnaire. Usually a five-point scale, this is named after the American Rensis Likert who developed the technique and so is spelt with a capital 'L'.

Limitations: All studies have their weaknesses. The researcher should identify those that may affect the outcome of the study and the interpretation of the results. This is usually found at the start of the discussion section.

Line graphs: Line graphs are often used to display change over time – it is portrayed as a series of data points connected by straight line segments on two axes. It encourages the reviewer to ascertain the relationship between two sets of values. Line graphs are drawn so that the independent data are on the horizontal x-axis (e.g. time) and the dependent data are on the vertical y-axis.

Literature review: An essential aspect of research studies where researchers place their study within the context of what is already known about the topic and the recent research that has been conducted. This should be critical in nature, and not simply a summary of previous work. Reviews of the literature, especially in their more systematic form, also play an important role in evidence-based practice and in producing standards for audit.

Lived experience: In phenomenological research, an attempt to understand a situation or health condition through the eyes of those experiencing it, so we can gain insights and understanding.

Longitudinal study: A type of research that follows a group of individuals over a long period of time to gain an understanding or measurement of any long-term changes, experiences or effects of a variable. Can take the form of a *panel study* where the same people are followed over time, or a *trend study* where different people from the same population are included at different points of time. The time period may range from weeks or months to years.

Manipulation: A feature of experimental design where the researcher introduces a change in the situation or to the subjects in the study. This is usually the introduction of the independent variable, or intervention.

Matching: A method of sampling in experimental design where individuals are matched by the researcher in terms of key characteristics that may have an undue influence or confounding effect on the study outcome. The aim is to divide those with possible confounding attributes such as age or sex equally between the different study groups so that the groups can be compared fairly. This reduces the effect of the confounding characteristic on the outcome, as it will affect each group equally.

Maturation: One of the threats to the validity of an experimental design, where the outcome could be influenced by changes to the individual, either physically or mentally, over the course of the measurement period.

Mean: The statistical term for an average. It relates to what is typical in the group and is part of a series of measures called *measures of central tendency*. The mean is calculated by adding up the scores and dividing the total by the number of scores

Measure of central tendency: A statistical term for the result of a procedure that attempts to establish a typical single value from a set of numbers. We usually talk about an average, but there are three such measures: *mean*, *mode* and *median*. Each of these can produce a very different result because of the way in which they are calculated.

Median: A measure of central tendency or 'average' in a set of results that identifies the value of a number that is midway along a set of values put in order from smallest to largest. Fifty percent of the values will be above that number and 50% below it. It is a stable measurement and is not unduly influenced by numbers that may be untypically large or small in the set.

MEDLINE: A database of medical journal articles, often accessed online.

Member check: Also called *respondent validation*. In qualitative research, the process of increasing credibility by getting those who provided data to check what has been written for accuracy.

Meta-analysis: A method of combining the results of a number of quantitative studies on the same topic, carried out in similar ways, in order to increase the total size of the study sample. If successful, this can increase the accuracy of the statistical procedures carried out on the data, and so increase the value of the prediction based on the combined outcomes.

Methodology or method: The overall design followed by researchers in carrying out their research, as in *survey method*, or *experimental method*. Each method will follow certain principles and set procedures. In everyday use, it is used as a heading in research reports under which the details of how the research was conducted are presented for scrutiny.

Mode: A measure of central tendency or 'average' that identifies the value of the unit that appears most often in a set of numbers. It is not a good indicator of what is typical in a set of numbers. If two numbers appear in a set the same number of times they form a *bimodal distribution*. If several numbers appear the same number of times, it is known as a *multi-modal distribution*.

Mortality: *See Study mortality.*

Naturalistic approach or paradigm: Used as an alternative description for qualitative research methods, where there is no attempt to control or manipulate, and the study takes places in a normal or natural setting rather than a carefully controlled laboratory setting. It represents a philosophical approach to thinking about the natural world and how it should be studied.

Nominal data: This is the most basic of the levels of measurement and relates to numbers that do not have a value in relation to quantity, but merely label a category with a number, e.g. primigravida=1, multigravida=2. It is not possible to carry out statistical procedures on nominal data apart from producing a frequency distribution, that is, how many were in each group.

Non-directional hypothesis: Here, a clear prediction is not made of the expected outcome between two groups in an experimental setting, only that a difference will be found. Unlike directional hypotheses that use such terms as 'greater than', 'smaller than' or 'more often than' in relation to the outcomes between the experimental and control group, non-directional hypotheses merely say there will be a difference. The nature of the difference and in which group it will be found is not stated.

Non-equivalent experimental designs: This indicates that those in a study have not been randomly allocated to the experimental or control group. This means that it is not possible to be certain that any differences are purely due to the independent variable; differences between those in the two groups could have influenced the outcome.

Non-experimental design: A study where the researcher does not introduce a variable and is not looking for a cause-and-effect relationship. It should not be inferred that research in this category is less worthy than experimental research, only that the intentions are different.

Non-maleficence: The ethical principle to do no harm in a study. This is one of the most powerful principles of ethical considerations.

Non-parametric statistics: A collection of statistical techniques to establish the likelihood of relationships amongst data that do not require the strict criteria of parametric statistics. This makes them easier to apply, but the results are not as widely accepted or as accurate as those in the parametric category.

Non-probability sampling methods: A collection of frequently used methods of selecting the sample in a study that includes opportunity/accidental, quota and purposive sampling strategies. It is not possible to say with any certainty how typical those selected are of the larger population using any of these methods. Their advantage is that they are relatively easy to use.

Non-significant result: This does not mean that the results of the research are not important; it means that in the case of a RCT the '*P*' value is too large to rule out the element of chance and therefore the null-hypothesis must not be rejected. In other words, no statistically significant difference between the results of the groups involved has been shown.

Normal distribution: This relates to a statistical pattern of the distribution of some variables such as height and blood pressure. If data on these variables were plotted on a graph for a sample group, they should produce a bell-shaped curve where most people are close to the mean, and others are in equal proportion on either side of the mean. In a normal distribution, the mean, mode and median all have the same value and graphically would be a single line dropping down from the apex of the frequency curve. A normal distribution allows the use of parametric statistical tests, making this an important statistical concept.

Null-hypothesis: This is the hypothesis of no difference, that is, it predicts that there will be no statistically significant differences between the outcome measures for the groups in the study. It is also called the statistical hypothesis. It is expressed in this way because it is easier to reject the null-hypothesis than it is to accept its opposite, the research hypothesis, which predicts a real difference between the results of the groups in the study. If the null-hypothesis is rejected, it leads to the automatic acceptance of the research or directional hypothesis.

Nuremberg code: Ethical principles applied to experimental research on humans. Designed to prevent inappropriate and dangerous research by protecting those involved, it is based on 10 principles, including informed consent.

Observation: Method of collecting research data through visible means using either the eye or a camera. This can be structured in the form of quantitative checklists, or unstructured, in the form of qualitative participant or non-participant observation.

Observer drift: Loss of concentration by the researcher in observation studies where observations are carried out over extended period. Shorter periods or time sampling may be a solution.

One-tailed hypothesis: Also called a directional hypothesis, this predicts a difference between two groups in the study and is indicated by the use of such words as 'more than' or 'less than'.

Open coding: The method of qualitative analysis where codes, or 'category headings' are given to the categories identified in the data.

Open (ended) questions: In questionnaire or interview designs, where respondents are encouraged to provide a response in their own words rather than choosing from a list of choices.

Operational definition: The way in which the researcher intends to measure or 'make operational' the variables under study.

Opportunity sampling: *See Convenience sampling.*

Ordinal level of measurement: The category that follows nominal data. Here, the numbers used relate to the position or order of the items along a simple measuring scale (first, second, etc.). As with nominal data, there are severe restrictions on the statistical procedures that can be carried out on them. Examples include Likert scales that go in order from 'strongly disagree' to 'strongly agree'.

Outliers: In a set of numeric measures, these are the values at the extreme ends of a distribution that are not necessarily typical of the others in the set, e.g. those untypically old or young in a group.

Overt observation: Where the research activities of an observer are clearly visible and known by those involved to be taking place. The opposite is covert observation, where those in the setting do not know they are being observed.

Panel study: This kind of longitudinal study takes the form of a survey where the same people are approached for information at two or more points over time. This provides information on how people, variables or experiences change over time.

Paradigm: A distinct way of looking at the world around us that colours all aspects of our understanding; it is a 'world view'. An example is the way obstetrics and medicine have been characterised as illustrating a different paradigm or view of the world compared to midwifery and nursing.

Participant: A person who voluntarily participates in a research study.

Participant observer: Where the researcher observes whilst carrying out similar activities in the setting as those being observed.

Phenomenology: A qualitative approach that seeks to uncover the 'lived experience' of people in a particular setting or with a particular health condition or status, e.g. the lived experience of parenting triplets.

Physiological measurement: A precise way of measuring some physiological factor or outcome, e.g. temperature or blood pressure.

Pilot study: A small-scale test to ensure that the tool of data collection is reliable and that there are no unforeseen or unanticipated practical difficulties in following the intended research method. The pilot is very much like a dress rehearsal and is an indication of rigour. The flexible nature of qualitative research means that pilots are mainly a feature of quantitative than qualitative research, although a small practice interview or observation may be used in the latter.

Placebo effect: The power of suggestion in drug trials where the belief in the effectiveness of a drug can produce perceived positive outcomes reported by subjects. To reduce this, a non-active drug or treatment is used to act as a measure against the drug or procedure being tested and concealment as to who has the active drug is applied to as many in the setting as possible, including clinical staff.

Population: A clearly defined group that shares common characteristics as specified by the researcher. The target population indicates those the researcher wants to say something about and the study population is the members of those groups that can be accessed to take part in the study.

Power analysis: Statistical procedure to calculate the size of a sample needed in a randomised control trial to ensure that the statistical calculations are sensitive and accurate.

Primary sources: A review of the literature in which the researcher consults the original authors and studies and does not depend on secondary sources, which are summaries or descriptions by other authors of someone's work.

Probability sampling methods: A collection of strategies for selecting a sample from a population that results in a highly representative group. Strategies include simple random sampling, stratified sampling, proportionate sampling and cluster sampling methods. A number of sophisticated statistical techniques can be used on such samples.

Probing: In interviewing, a way of gaining more in-depth data is by asking further questions to elaborate on points. This is not the same as prompting, where the interviewer offers a possible answer accepted by the respondent, although it may be inaccurate.

Proportionate random sampling: A method of ensuring that important subgroups in the sample are in the same proportions as those in the main population. This reduces the risk of bias through unevenly sized subgroups that might make a difference to the overall results.

Prospective study: A study where the data lies in the future at the start of the research. Newly occurring data are then collected as the study progresses. The opposite is a retrospective study, where the data already exist when the study is set up. Prospective studies have the advantage of greater control by the researcher, and therefore greater accuracy.

Purposive sampling: Sometimes also called judgemental sampling. This sampling strategy handpicks items or people on the basis of the researcher's prior knowledge of typical characteristics in the group. Despite sounding as though there is an element of

bias here, this type of sample can produce a typical or representative sample.

'P' value: This is the indicator that the researcher has statistically tested the results, particularly in RCTs, to establish the 'probability' that the differences could be due to chance, and not the intervention. The most common value used to indicate that the results are unlikely to have happened by chance is $P < .05$. Using this value means that there is less than a 5% probability that the results are not a matter of random chance. Another way of putting it is that there is more than a 95% chance that the results are *significant*.

Qualitative research: Broad heading for a number of research designs that are not concerned with numerical accuracy and the need to control or predict, but rather the need for insight and understanding. The findings are in the form of words and descriptions rather than numbers.

Quantitative research: Broad heading for a number of research designs to data gathering that produce numeric results. The concerns of this type of research centre on accuracy and to control and predict situations. Results from quantitative studies can be used to see patterns, make predictions, identify correlations, test causal relationships and make generalisations.

Quasi-experimental design: Used when random allocation may not be possible. This looks like an experimental study in that the researcher introduces an independent variable, but it uses groups that have not been randomly allocated. This means that the outcome might be due to factors other than the independent variable.

Questionnaire: Popular research method of collecting data. It usually involves participants answering a set of questions on a questionnaire and returning this to the researcher.

Quota sampling: A non-probability sampling strategy often used by market researchers where the researcher predetermines how many in the sample they will recruit with certain characteristics such as age or social class grouping. Once a particular quota is complete, emphasis is placed on the remaining categories.

Random allocation or Randomisation: The method of allocating those in a trial to the experimental or control group so that everyone has an equal chance of ending up in either group. Usually involves computer-generated random numbers, tables of random numbers and sampling frames (lists of those eligible for allocation). Other techniques, such as picking names out of a hat or using the last digits on a medical record, are less well accepted as achieving a high level of randomisation.

Random selection: This ensures that everyone in a target population has an equal chance of being selected for study. Where data are gathered from everyone selected, the findings should be highly accurate and representative of the population as a whole. A number of statistical tests assume data are taken from such a random selection of the population.

Reactivity: A change in behaviour due to the taking part in a study and not related to anything introduced by the research. This distortion has an adverse effect on results.

Reliability: The accuracy of the tool of data collection. This is usually subject to a number of tests to ensure consistency. A pilot study will also be used to examine the reliability of the tool of data collection unless a well-used tool is applied.

Replication study: A design based on a study that has previously been carried out to confirm the findings of the first. Can take a number of different forms, including replication of the sampling design, the tool of data collection and other testing procedures.

Research: Extending knowledge and understanding through the systematic collection of information that answers a specific question objectively and as accurately as possible.

Research governance: Framework of accountability to be met by organisations within which research is carried out. The purpose is to ensure high standards of research through meeting ethical, scientific and safety criteria in the conduct of research. Additional accountability includes ensuring that the results of studies are communicated and accessible to those who can benefit from them.

Research proposal: An outline of an intended piece of research. It is used to gain ethical approval, permission or funding. It also allows the researcher to think through the whole process and identify any weak areas.

Research question: Related to the aim of a study, this is the element that structures the research process, particularly data collection, as the results of a study should answer this question.

Respect for persons: Part of the ethical code that relates to ensuring individuals are treated as autonomous, e.g. must be given the freedom to determine whether or not to participate in research.

Respondent: Term describing someone taking part in a study, often used in relation to questionnaires and interviews.

Respondent Validation: Also called *member checking*. In qualitative research, the process of increasing credibility by getting those who provided data to check what has been written for accuracy.

Response rate: The number of those returning a questionnaire or agreeing to be interviewed, expressed as a proportion of the total sent out or approached.

Results: Usually applied to the numeric findings of a study produced by data collection.

Retrospective study: A study in which the data already exist when the study is set up. These data cannot be influenced by the researcher, which reduces bias. The disadvantage is the lack of control over the quality of the data. The opposite of a prospective study.

Review of the literature: *See Literature review.*

Rich Data: This data, usually in-depth and from small samples, is a feature of high-quality data in a qualitative study. It is data that reveals people's intricate emotions, ideas, stories and models of their world.

Rigour: The extent to which the researcher has actively sought to carry out the study to a high standard. This includes identifying possible pitfalls in the design of the study and reducing their effect as much as possible. The end result should be a study that is as accurate and professional as possible.

Risk versus benefit ratio: Ethical principle of assessing whether the risks inherent in the study design are outweighed by possible benefits. These should be made known to those invited to take part in a study, particularly where the risks are high or of an unknown magnitude.

Sample: A section of a defined population used in a study to provide data.

Sample mortality: In experimental designs or longitudinal survey designs, e.g. cohort studies. This refers to participants who, for one reason or another (not necessarily death), leave the study. If there is a high mortality rate in one or more of the groups in an experimental design, those remaining in a study may no longer produce a typical group, making comparisons between groups unreliable.

Sampling frame: A list of all those who are eligible to be included in a study according to the inclusion/exclusion criteria. Each 'unit' in the list is numbered and, using a table of random numbers or computer-generated random numbers, the researcher draws a predetermined set of numbers that are then matched against those in the sampling frame to provide the names or identities of those randomly selected.

Sampling strategy: Also referred to as a sampling plan. The choice of method used to select a sample for data collection.

Saturation: Also referred to as *'data saturation'*. In qualitative research, the point at which no new analytical categories or themes are arising from the data analysis, so the researcher ends data collection, as further data would be redundant.

Scientific approach: This is an ordered and objective method of collecting information in such a way as to provide verifiable data. Developed from the natural sciences, such as physics and chemistry, this approach has now been applied to human behaviour on the assumption that we are subject to similar constant patterns and influences. Those who favour a more humanistic approach, such as that of qualitative research, dispute this.

Secondary source: In reviewing the literature, where an author's original work is not consulted, only the work as cited, or outlined, by another author. There are dangers with this, as the primary source could be misquoted, or vital information omitted. The opposite of a primary source.

Selection bias: Where the sampling strategy used has not resulted in a representative group.

Self-report: Method of data collection that consists of asking people to provide information about themselves, such as in questionnaires, interviews or diaries. Built on the assumption that what people say they do is accurate, which might not always be the case.

Seminal study: Description of a study that was the first to tackle a topic and has become a 'classic'. It provided the 'seed' from which other studies have grown.

Semi-structured interview: A feature of qualitative interviews that contains some questions that are asked of everyone to ensure areas or topics of importance to the study are included; the remaining questions are more spontaneous and depend on the flow of conversation.

Simple random sample: A sampling strategy where everyone or every item has an equal chance of being selected. Requires a sampling frame and a table of random numbers or computer-generated random numbers.

Snowball sampling: Also known as 'chain', 'nominated' or 'network' sampling. A sampling strategy used in qualitative research when it is difficult to identify or locate suitable candidates for the study. The procedure depends on finding some appropriate members, and then asking them for the names of contacts who might be willing to take part. The disadvantage is that, as the nominated people will be socially close to the individual, the resultant sample may not be representative of the wider group.

Social desirability: Found in surveys when individuals answer inaccurately because they want to be seen in a good light and give socially approved responses.

Stability: Refers to a tool of data collection that is consistent in its ability to provide accurate measurements.

Standard deviation: In statistics, an indication of the spread of values around the mean.

Statistical significance: The extent to which the results of a study could have happened by chance rather than the result of an intervention or independent variable. This is indicated by the 'P' value.

Stratified random sampling: Method of dividing the sampling frame into appropriate subgroups and drawing the sample from within each one.

Structured interview: Type of interview that has a high degree of structure. Basically, the researcher reads from a questionnaire (called an interview schedule) and writes down the answers. The advantage is that people may be more willing to engage in this as opposed to finding time to completing and returning a questionnaire. It also makes the answers more easily comparable with the minimum of coding. The disadvantage is respondents can only follow the line of questioning and wording laid down in the schedule.

Structured observation: The use of a list of behaviours that will focus the observer's attention. This usually results in a quantitative analysis of the frequency with which events occurred.

Subject: Used to refer to someone in a study. Has overtones of 'using' and seeing people as objects.

Survey: A research method that commonly uses quantitative questionnaires or pre-set questions to collect data from a reasonably large sample or occasionally from the whole population: e.g. the national census. It is a useful method when a researcher aims to describe or explain the features of a large group and/ or identify trends.

Systematic sampling: Method of numbering all possible units in a sampling frame and then choosing units at a set interval, such as every tenth, to ensure that the entire range of the sample is included.

Theory: In quantitative research, the set of ideas about a situation that guides the construction of a study and its analysis. Hypotheses are developed from theories. In qualitative research using grounded theory, the findings may be used to construct a theory to explain them.

Thick data: In qualitative research, thick data refers to a large quantity of data. This may be from in-depth face-to-face interviews, for example, where participants talked at length about their experience. Thick data analysis can therefore be extremely time consuming. It may be very detailed data. It may contain *rich data* (see rich data).

Threats to internal or external validity: Factors that can provide an alternative explanation for the results of the study due to influences within the study (internal threats) or which reduce the ability to apply the results more widely (external threats).

Transferability: Also called fittingness. In qualitative research, the likelihood that the findings could provide insights into other situations.

Trend survey: This type of longitudinal study examines different groups of people from the same population at different times to identify any changes in the variable under study. This can include attitudes and experiences as well as physical, psychological or social changes. Following the same group over time would provide a '*panel*' study.

Triangulation: The use of more than one method of data collection in the same study in an attempt to produce more accurate information or understanding. This is called *method triangulation* and it is the most commonly referred to form of triangulation. However, triangulation may also refer to using more than one researcher (*researcher triangulation*), or multiple sampling strategies (*data triangulation*) or multiple methodologies (*theoretical triangulation*) as in mixed-methods studies.

Trustworthiness: In qualitative research, one of the criteria used in establishing the authenticity and accuracy of the information presented. Can be compared to the concepts of reliability and validity in quantitative research.

t-test: Statistical test that compares the means of two groups to establish if any differences between them could have happened by chance.

Two-tailed hypothesis: Also called a non-directional hypothesis, this predicts a difference between two groups in the study but does not indicate in which direction. It simply states there will be a difference.

Unstructured interview: Also called a non-standardised interview. In qualitative research, used as a way of gaining an insight into a situation from the other person's or insider's perspective (emic view) without enforcing the researcher's point of view on the situation. Broad questions and probing are used where necessary to maintain the flow of ideas.

Unstructured observation: An in-depth form of observation used in qualitative research, such as ethnographic studies, where the researcher tries to record as much of what is happening as possible.

Validity: The extent to which a tool of data collection has produced what it was intended to produce.

Variable: The item or 'thing' that forms the focus of the researcher's attention. Called a variable because such items vary in some way, e.g. temperature, pulse, age, gender, satisfaction with care or length of labour.

Vignette: Used in questionnaires or interviews. Takes the form of a story, pen portrait or scenario on which the respondents answer questions to reveal their attitude, knowledge or behaviour. The problem is knowing if such answers really predict what a person would do in the actual situation.

Visual Analogue Scale (VAS): Measuring instrument in the form of a straight line. Respondents indicate their location between the two points on the line, e.g. Most pain ever felt/No pain, extreme anxiety/No anxiety. The points on the scale are given numerical values to allow for statistical analysis.

Vulnerable subjects: In ethical considerations, those people who are especially at risk and may not be in a position to give true informed consent, e.g. women in painful labour asked to provide consent to a procedure to which they would not agree in normal circumstances. Other vulnerable groups include children, those who are distressed, those with a challenged mental capacity, those with language difficulties and the unconscious.

INDEX